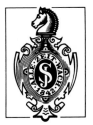

Werner Müller

The Knee

Form, Function, and Ligament Reconstruction

Foreword by J. C. Hughston

Translated by T. C. Telger

With 299 Figures
in 462 Partially Coloured Seperate Illustrations
Illustrations by R. Muspach

Springer-Verlag
Berlin Heidelberg New York 1983

PD Dr. Werner Müller
Universität Basel, CH-4056 Basel, and
Kantonsspital Bruderholz, CH-4101 Bruderholz

Translator:
Terry C. Telger
3054 Vaughn Avenue
Marina, CA 93933/USA

Translation of the German edition
Das Knie. Form, Funktion und ligamentäre
Wiederherstellungschirurgie
© Springer-Verlag Berlin Heidelberg 1982

ISBN 3-540-11716-4 Springer-Verlag Berlin Heidelberg New York
ISBN 0-387-11716-4 Springer-Verlag New York Heidelberg Berlin

Library of Congress Cataloging in Publication Data. Müller, Werner, 1933–. The knee–form, function, and ligament reconstruction. Translation of: Das Knie–Form, Funktion und Wiederherstellungschirurgie. Bibliography: p. Includes index. 1. Knee–Surgery. 2. Knee–Wounds and injuries. 3. Knee. I. Title. [DNLM: 1. Knee. 2. Knee–Surgery. 3. Ligaments–Surgery. WE 870 M947k] RD561.M8413 1983. 617'.582. 82-19425
ISBN 0-387-11716-4 (U.S.)

Typesetting, printing, and bookbinding: Konrad Triltsch, Graphischer Betrieb, 8700 Würzburg.
2124/3130-54321

For and with Ursi

Foreword

This new treatise is the most outstanding piece of work on the knee and its associated ligaments currently available. Never before have I seen such an extensive study of the biomechanics of the knee with such a comprehensive review of the literature.

The first section of the book, which deals with the functional anatomy (structure and biomechanics), immediately alerts the reader to the necessity of understanding the natural development and action of the related structures, clearly emphasizing that successful diagnosis and treatment cannot otherwise be expected; the many who want an easy standard approach to each classic problem may find this hard to accept. Study what Werner Müller has written and compare it with your own findings from repeated dissection of anatomical specimens.

The author goes on to stress that to have a real grasp of reconstructive surgery of the ligaments, one must be properly acquainted with the pathology and the repair of acute lesions. In no other way can one learn to recognize chronic problems. Once this step has been mastered it can be seen that the reconstructive procedures that Müller advocates do, for the most part, follow the laws of Nature rather than create the kind of abnormalities which often disrupt natural anatomical function.

However, I must state my reservations regarding the extent of his concern with the anterior cruciate ligament and the so-called anterior cruciate deficient knee, especially as expressed on page 12, although this has been the accepted opinion for years. Almost everyone in the field is aware that I do not believe the loss of an anterior cruciate ligament alone can be so disastrous. I am convinced that continued investigation and forthcoming long-term clinical studies will demonstrate that we have failed to recognize associated ligamentous lesions of a subclinical nature. In any case, the disorder should not be termed "anterior cruciate deficient knee", as this tells us no more than that the ligament is absent. The instabilities associated with this deficiency should be described according to the classification of knee ligaments, so that surgeons and researchers can efficiently communicate about them.

Werner Müller presents his solutions to knee ligament instability at the end, not at the beginning. The book should be studied from front to back; don't just turn quickly to the sections on operative procedures and expect to repeat his success in diagnosis and treatment.

The entire book bears witness to Dr. Müller's dedication and willingness to share his knowledge of the subject with others, who can thereby provide their patients with high-quality treatment.

JACK C. HUGHSTON, M.D.

Preface

The many injuries of the knee joint that can occur during working, driving and sports activities, together with their sequelae, create a host of problems that have not yet been adequately resolved. It is not unusual for multiple operations to be performed on a given knee joint without achieving a satisfactory result. Meniscectomies in particular have become notorious for their ability to damage athletic careers.

But if it is possible to restore patients to full soundness in the field of fracture surgery, why not in the surgery of knee injuries? My first meeting with Prof. Albert Trillat and his coworkers in 1972 gave me a new appreciation for the functional approach to knee surgery. Basically, this approach stresses the importance of maintaining the functional integrity of anatomic structures, even in major operations. By avoiding transverse and oblique incisions that disrupt tension-conveying structures, it is possible to reduce postoperative pain and speed rehabilitation.

Some years ago, I and the rest of my small surgical team instituted a systematic program of management and follow-up in patients treated for recent and old injuries of the knee. This ongoing quality control provides us with continual feedback as to which of our operative methods yields the best results in the short, intermediate and long term. It also forms the basis for our scientific documentation, in as much as our busy clinical practice kept us from conducting outside experimental studies. Nevertheless, the demands of clinical practice compelled us to make a detailed study of anatomic structures, and this taught us key relationships between form and function which then became an important basis for our clinical work.

I am greatly indebted to the anatomist, Prof. A. v. Hochstetter, whose anatomic preparations provided a vivid illustration of kinematic laws and of the integral relationship between form and function – a principle essential to the successful conduct of knee surgery.

It is hoped that with our discussions and many illustrations, we have succeeded in providing the physician, examiner and surgeon with a better understanding of the knee joint, enabling them to diagnose knee problems more accurately and treat them more effectively with a minimum of intervention.

At the same time, we have endeavored to combine the important discoveries of English and American authors such as Smillie, Slocum, O'Donoghue, Hughston, MacIntosh, Ellison, Kennedy and Marshall, as well as those of younger authors, with the major works of the French, Scandinavian and German-language literature. Much of our material is derived from conferences or gleaned from discussions. It is often difficult in retrospect to credit a particular author with a particular idea. Many ideas "evolve" over time and arise independently in several different locales. Others have a more unique provenance and significance.

I am indebted to Prof. K. S. Ludwig and to my colleagues at the Anatomical Institute of Basel University for their valuable support. University artist R. Muspach worked tirelessly to render our rough sketches into excellent didactic illustrations and thus has contributed greatly to the realization of this book.

Bruderholz, Fall, 1982   WERNER MÜLLER

Contents

Part I

List of Abbreviations

ACL	anterior cruciate ligament
AFCN	anterior femoral cutaneous nerve branch
AGM	articularis genus muscle
AH	adductor hiatus
AL	arcuate ligament
ALFTL	anterolateral femorotibial ligament
Am + IS	adductor magnus muscle and intermuscular septum
AMT	adductor magnus tendon
AT	adductor tubercle
ATM	anterior tibial muscle
Bi	biceps muscle
BT	biceps tendon
Caps	capsule
CI	condylar insertion
EDL	extensor digitorum longus muscle
Fa	fabella
FH	fibular head
FPG	femoral popliteal groove
Gr	gracilis muscle
IBSN	infrapatellar branch of the saphenous nerve
IFP	infrapatellar fat pad
IS	intermuscular septum
IT	impressio terminalis
ITT	iliotibial tract
LAI	linea aspera insertion
LCL	lateral collateral ligament
LCSN	lateral cutaneous sural nerve
LG	lateral gastrocnemius
LIS + VL	lateral intermuscular septum and vastus lateralis muscle
LLPR	lateral longitudinal patellar retinaculum
LM	lateral meniscus
LP	longitudinal portion of vastus medialis obliquus
LPo	oblique popliteal ligament
LTPR	lateral transverse patellar retinaculum
MAN	medial articular nerve
MCL	medial collateral ligament
MCSN	medial cutaneous sural nerve
Me	meniscus
MFC	medial femoral condyle
MG	medial gastrocnemius muscle
MLPR	medial longitudinal patellar retinaculum

MRMG	muscular ramus to medial gastrocnemius
MTPR	medial transverse patellar retinaculum
P	patella
PA	pes anserinus
PA + PV	popliteal artery and vein
PAI	pes anserinus insertion
PC	posterior capsule
PCL	posterior cruciate ligament
Pe, PN	peroneus nerve
PHLM	posterior horn of the lateral meniscus
PHMM	posterior horn of medial meniscus
Pl	plantaris muscle
PL	patellar ligament
PLB	peroneus longus and brevis muscle
PMFL	posterior meniscofemoral ligament
PML	patellomeniscal ligament
Po	popliteus muscle
POL	posterior oblique ligament
PP	planum popliteum
PT	popliteus tendon
QT	quadriceps tendon
RF	rectus femoris
Sa	sartorius muscle
SF	synovial fold
Sm	semimembranosus muscle
SmS	semimembranosus sulcus
So	soleus muscle
SP	suprapatellar pouch
SR	suprapatellar recess
St	semitendinosus muscle
TG	Tubercle of Gerdy
TL	transverse ligament
TN	tibial nerve
TP	transverse portion of the vastus medialis obliquus
TT	Tibial tuberosity
VL	vastus lateralis muscle
VM	vastus medialis muscle

Part I

Anatomy

The cornerstone of any reparative or reconstructive procedure is anatomy. Anatomic structures are never an end in themselves but are, by virtue of their size and strength, the expression of a corresponding function [226, 260, 261].

Individuality

Anatomy is always an individual matter. There is a large interindividual scatter, and anatomic variants are numerous. The functional systems remain unchanged, however.

Form, Function, and Synergisms

Noble [254] described congenital aplasia of the anterior cruciate in a knee with a medial ring meniscus. Among our patients, we know of three cases where the anterior cruciate ligament was lacking, and in its place was a kind of synovial septum which apparently was unable to guarantee mechanical strength.

Few anatomic structures bear the sole responsibility for a particular function. Nearly always, a structure will interact synergistically with other elements. Thus, in the present example, a ring meniscus or a meniscus with a bulky posterior horn and firm meniscotibial attachment [135, 136] can stabilize the tibia against anterior displacement, thereby partially assuming the function of an anterior cruciate ligament. This sheds light on the well-known problem of why progressive insufficiency of the anterior cruciate ligament can develop after meniscectomy [338]. The normal synergists of the anterior cruciate ligament are discussed elsewhere in their appropriate context (see p. 66 and 128 ff.).

On the lateral side, too, individual variants are numerous and common. The popliteus tendon, lateral collateral ligament and arcuate ligament complex (arcuate popliteal ligament) can vary greatly in their strength [21]. There are cases in which the popliteus tendon is extremely powerful, while the lateral collateral ligament and components of the arcuate popliteal ligament are quite poorly developed. Conversely, the latter structures may be quite powerful while the popliteus tendon appears weak next to the collateral ligament.

Many such examples of interrelationships can be cited. They will be discussed later on in their appropriate contexts.

The anatomical terms oblique *popliteal* ligament and arcuate *popliteal* ligament may seem somewhat confusing. Both structures are located in the posterior joint capsule facing the popliteal fossa, and so both share the designation "popliteal." However, the oblique popliteal ligament is in reality one of the five tendinous expansions of the semimembranosus muscle and belongs functionally to the "semimembranosus corner," while the arcuate popliteal ligament belongs to the tendon complex of the popliteus muscle and thus to the functional system of the "popliteus corner" (Figs. 1–5).

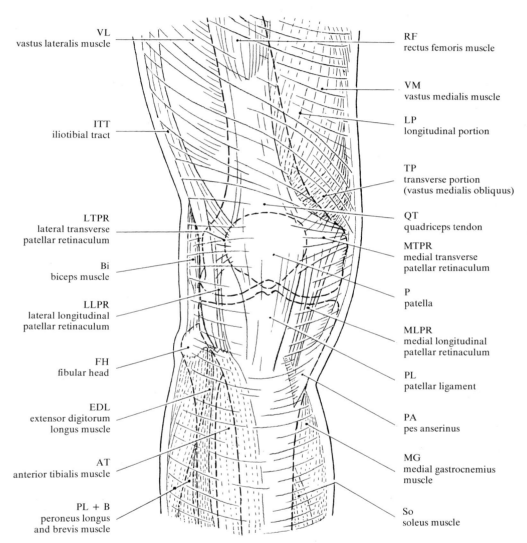

VL
vastus lateralis muscle

RF
rectus femoris muscle

ITT
iliotibial tract

VM
vastus medialis muscle

LP
longitudinal portion

TP
transverse portion
(vastus medialis obliquus)

LTPR
lateral transverse
patellar retinaculum

QT
quadriceps tendon

MTPR
medial transverse
patellar retinaculum

Bi
biceps muscle

P
patella

LLPR
lateral longitudinal
patellar retinaculum

MLPR
medial longitudinal
patellar retinaculum

FH
fibular head

PL
patellar ligament

EDL
extensor digitorum
longus muscle

PA
pes anserinus

AT
anterior tibialis muscle

MG
medial gastrocnemius
muscle

PL + B
peroneus longus
and brevis muscle

So
soleus muscle

Fig. 1. The knee joint and its main anatomic structures viewed from the anterior aspect

3

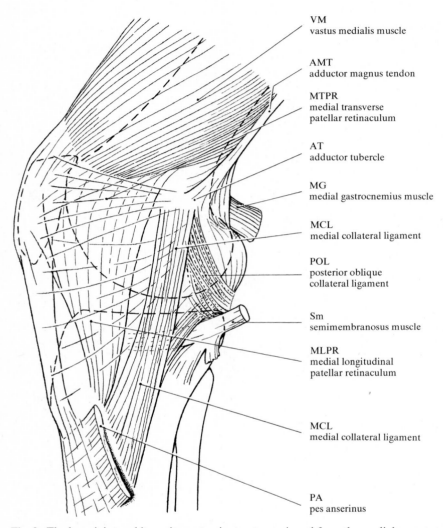

VM
vastus medialis muscle

AMT
adductor magnus tendon

MTPR
medial transverse
patellar retinaculum

AT
adductor tubercle

MG
medial gastrocnemius muscle

MCL
medial collateral ligament

POL
posterior oblique
collateral ligament

Sm
semimembranosus muscle

MLPR
medial longitudinal
patellar retinaculum

MCL
medial collateral ligament

PA
pes anserinus

Fig. 2. The knee joint and its main anatomic structures viewed from the medial aspect

4

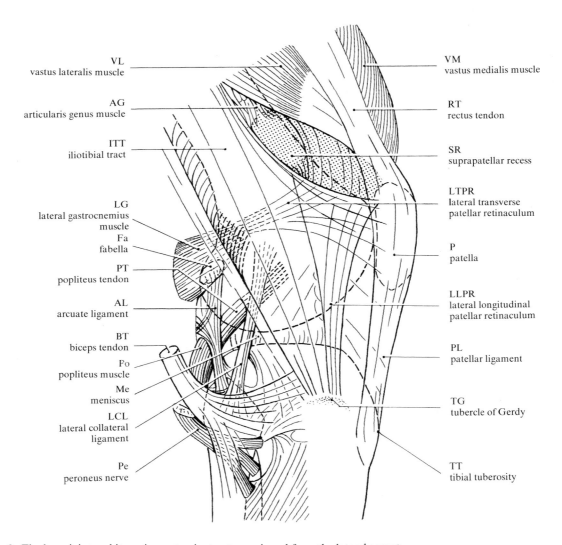

VL
vastus lateralis muscle

AG
articularis genus muscle

ITT
iliotibial tract

LG
lateral gastrocnemius
muscle
Fa
fabella

PT
popliteus tendon

AL
arcuate ligament

BT
biceps tendon

Po
popliteus muscle

Me
meniscus

LCL
lateral collateral
ligament

Pe
peroneus nerve

VM
vastus medialis muscle

RT
rectus tendon

SR
suprapatellar recess

LTPR
lateral transverse
patellar retinaculum

P
patella

LLPR
lateral longitudinal
patellar retinaculum

PL
patellar ligament

TG
tubercle of Gerdy

TT
tibial tuberosity

Fig. 3. The knee joint and its main anatomic structures viewed from the lateral aspect

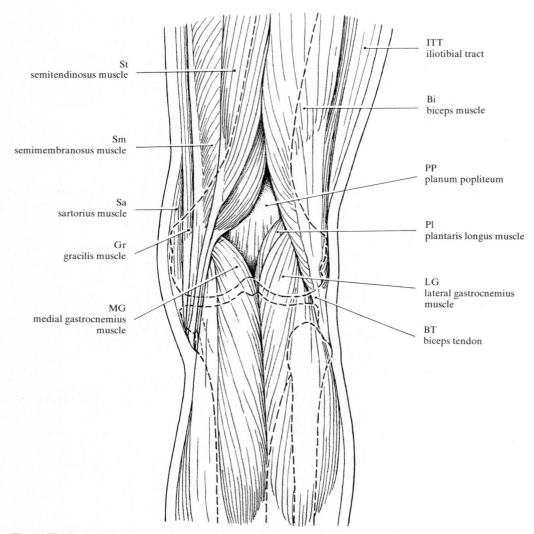

St
semitendinosus muscle

Sm
semimembranosus muscle

Sa
sartorius muscle

Gr
gracilis muscle

MG
medial gastrocnemius
muscle

ITT
iliotibial tract

Bi
biceps muscle

PP
planum popliteum

Pl
plantaris longus muscle

LG
lateral gastrocnemius
muscle

BT
biceps tendon

Fig. 4. The knee joint and its main anatomic structures viewed from the posterior aspect

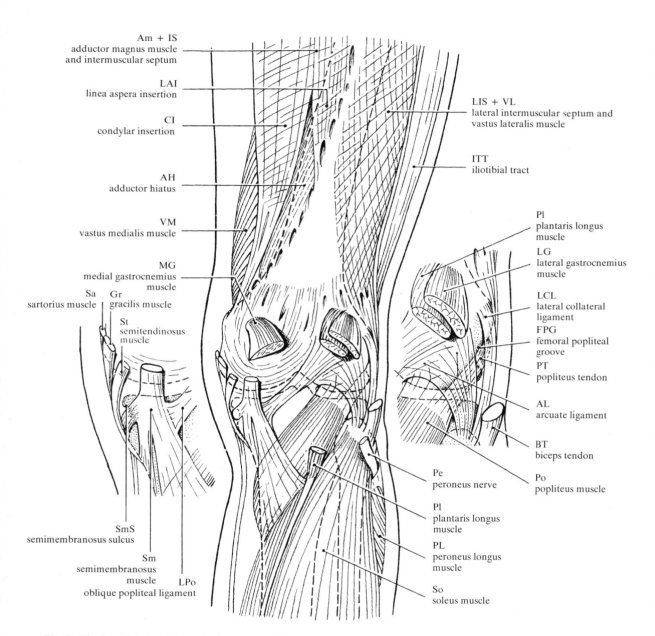

Fig. 5. The knee joint and its main deep anatomic structures viewed from the posterior aspect

Am + IS
adductor magnus muscle
and intermuscular septum

LAI
linea aspera insertion

CI
condylar insertion

AH
adductor hiatus

VM
vastus medialis muscle

MG
medial gastrocnemius
muscle

Sa
sartorius muscle

Gr
gracilis muscle

St
semitendinosus
muscle

SmS
semimembranosus sulcus

Sm
semimembranosus
muscle

LPo
oblique popliteal ligament

LIS + VL
lateral intermuscular septum and
vastus lateralis muscle

ITT
iliotibial tract

Pl
plantaris longus
muscle

LG
lateral gastrocnemius
muscle

LCL
lateral collateral
ligament

FPG
femoral popliteal
groove

PT
popliteus tendon

AL
arcuate ligament

BT
biceps tendon

Po
popliteus muscle

Pe
peroneus nerve

Pl
plantaris longus
muscle

PL
peroneus longus
muscle

So
soleus muscle

Kinematics

Kinematics of the Rolling-Gliding Principle

It is generally agreed that the Weber brothers [219–221, 336] were the first, in 1836, to describe the combination of rotational gliding and rolling in the tibiofemoral joint. Strasser [336] dealt exhaustively with this phenomenon in 1917, and in recent years Groh [116], Kapandji [164], Frankel [97, 98], Menschik [219–221], Huson [139], Nietert [253] and Goodfellow and O'Connor [109] have prompted refinements in our knowledge.

Interestingly, a long period elapsed between the painstaking studies of the 19th-century anatomists and present-day research. Apparently the findings of the anatomists, who focused on macrostructure and function, bore little relevance to practical medicine, including operative orthopedics, and so were largely forgotten during the subsequent period of microanatomic research. Only recently has the need for practical applications prompted researchers to reexamine these old findings. Thus, the work of Groh [116] on exoprostheses, of Nietert [253] on endoprostheses, of Kapandji [164] and Huson [139] on fundamental considerations, and of Menschik [219–221] and Goodfellow and O'Connor [109] on basic questions and special problems in endoprosthetics have served as an impetus for further research. Sports medicine and general traumatology can only profit from this in terms of the evaluation and management of the injured knee.

It is agreed that the basic mechanism of movement between the femur and tibia is a combination of rolling and gliding. On closer analysis, it becomes difficult to discern the

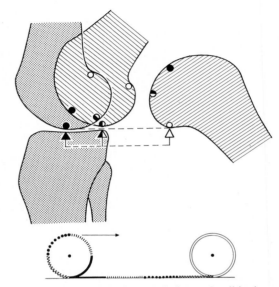

Fig. 6. Movement of the femur relative to the tibia during flexion, showing the theoretical contact points if a pure rolling motion were involved. The femur would roll off the tibial plateau. ▲ tibial and ● femoral contact point during extension; ▲ ◑ at about 45° flexion, △ ○ at 135° flexion

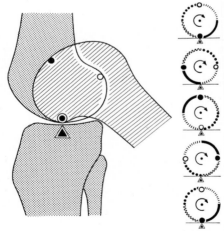

Fig. 7. Movement of the femur relative to the tibia during flexion, showing the single theoretical contact point if a purely gliding motion were involved. The metaphysis of the femur would engage on the posterior rim of the tibial plateau at 130° of flexion

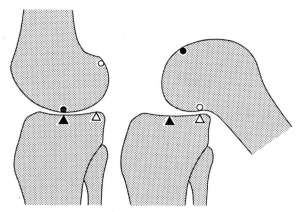

Fig. 8. Movement of the femur relative to the tibia during flexion, showing the contact points generated by a combination of rolling and gliding. This represents the true physiologic action of the tibiofemoral joint

exact mix of rolling and gliding in the individual phases of movement, because automatic initial and terminal rotation as well as voluntary rotation are superimposed upon the basic flexion and extension movements in the sagittal plane.

However, if we reduce the problem to one involving a single plane, the sagittal, it becomes easy to demonstrate and understand how the femoral condyle rolls (Fig. 6), glides (Fig. 7), and rolls and glides simultaneously (Fig. 8) on the tibia.

Model of the Crossed Four-Bar Linkage

As Kapandji [164], Huson [139] and Menschik [219–221] were able to show with diagrams, the basic kinematic principle of motion in the knee joint can be represented by the mechanism of the crossed four-bar linkage.

We can construct a simple apparatus consisting of a sheet of drawing paper on which two rods are hinged at one end like the hands of a clock. The two hinge points must lie on a line which intersects at a 40° angle the longitudinal axis through one of the points. One of the crossed rods is longer than the other, their length ratio being equal to that of the normal anterior cruciate ligament to the posterior cruciate. The free ends of the rods are linked by a movable rectangular Plexiglas bar. This bar forms the "coupler" of the linkage. A line can be drawn along the coupler as it is moved through its various positions to generate a set of tangents which delineate a curve. This "coupler envelope curve" (Fig. 9) approximates the contour of a sagittal section through the posterior half of the femoral condyle (Fig. 10).

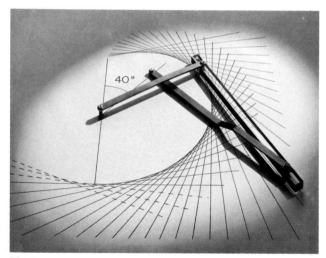

Fig. 9

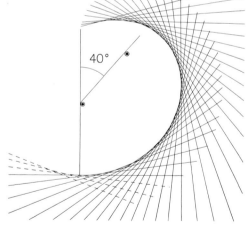

Fig. 10

Fig. 9. Model of a crossed four-bar linkage. The cruciate ligaments are represented by rigid rods that are hinged on a line set at a 40° angle to a given perpendicular. The tibial plateau is represented by the "coupler," which consists of a rectangular Plexiglas bar.

Successive lines drawn along the coupler as it passes through its range of motion describe a curve which approximates the contour of the posterior portion of the femoral condyle (photo Baur)

Fig. 10. The "coupler envelope curve" generated by the apparatus in Fig. 9 (photo Baur)

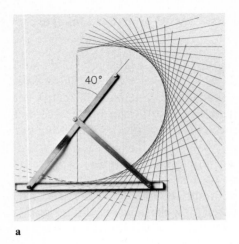

a

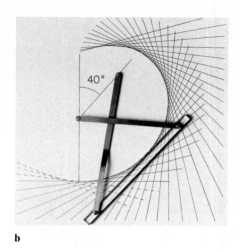

b

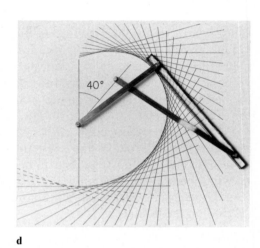

c

d

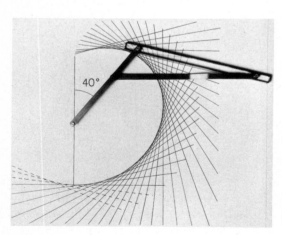

e

Fig. 11 a–e. Phases in the movement of the crossed four-bar linkage with a fixed vertical long axis (photo Baur)

10

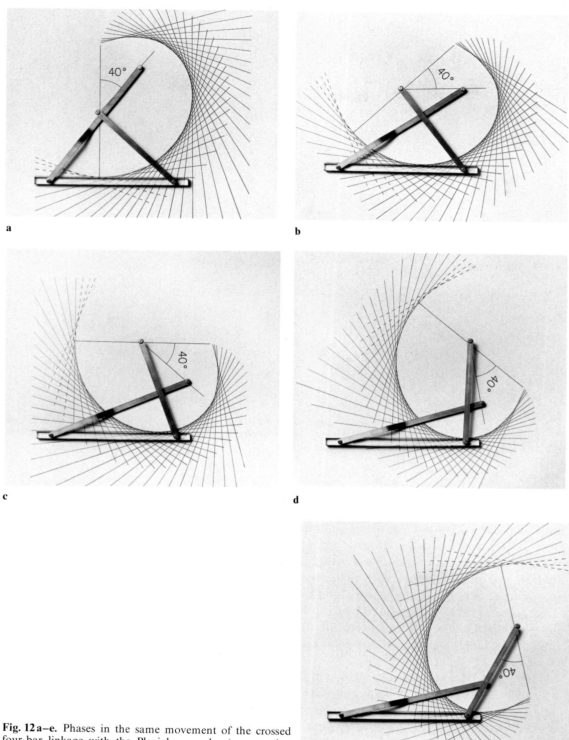

Fig. 12a–e. Phases in the same movement of the crossed four-bar linkage with the Plexiglas coupler (representing the tibial plateau) as the fixed member (photo Baur)

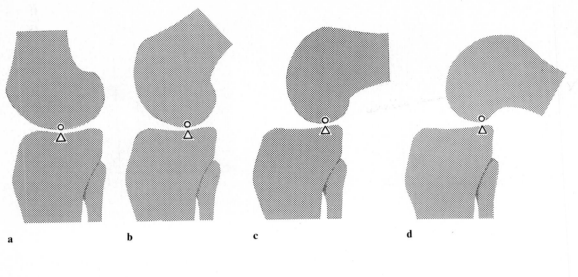

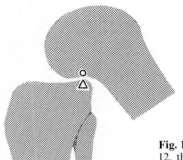

Fig. 13 a–e. In comparison with the model range of movement in Figs. 11 and 12, these drawings show the natural motion sequence with the varying positions of femorotibial contact

If, instead of a straight coupler, we were to use a concave or convex one corresponding more closely to the actual contour of the upper tibial surface, we would obtain a slightly different coupler envelope curve that would approximate very closely the natural contour of the femoral condyle. As stated previously, however, this holds only theoretically for motion in a single plane, without allowance for rotation.

With this model we can also demonstrate the obligatory shift of the contact points during articular motion. Whether we move the coupler itself (Fig. 11) or the envelope curve obtained with the coupler fixed horizontally (Fig. 12), the obligatory sequence remains unchanged. But with the coupler as the stationary member, the system-intrinsic backward shift of the contact point on the coupler becomes much more obvious. For

comparison, Fig. 13 shows the silhouettes of the tibia and femur indicating the natural posterior shift of the contact point of the articular surfaces during flexion. Under these circumstances the knee can be flexed without the femoral shaft impacting on the posterior tibial plateau at the end of flexion (cf. Fig. 7). As early as 1853, Meyer [226] was struck by the peculiar overhang of the posterior tibial plateau; now, with the obligatory shift of contact points understood, a convincing explanation for this phenomenon has been found.

Varying Ratio of Rolling to Gliding

An accurate plot of the contact points between femur and tibia reveals that the ratio of rolling to gliding does not remain con-

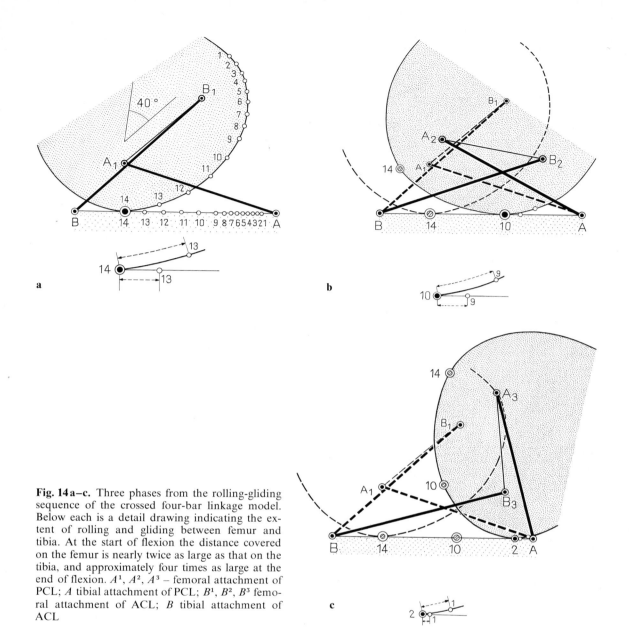

Fig. 14a–c. Three phases from the rolling-gliding sequence of the crossed four-bar linkage model. Below each is a detail drawing indicating the extent of rolling and gliding between femur and tibia. At the start of flexion the distance covered on the femur is nearly twice as large as that on the tibia, and approximately four times as large at the end of flexion. A^1, A^2, A^3 – femoral attachment of PCL; A tibial attachment of PCL; B^1, B^2, B^3 femoral attachment of ACL; B tibial attachment of ACL

stant through all degrees of flexion. This ratio is approximately 1:2 in early flexion and about 1:4 by the end of flexion (Fig. 14).

Kinematics and Anatomic Form of the Femoral Condyle

By a comparison of x-rays, it can be seen that actually only the posterior portion of the femoral condyle is subject to this law,

and that its validity ends where the femoropatellar joint surface begins (Fig. 15).

When hyperextension occurs, it is by angulation in the terminal sulcus of the femoral condyle between the femorotibial and femoropatellar articular surfaces, rather than by a continuation of rotational gliding (Fig. 16).

In ligamentous instability of the knee joint with anterior cruciate insufficiency and corresponding hyperextensibility, an impression often forms on the femoral condyle (either

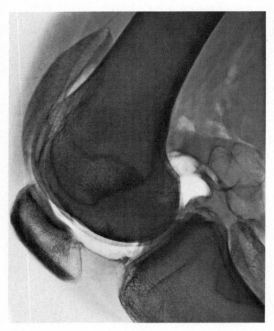
a

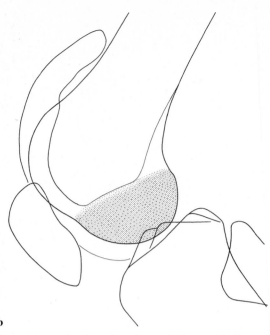
b

Fig. 15. a Roentgenogram and **b** corresponding positional drawing showing which part of the femoral condyle is subject to the law of the crossed four-bar linkage by virtue of its shape. This part corresponds precisely to the part of the femur that articulates with the tibia, while the more proximal portion that articulates with the patella has a shape that is dictated by different laws. Note also the extraarticular location of the patellar apex, whose point extends into the patellar ligament

a

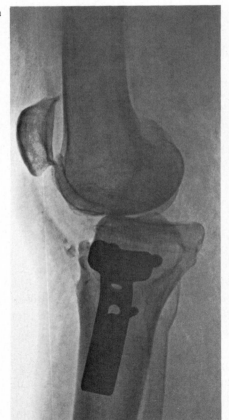

b

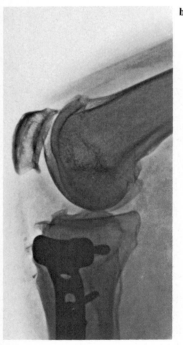

Fig. 16a, b. Roentgenograms of a post-traumatic genu recurvatum. Hyperextension does not involve a continuation of rotational gliding, but occurs by angulation at the terminal sulcus

14

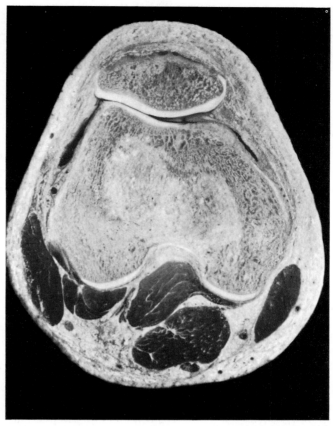

Fig. 17. Transverse section through the knee joint at the level of the femoral condyle showing the femoropatellar gliding surface. The patella in this specimen is not centered in the trochlea of the femur, but is subluxated laterally. (Ficat [88] describes this as "malposition externe de la rotule, MER.") The lateral part is generally un-der greater contact pressure than the medial facet. Occasionally a free space may even exist on the medial side between the femur and patella and may contain a special synovial fold, the plica alaris medialis (v. Hochstetter)

acutely or as a result of chronic pressure). This feature was first recognized in 1917 by Strasser [336], who called it the "impressio terminalis." An analogous phenomenon can be observed in knee joints with idiopathic laxity and hypermobility [328].

Superposition of the Patellar Gliding Surface on the Femoral Condyle

Anterior to the sulcus or the impressio terminalis is a cartilaginous area on the femur which articulates only with the patella and is fashioned like a trochlea. In the human knee, however, the patella articulates not

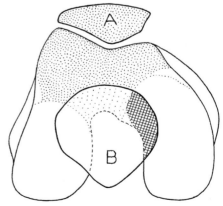

Fig. 18. Position of the patella in relation to the femoral articular surface. *A* In extension the patella articulates purely with the femoral patellar surface. *B* In full flexion it also articulates with portions of the femoral condyle in the true femorotibial area

15

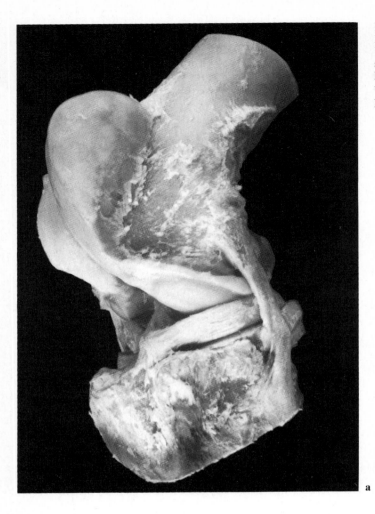

Fig. 19 a, b. Preparation of an equine knee demonstrating an hourglass-shaped boundary between the patellar and tibial surfaces of the femur. As in the human knee, the paired cruciate ligaments function according to the four-bar linkage principle (Boehnel)

a

just with the femoral patellar surface, but, beyond 90° of flexion, also with the cartilaginous surface of the femoral condyle that articulates with the tibia (Figs. 17 and 18), as Grant and Basmajian [113] demonstrated in 1965. In the horse knee, by contrast, the articular surfaces of the femur with the patella and with the tibia are entirely separate from each other (Fig. 19). Thus, the equine patella never comes in contact with the tibial articular surface of the femoral condyle.

The Cruciate Ligaments as the Foundation of Knee Joint Kinematics

The function of the cruciate ligaments and shape of the condyles are closely inter-related. Without the cruciate ligaments, knee joint kinematics could not exist in the form described. This raises the question of which is present first, the cruciate ligaments or the moving articular surfaces, and whether a knee joint can function normally after the loss or rupture of a cruciate ligament. Tillmann [340] showed in 1974 with histologic sections how the cruciate ligaments are formed in the human embryo, demonstrating their presence at 10 weeks and thus before the development of a joint space with freedom of movement. The basic contour of the femoral condyle is also apparent at this stage. Thus, the subsequent motion of the articular surfaces apparently is predetermined to a large degree by the early presence of the cruciate ligaments (Fig. 20). The

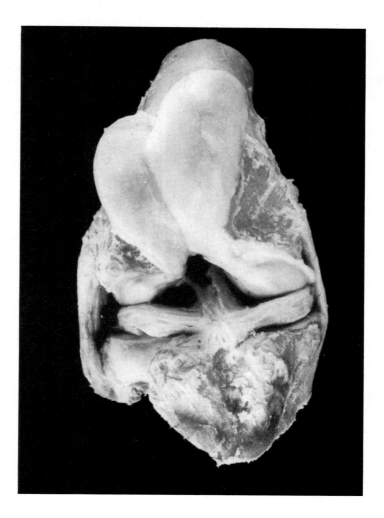

Fig. 19b

intercondylar roof angle of 40° is also evident in the 10-week-old embryo (see also Fig. 24). Distinct menisci are also present. They are still discoid in shape and are fused with the upper tibial surface. Only when joint motion begins must they separate from the tibia so that they can follow the excursions of the femur.

Thus, the functional importance of the cruciate ligaments has a very early origin. This functional congruence can be maintained in later life only if the ligaments continue to perform their function to a sufficient degree. They convert a simple rotational movement into a more complex movement of the "coupler." Hence, as Huson [139] and Menschik [219–221] point out, the cruciate ligaments perform the function of a true gear mechanism and form the nucleus of knee joint kinematics. Both Trillat and Menschik have confirmed in their films that the division of a cruciate ligament abolishes the gear mechanism, and that the latter cannot be satisfactorily replaced by the function of the peripheral ligaments and joint capsule.

Kinematics and Applied Physiology and Pathophysiology of the Ligaments

Cruciate Ligaments

If we adhere for the moment to our simple scheme of uniplanar motion, the cruciate ligaments, as radii of constant length, trace

17

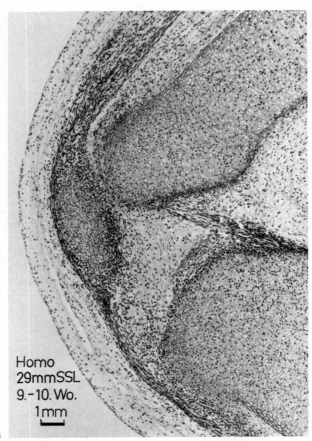

a

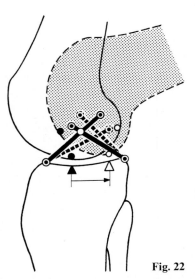

b

Fig. 20a, b. The two histologic sections from a human embryo at about 10 weeks' gestation in the frontal and sagittal planes already show the two cruciate ligaments in place, even before a true joint cavity is visible. The menisci are still discoid at this stage (Tillmann)

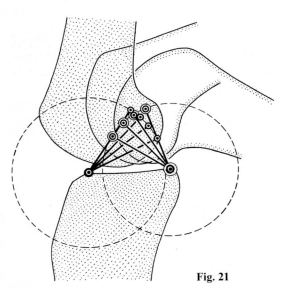

Fig. 21

Fig. 22

Fig. 21. Both cruciate ligaments move on circular arcs during flexion and extension, according to the principles of the crossed four-bar linkage, when motions are reduced schematically to a single plane

Fig. 22. Inherent in the motion of the cruciate attachments along circular arcs is an automatic posterior shift of the femorotibial contact point

18

out small circular arcs. With the tibia fixed, their end-points on the femur lie on a circular line (Fig. 21). Conversely, if the tibia is moved and the femur is fixed, the femoral end-point forms the center of the circle. Of course this model is valid only if we view the cruciate ligament as an ideal line. But of the many ligament fibers that are necessary for mechanical strength, not all can fit on the ideal line. The consequences of this are explored later on (see p. 31).

The laws of this cruciate "four-bar linkage," which determine the obligatory motion of the joint surfaces with the posterior shift of the contact point (Fig. 22), are solely responsible for this functional sequence. The sequence remains operative even if the collateral ligaments are lost and the extension and flexion movements between femur and tibia occur in one plane.

Cruciate Ligaments and Range of Joint Motion

The limits of knee joint motion are also determined by the arrangement of the cruciate ligaments. For example, if their proximal origins lay on a straight line at right angles to the long axis of the femur, the knee joint would have a mobility of 50°–0–70°, i.e., 50° of hypertension and only 70° of flexion (Fig. 23). To allow the normal mobility of 5°–0–145°, the femoral origins of the cruciate ligaments must lie on a line which forms a 40° angle with the long axis of the femur. As it happens, the roof of the intercondylar notch indeed forms a 40° angle with the long axis (Fig. 24).

Already we see, then, that the cruciate ligaments act to limit extension and prevent hyperextension. If the knee is forced into extension or hyperextension, the weaker anterior cruciate is placed in a critical situation, with the possibility of an acute lesion (see Fig. 30). Investigations of knee joints with chronic anterior cruciate insufficiency confirm that a pathologic hyperextensibility is always present in such cases. The posterior cruciate also engages on the vault of the intercondylar notch in maximum flexion. However, this contact in the terminal position does not carry as high a risk of injury to the posterior cruciate as hyperextension does to the anterior ligament (Fig. 25).

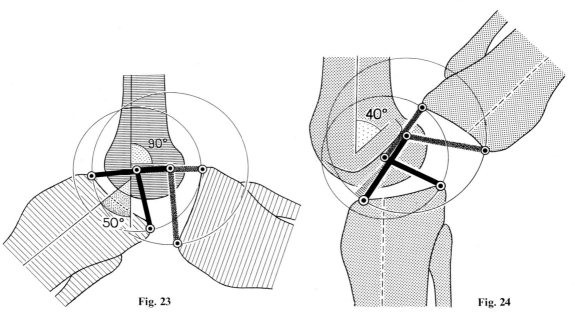

Fig. 23   **Fig. 24**

Fig. 23. If the femoral attachments of the cruciate ligaments lay on a line at right angles to the long axis of the femur, a mobility of 50°–0–70° would result (after Menschik [219])

Fig. 24. The normal knee mobility of 5°–0–145° is allowed only if the femoral attachments of the cruciate ligaments lie on a line forming a 40° angle with the long axis of the femur. The arc (– – –) anterior to the anterior cruciate ligament indicates the hyperextension problem associated with this ligament

19

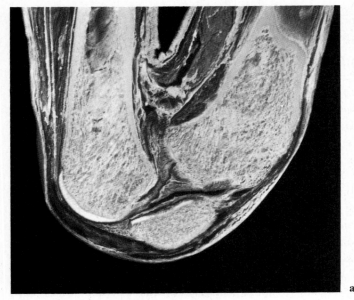
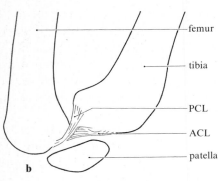

femur

tibia

PCL

ACL

patella

b

a

Fig. 25. a The anatomic section in the median sagittal plane (v. Hochstetter) and **b** positional drawing confirm the extreme position of the cruciate ligaments in maximum passive flexion, which causes some angulation of the posterior cruciate

The Consequences of Faulty Reinsertion of Avulsed Anterior Cruciate Ligaments

Not infrequently, a ruptured cruciate ligament is reinserted too far anteriorly in the vault of the intercondylar notch (Fig. 26). As a result of this, the anterior cruciate is too short during flexion and would prevent it were it not for the sizable forces generated by the muscles and lever arms. As the weakest member, the ligament must either rupture or elongate during flexion. This applies not just to the ligament, but to the fixation wire as well (Fig. 27). The wire frag-

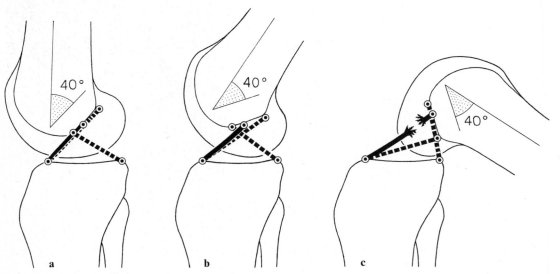

a   **b**   **c**

Fig. 26a–c. Improperly inserted, the cruciate ligaments cannot trace out circular arcs during flexion. Thus, an anterior cruciate ligament reinserted too far anteriorally (**a**) becomes lax at about 40° of flexion (**b**). At 120° of flexion it must tear due to insufficient length (**c**)

20

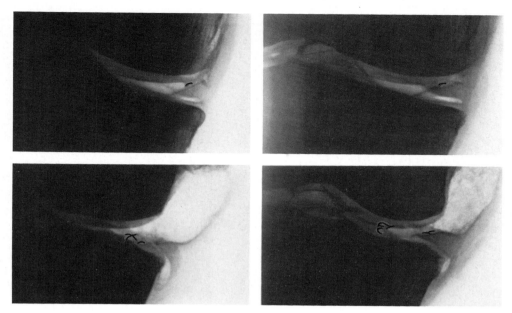

Fig. 27. Arthrograms of a knee joint with chronic hemorrhagic effusion and multiple metallic fragments from a ruptured cruciate ligament wire suture. The wire fragments lie on and beneath the meniscus

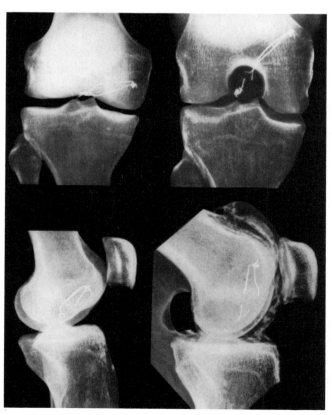

Fig. 28. Knee joint as in Fig. 27 with an improperly re-inserted anterior cruciate ligament. In extension the broken ends of the wire are in contact, i.e., the wire length is still sufficient for the reattached ligament in this position. In flexion, the wire is obviously too short as indicated by the marked separation of the torn ends (see also Fig. 26)

21

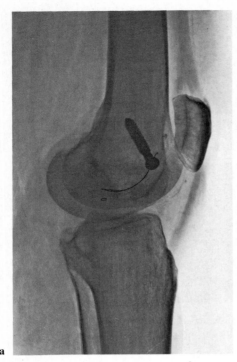

a

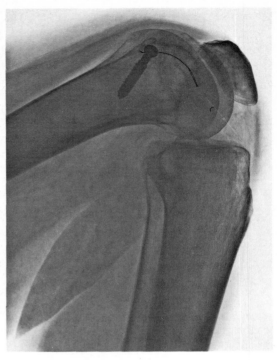

b

Fig. 29 a, b. Further documentation of an anterior cruciate ligament reinserted too far anteriorally and proximally, with a fatigue fracture of the wire suture. The torn ends are apposed in extension (**a**) and separated in flexion (**b**). Note also the femoropatellar relation in extension

ments then can enter the articular cavity, where they can cause chronic hemorrhagic effusion with corresponding secondary destruction of the cartilage [289].

The motion films for two such cases document the faulty action of the improperly reinserted cruciate ligament by means of the visible wire suture (Fig. 28). In extension (left of figure), the ruptured ends of the wire are in apposition, while in flexion they are widely separated (see also Fig. 26). We encountered a very similar situation (Fig. 29) in a patient who was prevented from engaging in her favorite sport, mountain climbing, by a serious anteromedial instability of the knee. At reoperation it was possible to restore stability by correct reattachment of the anterior cruciate ligament and secondary repair of the posterior oblique ligament, leaving only a mild residual instability that could be well compensated. One year after reoperation the patient is free of complaints and has been able to resume her former activities.

Hyperextension and the Anterior Cruciate Ligament

Active, violent hyperextension of the knee in internal rotation or hyperextension by passive violence can injure the anterior cruciate ligament at the anterior border of the intercondylar roof (Fig. 30). At that location, according to Grant and Basmajian [113], there is a notch into which the anterior cruciate fits on extension of the knee. In hyperextension this ligament can become kinked and torn at the edge of this "notch of Grant"; the synergistic ligament structures in the semimembranosus corner on the medial side and popliteus corner on the lateral side can only become stretched.

The Anterior Cruciate Ligament and the Menisci

The two sagittal sections through the medial and lateral compartments (Figs. 31 and 33) demonstrate the lack of congruence of the

22

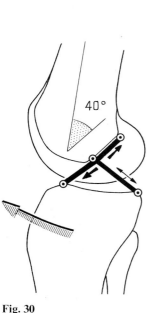

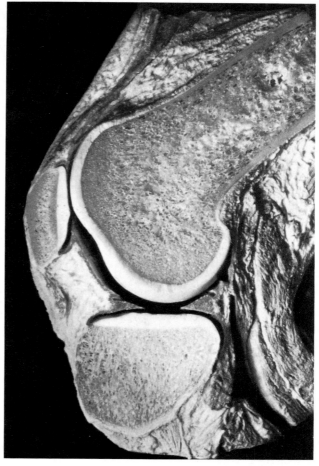

Fig. 30   **Fig. 31**

Fig. 30. Violent hyperextension of the knee (*large arrow*), especially in IR, causes extreme tensile forces to act on the anterior cruciate ligament (*short, thick ar-* *row*), which is also increasingly stretched over the anterior edge of the intercondylar notch. The posterior cruciate ligament is also tightened (*thin arrow*)

Fig. 31. Sagittal section through the medial half of the knee joint, showing the "point" contact area between the femur and tibia. This specimen also demonstrates how the stability of the knee derives not from the bone contours or congruence of the joint surfaces, but entire- ly from the ligamentous system. Note the location of the menisci and fat pad, the sulcus between the femoro- patellar and femorotibial joint surfaces, and the area of patellar contact with the femur (v. Hochstetter)

articular surfaces of the knee. The congruence that exists is a purely functional one, deriving chiefly from the gear-like mechanism of the cruciate ligaments. All other passive and dynamic structures are oriented toward this fact, including the menisci. The menisci improve the instantaneous joint congruence but must move out of the way of the femoral condyles during knee motion so that they will not become "caught beneath the wheels" as the contact point moves anteriorly or posteriorly.

Cruciate Insufficiency and Meniscal Lesions

As Artmann and Wirth [14] were able to demonstrate in 1974, *anterior cruciate insufficiency* actually results in a *disintegration of the rolling-gliding movement,* causing the femoral condyle to roll excessively before it glides.

If the anterior cruciate ligament is torn, the femur rolls up onto the meniscus and its posterior horn with flexion and then skids back (Fig. 32). This leads to the well-known

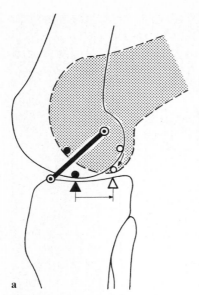
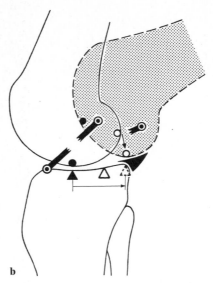

a

b

Fig. 32. a Function of the intact anterior cruciate ligament. **b** *The loss of its function* leads to excessive femoral rolling, resulting in an abnormal posterior shift of the femoral contact point on both the medial and lateral sides. The posterior horns of the menisci are severely stressed as they act to brake this rolling movement and are subject to chronic attrition. △ Normal contact point in flexion; ▵ abnormal contact points in anterior cruciate insufficiency

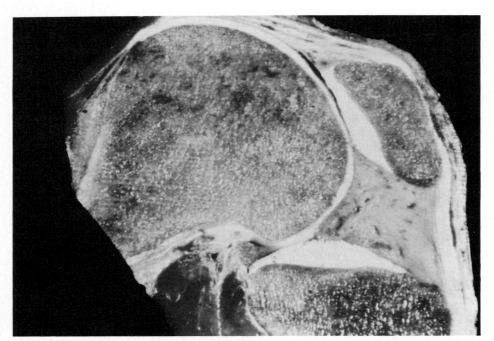

Fig. 33. Sagittal section through the lateral half of the knee joint. Note the relation of the posterior meniscus horn to the femoral condyle and tibial plateau in full flexion and the extreme posterior position of the femorotibial contact point. The convexity of the lateral tibial "plateau" is clearly visible, as is the very thick layer of articular cartilage on the lateral tibia and patella (McIntosh)

24

pattern of clinical deterioration described by Chalandre [48] in 1977: First meniscal symptoms appear on one side, with subsequent tearing. A meniscectomy on this side is frequently followed in the next phase by the appearance of meniscal symptoms with a tear on the opposite side. Finally this second meniscus is also excised, resulting in the unhappy situation of a knee joint with bilateral meniscectomy, anterior cruciate insufficiency and progressive cartilage damage. Typically at this stage, some type of ligamentous repair is done [66].

The breakdown of functional congruity in anterior cruciate rupture, as described by Olsson et al. [277] 1972 in studies on dogs, leads to the formation of reactive degenerative osteophytes. A vicious cycle develops, with progression from insufficiency to late changes to arthrosis.

In 1972 Gudde and Wagenknecht [119] reported very poor results in 50 patients who underwent medial meniscectomy but had untreated anterior cruciate lesions. On follow-up they found abnormal passive hyperextensibility, an anterior drawer sign of 10–20 mm, and degenerative osteophytes.

The experiences of these authors agree closely with our own observations in earlier cases as well as in late referred cases.

Anterior Cruciate Insufficiency and the Lateral Pivot Shift Phenomenon

Slocum and Larson [324] pointed out in 1968 the abnormal freedom of rotation in complex instabilities, thereby adding a new dimension to the study of the effects of individual ligamentous ruptures.

Today the names McIntosh and Galway are closely associated with the concept of "lateral pivot shift." In 1972 Galway [102] wrote his now-famous report, and in 1974 Kostuik (personal communication) gave the first lecture-demonstration at our clinic in Basel, Switzerland.

It was strongly suspected that insufficiency of the anterior cruciate ligament was responsible for this subluxation phenomenon, which can give rise to a whole syndrome of associated changes, such as flattening of the femoral condyle, cartilage erosion and lateral meniscal ruptures. Ségal et al. [314] gave in 1980 a topographic and chronographic description of the inevitable progress of these secondary changes.

Jakob and Noesberger [49] demonstrated in 1977 in the stable cadaveric knee that the division of the anterior cruciate was the key to eliciting the lateral pivot shift phenomenon. Simultaneous division of the medial deep posterior ligament (semimembranosus corner) and lateral structures accentuated the phenomenon.

On complete division of the deep and long ligaments of the medial side, the phenomenon could no longer be elicited, because the knee could no longer be subjected to the valgus stress necessary for the test. Galway et al. [103] also spoke of an anterior cruciate insufficiency syndrome in 1979.

To explain the phenomenon further, we must recount briefly the McIntosh test.

When the anterior cruciate ligament is incompetent, a distinct "subluxation snap" occurs when the extended knee is slowly brought to about 30–40° of flexion under valgus stress and internal rotation.

Observing the knee joint shortly before the snapping point is reached, one will note an increasing anterior subluxation of the tibia which reduces abruptly when the snap occurs. After this reduction the femur and tibia are once again in normal relation to each other for the degree of flexion attained. The phenomenon clearly demonstrates the disintegration of the rolling-gliding movement as a consequence of the anterior cruciate insufficiency.

Wirth and Artmann [389] in 1974 demonstrated this disintegration in a different context and thus proved the possibility of its occurrence in anterior cruciate insufficiency. In the present situation, the disintegration means that the femur rolls without gliding through up to 30° of flexion and thus comes to lie too far posteriorly on the tibial plateau (Figs. 36 and 37). This is aided by the superior convexity of the lateral tibial pla-

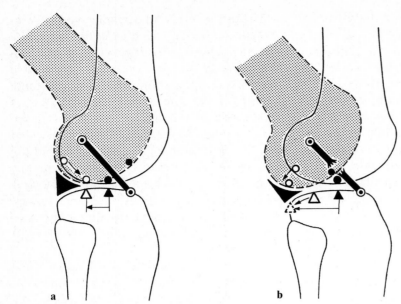

Fig. 34a, b. If the anterior cruciate ligament is insufficient, the femur can easily roll down beyond the posterior half of the tibial plateau. This phenomenon also underlies the "lateral pivot shift," a clinical sign of anterior cruciate insufficiency

teau, and the phenomenon is driven by the strong valgus pressure, favoring rolling over gliding, when the iliotibial tract is stretched taut by the internal rotation of the tibia (Fig. 35). The tract, with its Y-shaped expansion directed posteriorly, pushes the lateral femoral condyle backward on the tibia as it rolls, until it has crossed, at 30–40° of flex-ion, the culmination point of the femoral condyle and the momentary flexion axis. At that moment the femur can snap back forward into its normal position relative to the tibia. Because the femur is joined with the trunk via the hip joint, it is the tibia that actually snaps back into place relative to the femur (Figs. 38 and 39).

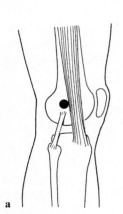
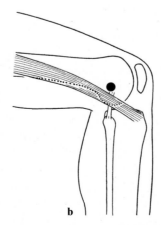

Fig. 35a, b. The iliotibial tract is a combined active and passive stabilizer. As such, it lies on the extensor side of the flexion axis between 0° and about 40° of flexion (**a**). As the knee is flexed further, the tract glides posterior-ally across the rotational axis and thus across the lateral femoral condyle and acts as a synergist of the flexors (**b**). This circumstance also plays a role in the pathogenesis of the lateral pivot shift phenomenon

26

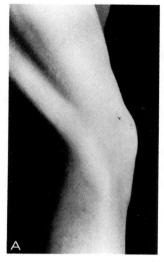
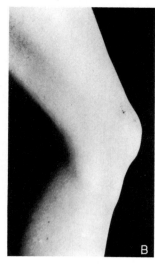

Fig. 36a, b. Phases of the lateral pivot shift phenomenon as viewed from the lateral side. Under general anesthesia the knee was flexed preoperatively in the McIntosh test to the point just short of eliciting the snapping phenomenon. **a** Here the iliotibial tract is in extreme tension and still passes anterior to the flexion axis; the tibia is in the anterior drawer position. **b** In this photo the knee has been flexed a few degrees farther, and the tibia has snapped back into its normal position relative to the femur. The silhouette also shows clearly that the iliotibial tract now passes behind the transverse flexion axis

At this point it is important to elaborate on a further peculiarity of knee physiology, without which this phenomenon could scarcely be elicited in the manner described.

The iliotibial tract has a complex task and, accordingly, performs multiple functions. As the tendon of the tensor fasciae latae muscle, it acts as an extensor when the knee is in 0–30° flexion, and becomes a flexor when the knee is flexed to 40–145°. Passage of the momentary transverse flexion axis occurs at 30–40° of flexion. This neutral role of the iliotibial tract is also exploited in Slocum's test (see p. 134) for anterior and posterior drawer sign.

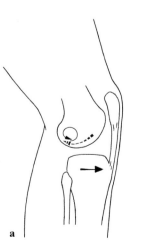
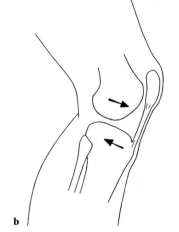

a   b

Fig. 37a. The drawing shows the increased posterior rolling (*circular arrow* and *dashed arrow*) of the femur with the relative spontaneous reduction of the joint members at the moment the snap occurs (**b**)

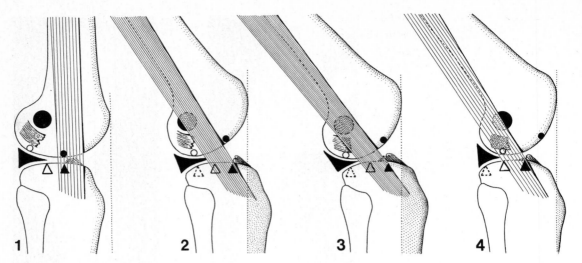

1   2   3   4

Fig. 38. Four-phase schematic representation of the lateral pivot shift phenomenon in anterior cruciate insufficiency. *Phase 1.* Normal starting position in extension. *Phase 2.* Increased posterior rolling of the femur due to anterior cruciate insufficiency. The iliotibial tract is still in front of the transverse flexion axis and lateral epicondyle. The tibia is in the anterior drawer position. *Phase 3.* At this moment the iliotibial tract snaps across the flexion axis and epicondyle. The tract is under maximum tension, and anterior displacement of the tibia is also maximal. *Phase 4.* The tract is now behind the transverse flexion axis and epicondyle. The femur was able to snap back anteriorly, occupying a position on the tibia appropriate for the angle of flexion. The tibia has performed an opposite movement, snapping back from its anterior drawer position into a normal relation with the femur; this movement is more obvious than that of the femur. The superior convexity of the lateral tibial plateau (Fig. 33) is recognized as another enabling factor in the pivot shift phenomenon, together with anterior cruciate insufficiency and the pathophysiology of the iliotibial tract; ●symbol for flexion axis

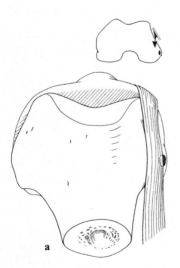 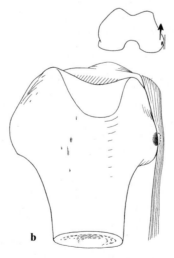

a   b

Fig. 39a, b. The iliotibial tract during the pivot shift phenomenon (transverse section). During the first 40° of flexion in which the knee is slowly flexed manually in IR and under a valgus stress, the tract pushes the V-shaped condyle backward and forces it into a purely rolling movement, as may occur in anterior cruciate insufficiency. As soon as flexion has passed the critical angle between 40 and 50°, the tract passes the summit of the lateral femoral epicondyle, allowing it to snap back into its normal, unforced position. In such cases the ligamentous portion of the tract is no longer properly attached to the lateral condyle via the intermuscular septum

At the same time, the iliotibial tract is an excellent example of a "dynamized" ligament. It incorporates extensions of the intermuscular septum – femorotibial ligamentous fibers that extend from the proximal part of the femoral condyle to the tubercle of Gerdy.[1] This ligamentous extension is no longer competent in anterolateral instability of the knee and is another enabling factor in the lateral pivot shift phenomenon. More will be said about this "lateral femorotibial ligament" and its physiologic importance in a later chapter.

For an adequate discussion of the lateral pivot shift phenomenon, it is important to note further that the greater the anterior cruciate insufficiency and the less competent the femorotibial component of the iliotibial tract, the farther posteriorly the femur can roll and thus subluxate. Additional tests of Hughston and Losee relating to the same problem are discussed under Examination (see p. 134).

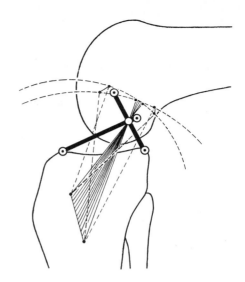

Fig. 40. Like the insertion points of the ideal cruciate ligaments, the insertion points of the collateral ligament fibers also follow circular paths in the ideal case. The broken lines indicate the terminal positions of the collateral ligaments in extension and flexion

Collateral Ligaments

As in the case of the cruciate ligaments, which can be ideally represented as a crossed four-bar linkage, there is also an ideal construct for the collateral ligaments. They, too, can follow an approximately circular path during the kinematic sequence. This path corresponds to a short circular arc when the femur is in motion (Fig. 40, 41) and to a somewhat larger arc when the tibia is moved.

Subsequent to his work at the Technical College of Vienna, Menschik [219–221] described in 1974 the "Burmester curve" and quotes [in 49] from the *Lehrbuch der Kinematik* ("Textbook of Kinematics") written by the Munich mathematician Burmester and published in 1888.

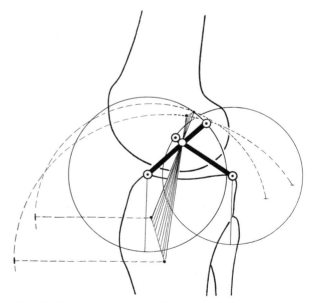

Fig. 41. The circular paths of motion of the cruciate ligaments are indicated by solid lines. The smaller circle is traced out by the shorter posterior cruciate ligament, and the larger circle by the longer anterior cruciate. The broken lines show the paths of the anterior and posterior edges of the medial collateral ligament and indicate a smaller circle for the fibers that insert anteriorly on the tibia and a larger circle for those that insert posteriorly

---

1 In official nomenclature the tubercle of Gerdy is the "tuberosity of the iliotibial tract." But the former term, after the French anatomist, is preferred because it helps avoid confusion with the adjacent tibial tuberosity

29

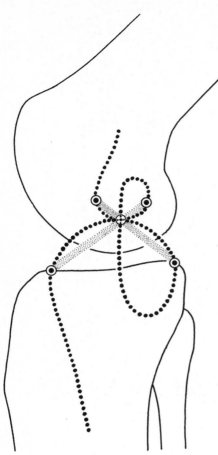

Fig. 42. The Burmester curve forms an important part of the kinematics of the four-bar linkage. It is comprised of the pivot cubic and the vertex cubic. A point on the pivot cubic that is connected by a straight line through the center with an opposite point on the vertex cubic follows an approximately circular path about the latter point when the linkage is moved (see also Figs. 62 and 63)

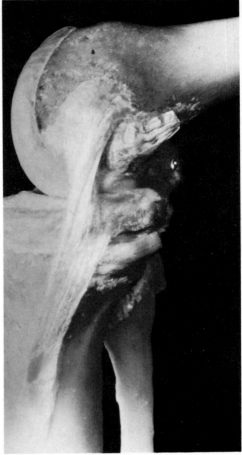

Fig. 43. Anatomic preparation of the medial collateral ligament. Note that ⅓ of the course of the ligament is femoral, and ⅔ is tibial. The shape and position of the ligament conform almost perfectly to the conditions of the Burmester curve

According to Burmester, there is a curve which is comprised of two third-order curves called the "vertex cubic" and the "pivot cubic" (Fig. 42). The Burmester curve is of fundamental importance with regard to the sites of ligament insertion on the knee. If we draw a straight line from a point on the vertex cubic through the crossing point P of the four-bar linkage to a point on the pivot cubic, the two points will follow approximately circular paths when the linkage is moved, such that their distance from each other on the straight line remains practically constant. It is unclear whether these points follow true circular arcs or whether their paths are only approximately circular. We have approached physicists with this problem, but they have yet to furnish us with a definitive answer.

But whether the paths are precisely circular or not does not really concern us here, inasmuch as nature has confirmed the validity of the laws by the actual sites of the ligament insertions. The ligaments insert at the sites that theory would predict, and the course of the ligaments also conforms to theory (Fig. 43).

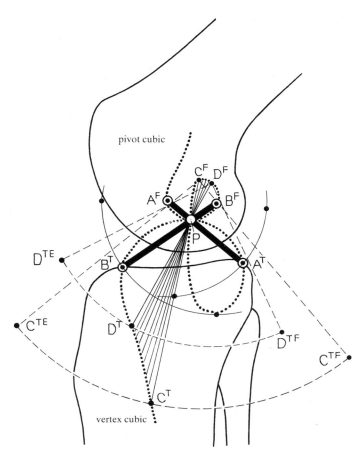

Fig. 44. The theoretical course of the medial collateral ligament and its position in relation to the Burmester curve. In our simplified scheme after Menschik [220], the tibia is moved relative to the stationary femur. If a point C^F on the pivot cubic is connected with a point C^T on the vertex cubic through the center P, the point C^T will follow an approximately circular path when the tibia is moved. (Hereafter we will assume this path is circu- lar to simplify the drawings.) Thus, the point C^T (tibia) belonging to C^F (femur) traces out a circular arc when passing from C^{TE} (extension) to C^{TF} (flexion). An analogous path is followed by the boundary points D of the collateral ligament. The end-points of the cruciate ligaments on the tibia, A^T and B^T, also follow circular paths in the present uniplanar scheme of motion (without rotation)

Medial Collateral Ligament

If, in 43° of flexion [219–221], we connect several points on the culmination of the loop of the pivot cubic through center P with corresponding points on the descending limb of the vertex cubic, we obtain a construction which corresponds closely to the natural form and length of the medial collateral ligament (Fig. 44). It even possesses the decussation characteristic of the medial collateral fibers (Fig. 43). One gains the impression that we are again dealing with a type of crossed four-bar linkage system.

Inevitable Placement of Some Ligament Fibers Outside the Theoretical Ideal Line

The numerous collagenous fibers necessary for imparting mechanical strength to the ligament cannot all fit on the ideal line of the Burmester curve. Where, then, can these "odd" fibers insert?

Ligament Fibers Within the Loop

If we draw fiber insertion points within the loop portion of the pivot cubic over the sil-

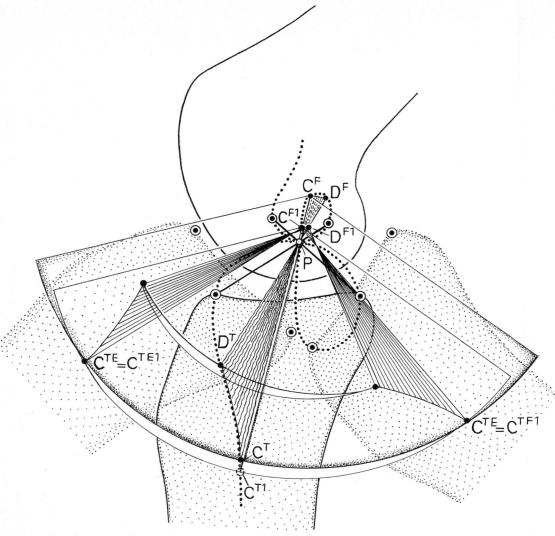

Fig. 45. All the collateral ligament fibers cannot fit on the ideal Burmester line, due to the large number necessary to ensure passive stability. A large portion of them must insert alongside the Burmester curve. Points C^F and D^F are located on the ideal line, while the circled points C^{F1} and D^{F1} are not on this line, yet lie within the pivot cubic of the curve and are still within the theoretical area of expansion of the collateral ligament. We may assume that the ligament fibers which originate at C^F and C^{F1} on the femur are rigid and, in extension, insert on the tibia at point C^{TE}, which thus coincides with point C^{TE1}. During joint motion the ligament fiber C^F–C^{TE} describes a circular arc from C^{TE} through C^T to point C^{TF}. The arc for the fiber C^{F1}–C^{TE1}, passing from C^{TE} to C^{TF}, extends beyond the arc of the fiber C^F–C^T. At point C^T, therefore, both fibers (C^F–C^T and C^{F1}–C^{T1}) can no longer be taut. If we assume that the fiber C^F–C^T remains taut, then the fiber C^{F1}–C^{T1} will not come under full tension at the position C^{F1}–C^{T1}. It remains lax in a position of intermediate flexion (see also Fig. 47). The model has several interesting implications. For example, let us assume that there are ligamentous fibers which are still slightly lax in intermediate flexion by an amount equal to exactly 1% of their length. Now if tension is applied to the ligament causing fiber C^F–C^T to elongate by 1%, the fibers within the pivot cubic with a 1% "reserve" will immediately become tense. With increasing elongation of fiber C^F–C^T, progressively more of the lax fibers will become tense, thereby increasing the resistance to further deformation. As a result of this fluid transmission of forces, the ligament will not snap like a metal chain under excessive stress or suddenly tear from the bone, but will behave more like an elastic band, developing interstitial tears as the stress builds. The rate of deformation will influence the manner in which the tearing occurs. The more rapid the deformation, the greater the likelihood of a bony avulsion or smooth rupture, whereas a gradual deformation will cause considerable elongation of the ligament with cascade ruptures at the microstructural level (adapted from Menschik [220])

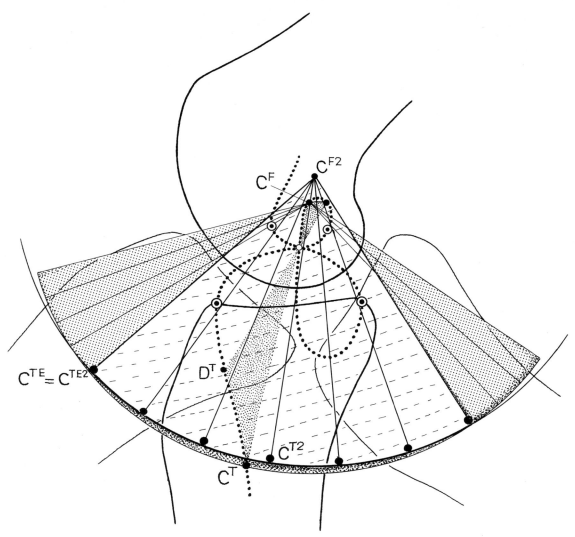

Fig. 46. If a ligamentous fiber were attached at point C^{F2} proximal to the loop of the pivot cubic and then moved through a circular arc like a pendulum such that, as in Fig. 45, the points C^{TE} and C^{TE2} coincide in extension (i.e., the real fiber attached at C^F and the hypothetical one at C^{F2} are taut in extension), then the hypothetical fiber would be too short in intermediate flexion, since its arc lies within that required for a normal ligament length. The too-short fiber would inhibit joint movement. Comparing theory with reality, we find that indeed there are no femorotibial ligamentous connections proximal to the loop of the pivot cubic. The only collagenous fibers that can be found in this area and still extend in the direction of the tibia are not attached to the femur itself, but terminate partly in the adductor fascia and tendon and partly in the fascia and distal tendinous end of the vastus medialis muscle. In this way they are "dynamized," i.e., actively tensed and relaxed, during joint motion. In reality we find that these dynamized fibers are very often blended with the most superficial layer of the medial collateral ligament system. They form an important element of active stabilization

houette of the natural course of the ligament, we can construct circular arcs for these points with the fiber length as radius (Figs. 45 and 47). If we assume that these shorter fibers are taut in extension, like the fibers on the ideal line, then the arcs must intersect in that position. In 45° of flexion this second arc overlaps the "ideal" arc, owing to its smaller radius of curvature. This means that these shorter fibers inserting within the loop of the pivot cubic are not stretched taut at this flexion angle and so are lax. Menschik [219–221] sees this as the reason for the laxness of the joint in moderate flexion.

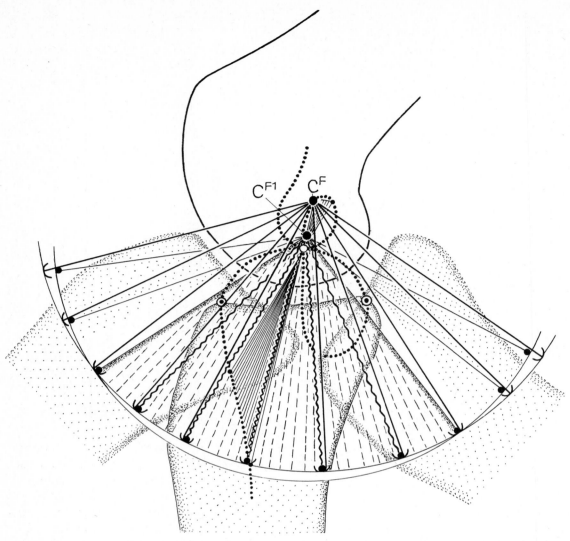

Fig. 47. The ligamentous fibers attaching at C^F and C^{F1}, if tight in extension, describe different arcs of motion. In intermediate flexion the arc centered at C^{F1} sweeps beyond the arc centered at C^F by the *crescent-shaped white sector*. If we imagine two swinging pendulums anchored at C^F and C^{F1}, and that a cup is attached to the end of the C^F pendulum while a ball is attached to the C^{F1} pendulum, then the cup of the C^F pendulum would momentarily catch the ball of the C^{F1} pendulum in the range of intermediate flexion; at 45° of flexion this would cause the C^{F1} pendulum to shorten by the distance between the outer and inner arcs of the *crescent-shaped white sector*. Although our analogy with two unequal-length pendulums falters somewhat due to the different period lengths, it is useful in explaining the entrainment of ligamentous fibers in different states of tension

Although the paths of fiber motion do not coincide for the case described, the shorter fibers from the more central area within the pivot cubic are nevertheless "allowed to exist," since they are not overstretched in any degree of flexion. According to Noyes and Grood [258] and Noyes et al. [259–261], collagenous ligament fibers can be stretched by no more than 5% of their length; other authors state a limit of 6%.

In the present model, critical overstretching of the fibers could occur only beyond 90° of flexion. At this degree of flexion, however, there is an automatic internal rotation

(IR) of the knee with increasing varus, departing from the valgus-external rotation of early flexion. This IR also leads automatically to a relief of tension on the collateral ligaments and in this way checks unphysiologic stretching of the collagenous ligament fibers.

Ligament Fibers Outside the Loop

If we similarly construct the arc of motion for a theoretical ligament insertion point located farther proximally on the femur, outside the loop of the pivot cubic, the associated ligament fibers would be too short in intermediate flexion and would either block joint motion or become excessively stretched (Fig. 46). Such fibers cannot exist if they are stressed beyond the 5–6% elastic reserve of the collagenous fibers. Warren et al. [380] found elongations up to 10% in their calculations of collateral ligament movements, but we believe this value is incompatible with the physiology of the collagenous fibers and is probably attributable to the measuring technique. Indeed, we have found no medial collateral ligament insertions lying outside the Burmester curve either in our clinical cases or in specimens.

The described laxness of the knee joint in moderate flexion simultaneously gives the ligament system the desired elastic reserve, which is important for rotation. With the ligament unstressed, only the ligament fibers situated on the ideal line are taut; the others occupy a "waiting position" under little or no tension. If, under a tensile stress, the "ideal" fibers are lengthened by 1%, then theoretically the fibers that are 1% shorter will immediately come under full tension. As a result of this, the mechanical resistance to tension increases with the degree of tensile stress applied. This recruitment of tensile strength enables a smooth transmission of forces, so that the ligament will not suddenly reach its limit of deformation.

If this limit were to be reached abruptly and then almost simultaneously surpassed, the instantaneous peak forces could not be adequately absorbed and neutralized. The risk of injury to all involved tissues and especially the delicate cartilage would then be considerably greater, and the ligaments would rupture almost explosively. Very heavy loading, as in competitive athletics, would carry an exorbitant risk of attrition and permanent damage. The relationships between ligament strength, stability and articular surface pressure have been well represented schematically by Goodfellow and O'Connor [109].

The Ideal Lines of Ligament Insertion and the "Dynamization" of Articular Ligaments

Since we became aware of the principles that govern ligament insertions, we have viewed every reparative procedure performed for recent and old injuries as an experiment in which we could compare reality with kinematic laws.

We have made several interesting observations:

1. A ligament that became lax or torn during trial flexion and extension had not been reinserted at the correct site. By reattaching the ligament at a topographically better site, isometric tension conditions could be obtained throughout the range of motion.

2. The actual ligaments always inserted on the theoretical ideal lines.

3. Outside the ideal lines, it was impossible to place a suture that would not tear or become lax during motion testing.

4. On the femur there are ligamentous collagenous fibers which *can be traced beyond the ideal lines.* They are in close association with the normal ligament and even appear to be blended with it over part of their course, but *they all terminate directly or indirectly* on the vastus medialis muscle or on the fascia and tendon of the adductors. These fibers are protected from possible overstretching by attaching not directly to the bone, but to a dynamic, mobile part, i.e., either directly or indirectly, via fascia, to the muscle.

We found marked individual differences in the numerical relationship between the rigid, passive ligament fibers passing from bone to bone and the "dynamized" (dynamically stabilized) fibers passing from bone to tendon and muscle. In some cases the dynamized fibers were quite numerous, even outnumbering the passive fibers, while in other cases the latter were far more numerous.

The existence of these dynamized ligaments can account for the well-known fact that good muscular function can successfully overcome passive instabilities that have been objectively diagnosed. It further explains why this mode of stabilization is not successful in all cases, and why instabilities are particularly disabling in individuals with poor muscular strength and especially in patients with paralysis. One gains the impression, in fact, that postpoliomyelitic flail knee is a consequence of laxity of the "rigid" ligaments brought about by chronic overstretching, when they can no longer be protected from excessive stress by an actively dynamized ligament component.

5. Those ligamentous fibers that cannot behave isometrically in an AP direction during flexion-extension are attached to the semimembranosus muscle, which can keep these fibers taut even when the knee is flexed (see Fig. 96).

All these dynamized fibers of the medial ligamentous apparatus (vastus medialis, adductor and semimembranosus muscles) are located in the most superficial layer of the medial collateral ligament and form a coherent system which Warren and Marshall [379] call the "supporting structures and layers." The "superficial arm" of the posterior oblique ligament of Hughston and Eiler [136] also belongs functionally to this system.

6. The almost limitless ability of the dynamized component of the ligament fibers to be strengthened by training may underlie the capability to adapt to higher performance. It also explains why well trained athletes suffer fewer injuries than poorly trained ones [193, 194].

The supporting structures and layers of Warren and Marshall [379] may be viewed in a similar light. Superficially, there are various differences that relate mainly to the numerical distribution of the fibers in the various layers. The form and principle are similar, however.

The Retinaculum and Pes Anserinus as "Dynamized Ligaments"

The Longitudinal Medial Patellar Retinaculum as a Dynamic Anteromedial Longitudinal Stabilizer

Our investigations of ligament insertion sites have consistently shown that the distal, tibial end of the medial collateral ligament is sharply delineated along the ideal line, in conformance with the vertex cubic described earlier. The extension of this line in an anteroproximal direction regularly forms the site of insertion for ligamentous fibers that often are scarcely distinguishable from the true collateral ligament. These fibers bridge the anterior half of the joint in a proximal direction, in the manner of a ligament. But since the fibers cannot insert on the femur under conditions of isometry, they radiate broadly into the fascia of the vastus medialis and the quadriceps tendon. Thus, they perform the function of active medial stabilizers. Because they are situated in front of the axis of knee flexion, they also act as extensors, thus accounting for the name "reserve extensor apparatus." This term is not entirely descriptive, however, for these fibers play at least an equal role as active stabilizers of the medial side. The fact that this retinaculum also has its tibial insertion on the Burmester curve underscores the importance of this line in the kinematics and fiber physiology of the knee.

The Pes Anserinus as an Active Auxiliary Stabilizer on the Medial Side

Like the retinaculum, the pes anserinus bears a functional relationship to the medial collateral ligament.

The collateral ligament inserts on the tibia directly on the vertex cubic. The pes anserinus inserts no more than 1 mm from the collateral ligament, lying parallel and immediately anterior to it. With the knee in extension, it rides directly on and parallel to the medial collateral ligament, forming an external layer. Thus, one might envision the pes anserinus as an active duplication of the medial ligament which, like the retinaculum, can have no ideal insertion on the femur, but instead has its own muscle bellies that enable it to exert dynamic stabilization reinforcing that of the ligament. Besides its ligament-protecting function in extension, the pes anserinus also acts synergistically with the medial collateral ligament in flexion, where it resists external rotation (ER); this function will be discussed later in more detail.

The Medial Ligament System During Movement

The often-quoted studies of Palmer [279] in 1938, Brantigan and Voshell [34, 35] in 1941 and 1943 and Abbott et al. [2] in 1944 are among the pioneering works that later were supplemented by Kaplan [170], Smillie [328], Wang et al. [375], Warren et al. [379, 380] and Bartel et al. [20].

In these works, variations in ligament tension are discussed as a function of the degree of flexion. Some reports are contradictory. Horwitz (quoted in [380]), for example, found the long medial collateral ligament fibers to be more tense in 90° flexion than in extension.

None of the examination methods proposed were entirely satisfactory in terms of the results obtained. The assigned end-points of the ligaments may not correspond to the end-points of the fibers in the interior of the ligaments.

Length changes of 10–20%, such as reported by Wang et al. [375], appear unrealistic. Such ligaments may exist only if they are "dynamized," i.e., have at least one end

that inserts on the bone via an intermediate elastic or mobile element in the form of fascia, tendon or muscle.

A normal, effusion-free knee joint is stable throughout its range of motion. Nevertheless, its stability is not constant, for the number of ligaments involved in passive reinforcement varies from one position to the next. In extension, for example, all the ligaments and the posterior capsule with its tendinous extensions are taut. The muscles stabilize the joint synergistically; the only freedom is in the direction of flexion. In moderate flexion, on the other hand, the knee is free to rotate internally and externally as well as alter its flexion angle in two directions. The superior convexity of the lateral tibial plateau also allows slipping of the lateral femoral condyle with changes in the distance relation between the femur and tibia, causing variations in the stress on the ligaments. These circumstances can easily create the impression of laxity and instability, when actually they reflect the enhanced functional potential of the knee joint in flexion. As a result of this, the dynamic stabilizers become considerably more important in the flexed knee.

The paired cruciate ligaments and collateral ligaments jointly stabilize the knee during rotation and on varus or valgus loading. They also check anterior and posterior displacement of the articular surfaces.

The mode of action of these ligaments in stabilizing the knee varies significantly with the direction of the mechanical loads and the functional position of the knee.

In ER the collateral ligaments are more tense and resist varus or valgus rocking, while the cruciate ligaments are lax. Conversely, in IR the collateral ligaments are lax while the twisted cruciates pull the joint surfaces together from the center and thus resist varus or valgus rocking. There are, of course, many possible stress configurations, but the possible combinations of ligamentous actions are equally numerous. Thus, if lateral stability is tested in moderate IR in a patient with cruciate ligament damage, a relative varus or valgus laxity will be noted. This supports Smillie's statement [328] that all ligaments act in concert to maintain stability, and that individual ligaments are difficult to isolate in terms of their function.

Special Conditions for the Anterior Fibers of the Medial Collateral Ligament

During flexion, those fibers located farthest anteriorly that can still be considered true ligament fibers undergo a kind of winding around the oval loop portion of the pivot cubic on the medial side of the femoral condyle (Figs. 48–50). This special behavior of the "leading edge" of the collateral ligament has already been described in the still-important works of Brantigan and Voshell [34, 35] and by Kaplan [170]. A similar winding occurs in the fibers that insert posteriorly on the femur and are located somewhat outside the loop of the pivot cubic. During flexion this posterior part of the ligament disappears beneath the longer, more superficial ligament fibers anterior to it.

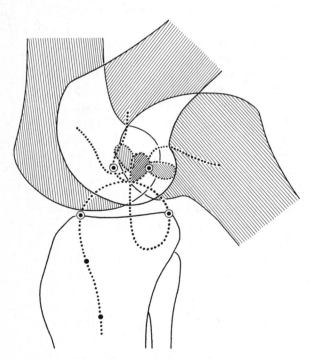

Fig. 48. The behavior of the femoral ligamentous attachment within the pivot cubic during flexion-extension (adapted from Menschik [220])

These processes cast doubt on the value of such procedures as the five-one reconstruction, in which the suturing of the layers is contrary to physiologic conditions, i.e., the posterior layer is sutured over the anterior layer [252]. With the posterior part of the ligament thus advanced anteriorly over the long ligamentous strands, it is no longer able to slip beneath these strands when the knee is flexed.

Mobility of the Medial Collateral Ligament Relative to the Tibial Plateau

The femur moves posteriorly on the tibia with increasing flexion. The oval insertion of the ligament on the medial femoral condyle follows this movement. As a result, the long fibers of the main ligament slide backward along the tibial plateau during flexion. Thus, the true medial collateral ligament can have no ligamentous attachment to the medial meniscus, for both parts – the deep layer with the meniscus and the long ligament – perform separate and distinct movements within the system.

Behind the superficial ligament, where the superficial and deep layers join, as demonstrated by Warren and Marshall [379], there is an area in the system where the border of the meniscus and the overlying posterior medial ligament move in the same direction during knee motion. There the peripheral fiber system of the medial meniscus is intimately blended with the posterior oblique ligament described by Meyer [226] (cross-hatched area in Figs. 49 and 50).

If we trace the course of the deep fibers beneath the long medial collateral ligament (Figs. 51 and 52), we can appreciate clearly the opposite directions of movement of the two layers. In extension the deep femoromeniscal ligamentous fibers run almost parallel to the anterior cruciate. Because this ligament is one of the principal kinematic guides, it stands to reason that fibers running parallel to it must follow the same kinematic principles.

Despite their considerable displacement in space and change of position, the fibers of

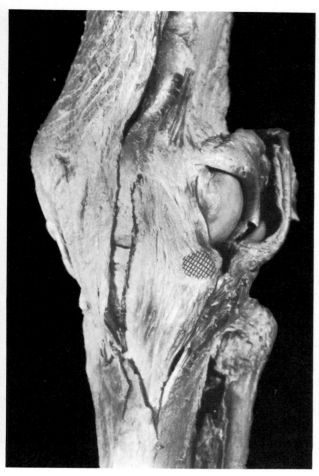
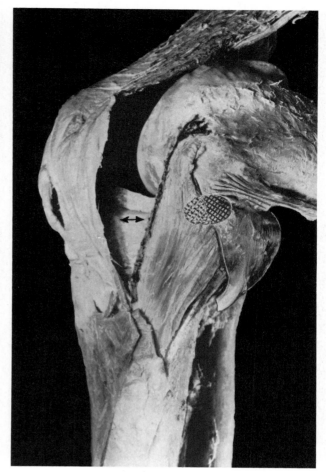

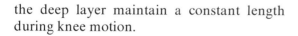

Fig. 49. View of the medial collateral ligament system and raised quadriceps extensor apparatus in extension. The area of attachment of the POL to the posterior meniscus horn and the tibia is *cross-hatched.* The anterior edge of the MCL is colored *dark* in order to emphasize its displacement relative to the upper tibia and the "winding" mechanism of its anterior fibers (see also Fig. 50) (v. Hochstetter)

Fig. 50. The quadriceps extensor apparatus was left in its original position during flexion of the femur in order to demonstrate the backward shift of the femur during flexion and the associated backward shift of the MCL (*arrows*) along the side of the upper tibia. Only the posterior portions of the ligament system (*cross-hatched*) are firmly attached to the tibia and meniscus and move only in association with the posterior shift of the medial meniscus (v. Hochstetter)

the deep layer maintain a constant length during knee motion.

The Lateral Collateral Ligament

Returning to the Burmester curve [219–221], if this time we draw lines through the crossing point of the four-bar linkage connecting points on the distal loop of the vertex cubic with corresponding points on the ascending limb of the pivot cubic, we obtain a structure having the approximate form, length and

position of the fibular collateral ligament. This ligament runs obliquely inferiorly and posteriorly and so crosses in space the direction of the medial collateral ligament (Fig. 53).

The Deep Ligamentous Structures of the Lateral Side

Individual ligamentous elements are more easily distinguished on the lateral side than on the medial side, although anatomic vari-

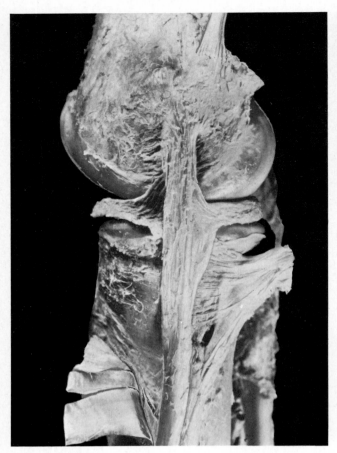

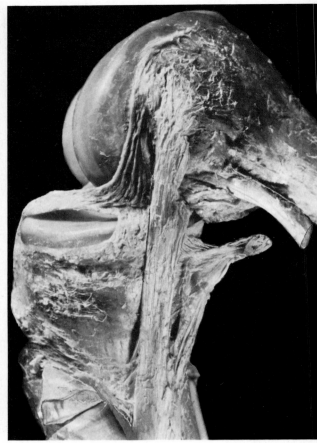

Fig. 51. The deep femoromeniscal ligamentous structures lie beneath the MCL, which at this level is not adherent to the meniscus and can move relative to it and the upper tibia. The fiber orientation of the deep ligamentous structures is comparable to that of the anterior cruciate ligament (v. Hochstetter)

Fig. 52. In flexion these fibers are stretched to their full length and can follow the movement of the joint in this state. There is a corresponding posterior shift of the meniscus which enables these fibers to maintain isometry. The attachment of the posterior part of the MCL to the semimembranosus tendon is clearly visible (v. Hochstetter)

ants are more frequent. This question is still being investigated in systematic studies of anatomic material. Just as Lahlaidi [187] reported a wide range of variation for the meniscofemoral ligament extending from the posterior meniscus horn to the posterior cruciate ligament, the entire posterolateral aspect of the joint is subject to great variability. A fabella is present in only about 20% of the population. Just as the patella lies at the anterior intersection of transverse and longitudinal tensile stresses, the fabella is located at a posterior site where lines of tensile stress intersect. It lies at the end-point of the oblique popliteal ligament (extension of semimembranosus) in the posterior capsule and gastrocnemius tendon, where an arm of the arcuate ligament terminates as the "fabellofibular ligament" [170]. Vallois [362] and Basmajian and Lovejoy [21] consider this part of the arcuate ligament to be a variant of insertion of the popliteus muscle into the fibular head, while Meyer [226] calls it a posterior extension of the lateral collateral ligament ("posterior lateral collateral ligament," analogous to his term "posterior medial collateral ligament" for the posterior oblique ligament).

There is no femorotibial ligamentous connection in the anterior half of the deep lat-

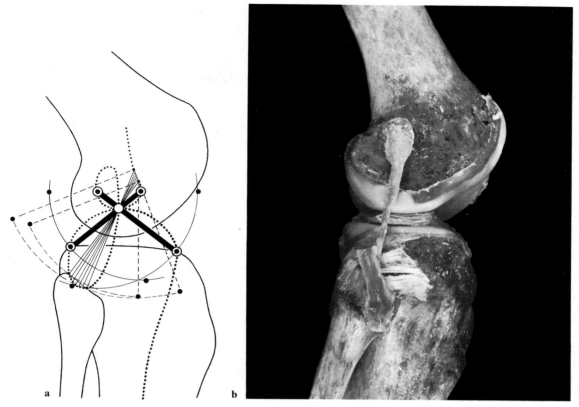

Fig. 53. a Theoretical and actual orientation of the LCL according to the principles of the Burmester curve and **b** in an anatomic specimen (Institute of Anatomy, University of Basel)

eral capsule. The deep structures are most clearly demonstrated by retracting the iliotibial tract together with its tubercle of insertion upward to its attachment on the femoral condyle. The detachment of Gerdy's tubercle in itself has two immediate consequences:

1. lateral looseness under varus stress;
2. extreme anterolateral rotatory instability.

The degree of these instabilities may be 1 cm or more. The underlying anterior capsule is generally thin and delicate like a synovial duplication and stretches elastically on stability testing with the iliotibial tract detached. This deep capsule, which is continuous with the fat pad anteriorally and is firmly adherent to the meniscus, is freely mobile relative to the tract. We found no mechanically effective ligamentous structure in its anterior half other than the occasional connection of the meniscopatellar ligament

[161–170]. Only in the posterior half of the lateral capsule do stronger femorotibial structures occur. The avulsion fragment described by Segond [316] on the lateral tibial plateau just below the articular cartilage and above the fibular head (see Figs. 230 e–231 a) is proof of the existence of tension-resistant collagenous fibers in the lateral capsule.

Besides these structures, which are somewhat difficult to define, the popliteus muscle with its tendon is the most important stabilizing element of the deep layer. Its quantitative features, like those of the arcuate popliteal ligament, are subject to much variation. One gains the impression that the *summation* of ligamentous strengths in this corner is much more important than the strengths of its individual components. Nevertheless, the popliteus muscle remains important. According to Basmajian, it pulls

41

the lateral meniscus backward during flexion and IR, stabilizes the femur against rotation on the tibia, and is the major posterolateral synergist of the posterior cruciate ligament. Viewed laterally, the popliteus muscle and tendon run parallel to the posterior cruciate ligament. As on the medial side, there are structures that run parallel to a cruciate ligament and thus are not only correctly placed kinematically to maintain isometry during movement, but also act as synergists of the cruciate ligament.

These facts also explain the classic combination of ligamentous injuries. It is little wonder why, in about 80% of cases [359], a lesion of the posterior cruciate ligament is associated with a lesion of the posterolateral side, or a lesion of the medial ligamentous structures with an injury of the anterior cruciate ligament. The remaining 20% of lesions involve other possible combinations based on less common mechanisms of injury.

The Lateral Ligament System During Movement

If we view the lateral side after removing the femorotibial elements of the iliotibial tract (Fig. 54) and reflecting the biceps muscle downward (Fib. 55), we are left with the fibular collateral ligament and deep ligament. In the case depicted, we could adopt Meyer's description of a "posterior lateral

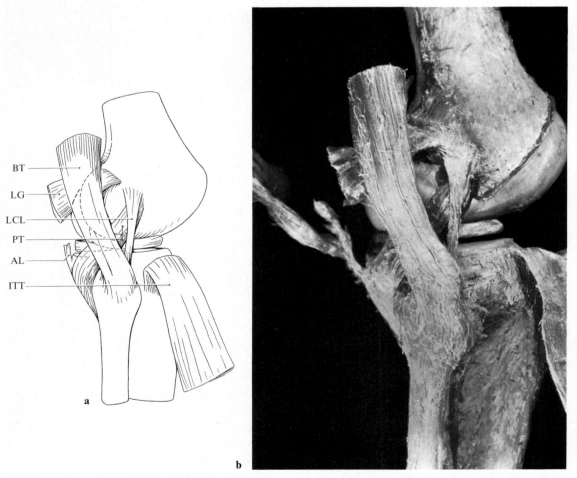

BT
LG
LCL
PT
AL
ITT

a

b

Fig. 54. a Positional drawing and **b** anatomic specimen of the lateral deep elements associated with the LCL, biceps tendon, lateral gastrocnemius and iliotibial tract.

The segment of popliteus tendon in this specimen is largely blended with the capsular fiber system (v. Hochstetter)

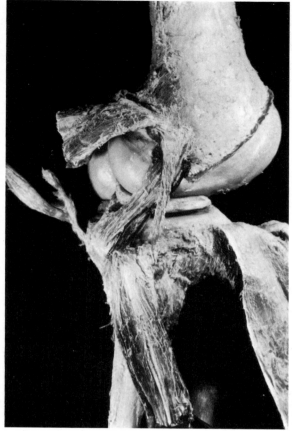

b

	LG
	LCL
	PMFL
	IT
	LM
	PT
	AL
	MM
	ITT
	BT

a

Fig. 55. a Specimen (v. Hochstetter) with **b** positional drawing after the biceps muscle has been reflected downward. The major deep structures have an orientation similar to the posterior cruciate ligament, if we consider the system in one plane. IT = impressio terminalis. PMFL = ligament of Wrisberg, now called the posterior meniscofemoral ligament

collateral ligament" [226], for here the popliteus tendon is indeed replaced for the most part by a powerful collagenous band stretching from femur to tibia. In most other cases we find at this site a powerful popliteus tendon and weaker ligament. This example is only one of several possible variants. However, ligament or tendon, it may run in *one* direction only, as dictated by kinematic laws.

As on the medial side, the deep posterior ligamentous layer is "wound up" somewhat below the lateral ligament on the femoral condyle during flexion (Fig. 56). Due to the great displacement of the lateral plateau during voluntary rotation, fiber isometry is maintained far less well than on the medial side. Dynamized structures are more numerous on the lateral side, therefore. In a broad sense these include the biceps muscle, and in a narrower sense the popliteus muscle and iliotibial tract (tensor fasciae latae).

The Iliotibial Tract as a Direct Femorotibial Collateral Ligament

As mentioned earlier, detachment of the tract by its bony tibial insertion results in an immediate and pronounced varus laxity of the joint. At the same time, the lateral tibial plateau can be pulled some distance forward in IR. This represents a first stage of anterolateral instability.

If we now attempt to retract the detached iliotibial tract farther upward toward the hip, we are unable to do so, because the tract

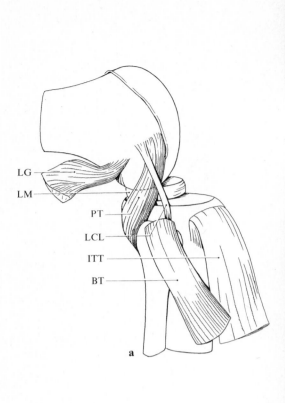

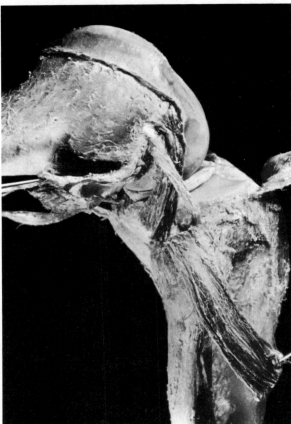

Fig. 56 a, b. The specimen in flexion. Note that the deep posterior ligamentous structures, too, have maintained isometry during the movement. The popliteus tendon could not be isolated in this specimen, but the course of the accompanying fibers corresponds entirely to that of the tendon

is firmly adherent to the system of the lateral intermuscular septum on the proximal part of the lateral femoral condyle.

This anatomic fact, the presence of instability after the detachment of Gerdy's tubercle, and the clinical observation [167] of similar, severe lateral varus instabilities following substitution operations with strips of the iliotibial tract by the technique of MacIntosh and Darby [215] or Ellison et al. [76] are proof that the tract functions as a femorotibial ligament. It should be mentioned that we have repeatedly found the tract to be freshly sheared from the lateral femoral condyle in recent injuries of the "unhappy triad" type.

Comparing the position and orientation of this ligament-like segment of the tract with the position of the Burmester curve, it is seen at once that this ligament runs obliquely inferiorly and anteriorly from the femur to the tibia in a manner analogous to the medial collateral ligament. It may be described, therefore, as a femorotibial collateral ligament (Fig. 57). If the lines of insertion of the femorotibial ligamentous connection do not conform as strictly to the requirements of the Burmester curve as on the medial side, it is because of the much greater anterior and posterior freedom of motion of the lateral tibial plateau during voluntary rotations, whose longitudinal axis lies more in the medial half of the joint (see also Figs. 90 and 91).

Kapandji [164] mentions this disparity in the motions of the lateral and medial halves of the joint, noting that the lateral femoral condyle recedes a distance of 10–12 mm at

44

Fig. 57. The deep posterior portions of the iliotibial tract which are attached to the intermuscular septum proximal to the LCL on the femoral condyle contain femorotibial ligamentous fibers whose insertion points lie for the most part on the Burmester curve. We call this "ligament," which is roughly parallel to the MCL, the anterolateral femorotibial ligament (ALFTL)

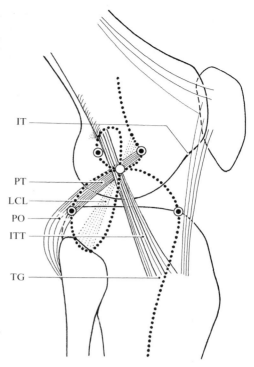

the start of flexion while the medial condyle recedes only 5–6 mm. This disparity ends at about 20° of flexion, at which point the movements equalize (see also Initial Rotation, p. 47).

For the same reason, a large part of the iliotibial tract must perform its ligament function dynamically. It is dynamized from the proximal direction by the tensor fasciae latae muscle. Interestingly, many fibers extend across the tubercle of Gerdy in a dense, flat band to merge with the aponeurosis of the anterior tibial muscle. This muscle has dense muscle-fiber connections with this aponeurosis, which thins out to become the fascia of the anterior compartment. Thus, it appears that the ligament is dynamized from the distal side as well. This latter mechanism may be more important as a lateral "tension band" against external varus forces.

The Theoretical Interplay of the Cruciate and Collateral Ligaments

According to Menschik's model [219–221], the fibrous strands of these ligaments always intersect at the "pole," or instant center, which is located on the transverse flexion axis. Viewing these bands through the transparent femur (Figs. 58 and 59), we see that they radiate out from the center like the spokes of a wheel. These spokes are distributed somewhat unevenly, with the medial collateral ligament and anterior cruciate ligament grouped on one side, and the lateral collateral ligament and posterior cruciate ligament on the other. This is one reason why in combined injuries the anterior cruciate ligament is torn along with the medial collateral ligament, and the posterior cruciate ligament along with the lateral collateral ligament.

Groh [116], Frankel [97, 98] and Nietert [253] calculated the position of the flexion axis and instant center differently and represented them with different models than Menschik. But topographically their axes are located very close to the center of motion in the Menschik model. Thus, the spoked-wheel principle is well described by all these theories.

There is an essential difference between the work of Menschik and the others, how-

45

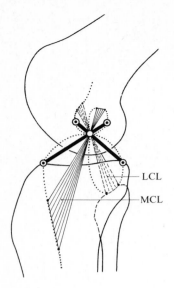

Fig. 58. Here the cruciate ligaments are represented by a crossed four-bar linkage, and the medial and lateral collateral ligaments by the principles of the Burmester curve. All elements intersect at the crossing point of the four-bar linkage (after Menschik [220])

ever. Menschik's model provides a unique solution for each individual knee. Different length relations of the two cruciate ligaments, as described by Beauchamp et al. [23], necessarily result in different condylar profiles. Both together, in turn, yield a unique position of the Burmester curve. Thus, the length and position of the collateral ligaments also vary in each individual. This is confirmed clinically by the marked variations of condylar shape that are observed in x-rays. These individual differences are also an important consideration during surgical repairs.

Groh and Nietert attempted in their research to find an average flexion axis, with the object of developing standardized replacement joints for exoprosthetic (Groh) and endoprosthetic (Nietert) applications. Thus, the goals of these studies were quite different from those of Menschik, and these authors were able to neglect rotation in their radiographic analysis of knee flexion.

Both approaches have their justification. Prosthetic devices must employ standard forms having an optimum functional design. On the other hand, the prime concern in the repair of soft tissues is the individuality of

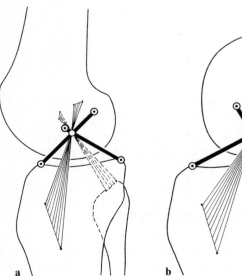

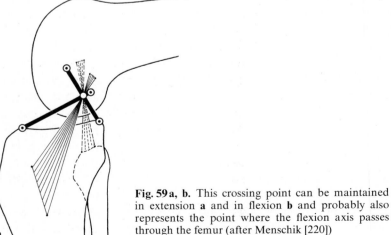

Fig. 59a, b. This crossing point can be maintained in extension **a** and in flexion **b** and probably also represents the point where the flexion axis passes through the femur (after Menschik [220])

46

each knee joint. With the axis of rotation located in the medial half of the knee, producing a greater freedom of movement on the lateral side, one consideration in such surgery is that the freedom of rotation in flexion causes some variations in the rolling-gliding pattern of the lateral femoral condyle [389], although it remains comparable on the whole to the rolling-gliding principle of the medial side.

(Figs. 62 and 63). A falsely placed suture will promptly tear.

Compared to a normal ligament with a crossed fiber structure, a rectangular ligament can no longer maintain fiber isometry during knee movements (Fig. 64). The anterior edge of the ligament is overstretched, while the posterior edge is lax. Muller [243] and Bartel et al. [20] concluded in 1977 that a proposed proximal advancement of the

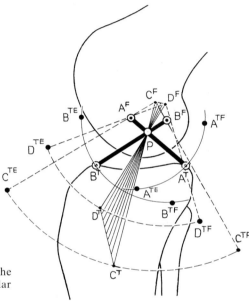

Fig. 60. During normal movement the points of attachment of the cruciate and collateral ligaments follow approximately circular paths (– – –) (after Menschik [220])

Loss of Isometry from Faulty Ligament Insertion

With the aid of Menschik's model (Fig. 60), we can appreciate the serious consequences of shifting the ligament insertion just 1 cm anteriorly in terms of ligament length changes during flexion and extension (Fig. 61).

In the example shown (Fig. 61c), the falsely inserted ligament is stretched by 1/6 (16.7%). Even during surgery, it can be confirmed experimentally that sutures will withstand trial flexion and extension only if they have been placed on the correct line

ligament insertion was unsound due to the resultant deformation of the ligament on flexion. The theoretical deformation curves become even more unfavorable if the tibial insertion is too short and too broad (Fig. 65).

Thus, operations of the type recommended by Mauck [212] or Lange [190] must be considered unphysiologic and thus of dubious value.

The Resting and Motion Pole Curves

If the femur is held stationary while the tibia is moved from extension to flexion, the suc-

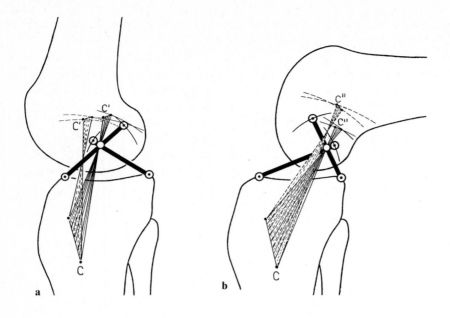

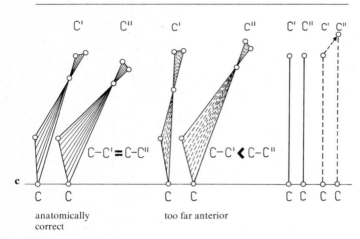

Extension – flexion C′ c′ at 0°
C″ c″ bei 90°

C–C′ = C–C″

C–C″ < C–C″

anatomically
correct

too far anterior

Fig. 61 a–c. If we mistakenly reinsert the MCL too far forward on the femur, as represented by the ligament (– – –) in the left half of Fig. **a**, it violates the law of the Burmester curve and becomes overstretched during flexion

cessive instant centers trace out a curve which we call the *resting pole curve* (Fig. 66).

If the tibia is fixed while the femur is moved, a different curve is traced by the instant centers; we call this the *motion pole curve* (Fig. 67) [139]. Interestingly, both curves are of precisely the same length, and one can be rolled off on the other (Fig. 68). The "gear" function of the cruciate liga-ments is stressed in particular by Menschik and Huson. For completeness, it should be noted that the evolute of the various centers of curvature of the posterior half of the femoral condyle no longer has anything to do with the gear kinematics and thus retains only a geometrically described value (Fig. 69).

48

Fig. 62. Reference drawing showing normal collateral fiber insertions and arc segments, for comparison with faulty collateral ligament configurations and reconstruction techniques, such as those still advocated for plastic operations ► (Fig. 63 ff.)

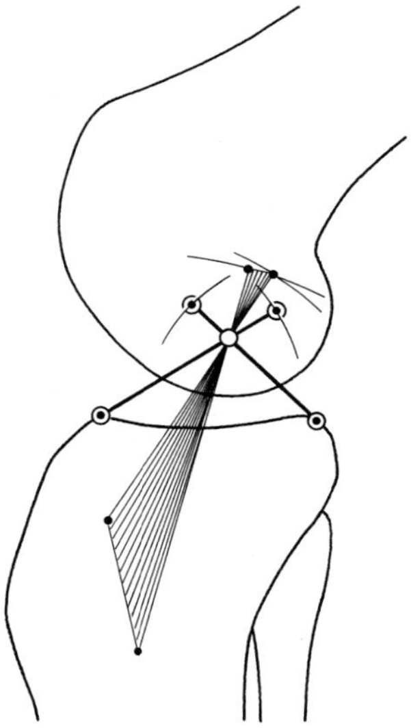

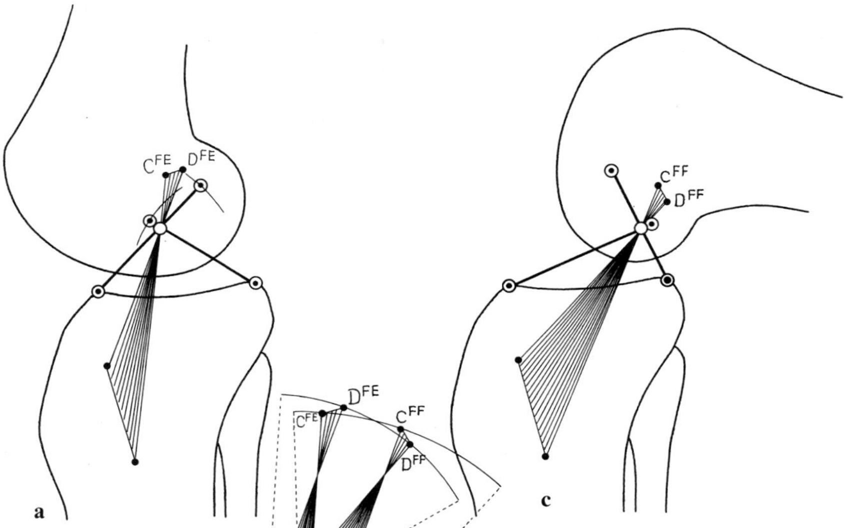

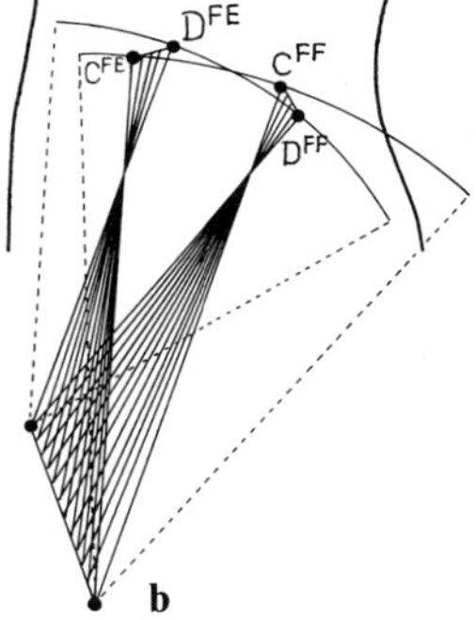

Fig. 63 a–c. Motion sequence in a knee with normal ligament insertions

Automatic Rotation, Terminal Rotation, Initial Rotation

As early as 1853, Meyer [226] observed the phenomenon of automatic rotation at the beginning of flexion and end of extension. Strasser [336] found in 1917 that the cruciate ligaments do not lie simply in the sagittal plane, but occupy a plane set at about a 15° angle to it. Menschik marked the cruciate ligaments with contrast material and followed their movement during terminal extension by means of axial x-rays. In this way he determined a shift of the marked cruciate ligaments of 15° – a shift which corresponds exactly to the known degree of terminal ro-

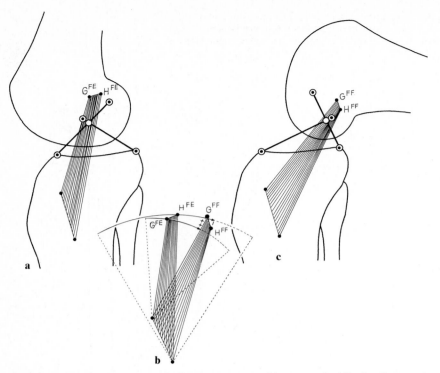

Fig. 64 a–c. Motion sequence of a ligament system with an uncrossed internal fiber architecture. The anterior edge is too short during flexion and must be over-stretched by the distance (+ +) to assume the necessary position. The posterior edge is too long by the distance (−) and is lax in flexion

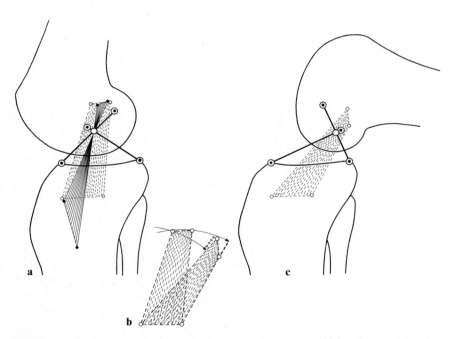

Fig. 65 a–c. Practical example of a plastic substitute for the MCL that is still employed today. The substitute is unable to follow flexion-extension without considerable distortion. In the example shown, the anterior edge would be elongated by almost ⅕ during flexion, while the posterior edge would be more than ⅕ too long in flexion and thus completely lax and useless

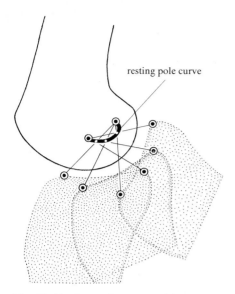

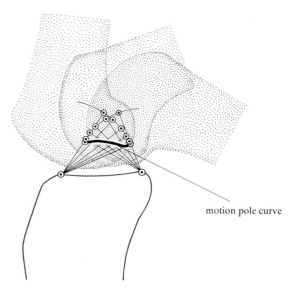

Fig. 66. Resting pole curve. This curve represents the locus of all crossing points of the cruciate ligaments when the tibia is moved from extension to flexion while the femur is fixed (after Menschik [219] and Huson [139])

Fig. 67. Motion pole curve. This curve represents the locus of all crossing points of the cruciate ligaments when the femur is moved from extension to flexion while the tibia is fixed (after Menschik [219] and Huson [139])

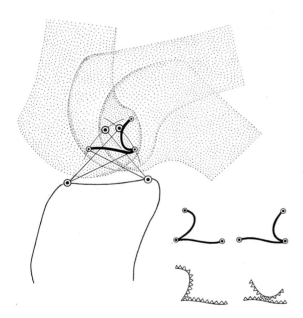

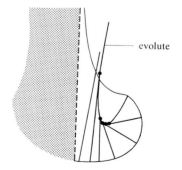

Fig. 68. The resting and motion pole curves are exactly the same length, and either can be rolled off on the other without sliding; if toothed like gears, both would "mesh" precisely (after Menschik [219] and Huson [139])

Fig. 69. Evolute: The locus of all centers of curvature of the posterior (femorotibial) condylar joint surface (after Menschik [221])

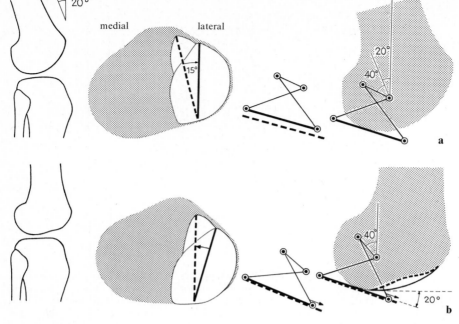

Fig. 70a, b. The automatic rotation that occurs during the last 20° of extension ("terminal rotation") leads to a typical shape modification of the lateral femoral condyle. **a** At a flexion angle of 20°, the solid sagittal line in the lateral portion of the tibial joint acts as a "coupler," and its length determines the shape of the coupler envelope curve, i.e., the shape of the femoral condyle. **b** Here is the situation after the 15° automatic ER that accompanies terminal extension. The tibial plateau has rotated 15°, and the broken line has now become the coupler. It now lies in the sagittal plane. Because this lateral plateau diameter (– – –) is longer than the other diameter (——), movement of the coupler in the four-bar linkage system generates a different coupler envelope curve. This results in the characteristic indendation of the lateral femoral condyle at the anterior limit of the femorotibial articulation, called the terminal sulcus or impressio terminalis (after Menschik [221])

tation. This terminal rotation occurs automatically during the final 20° of flexion and so is commonly called the *automatic* rotation of the knee. At the beginning of flexion this rotation occurs in reverse and is called initial rotation.

This automatic rotation influences the anatomy of the knee joint in important ways.

The 15° rotation of the tibial plateau during terminal extension effects a change in the length and shape of the coupler on the lateral side, which in turn alters the coupler envelope curve and thus the profile of the lateral femoral condyle (Fig. 70).

The change in coupler length with practically no change in the length of the cruciate ligaments leads, even in our model diagram, to an indentation of the femoral condyle at the anterior limit of the femorotibial joint surface. We regularly find this terminal de-

pression during arthrotomies, though its depth varies greatly from one individual to the next. This accounts for the use of the terms "sulcus terminalis" by Meyer [226] and Fick [92] and "impressio terminalis" by Strasser [336] in the older nomenclature.

This depression is always deepened (forming a true "impressio terminalis") in cases of chronic cruciate ligament insufficiency. Unilateral post-traumatic genu recurvatum is an accompanying symptom of chronic anterior instability.

We have also seen fresh, true impressions with cartilage fractures in major combined injuries of the "unhappy triad" type with anterior cruciate rupture. A hyperextension trauma is not always responsible for the injury. Idiopathic genu recurvatum can also cause a marked sulcus to form. Since a general weakness of the ligaments is present in most cases, extension is checked inadequately or too late, and the condyle continues to move violently forward to the edge of the plateau. This leads to a pressure lesion that may take the form of an "impressio terminalis," as Morscher [230c] has repeatedly emphasized. All knee-joint prostheses of the hinge type lack this terminal rotation with its checking effect. As a result, the patient feels an unpleasant, often audible impact as the prosthetic components strike each other in extension. This repeated concussion is one reason for the premature loosening of such implants.

The Unequal Profile Lengths of the Femoral Condyles and Automatic Rotation

The unequal profile lengths of the femoral condyles is described even in historical writings.

Viewing the femur axially from below, one is struck at once by its asymmetry. As a rule, the medial condyle is distinguished by the presence of an extra area of bearing surface in the form of an annular sector of about 50–60° (Fig. 71). Viewing an anteriorly exposed knee in 90° flexion, we find that the posterior cruciate ligament forms a similar angle to the horizontal. Its fibers pass upward to the femur like radii of the annular sector (Fig. 72). According to Menschik [219–221], the femoral attachments of the cruciate ligaments also form a 50–60° angle to each other (Figs. 73–75).

The shape of the medial femoral condyle with its extra bearing surface prompted us to study automatic rotation, i.e., initial and terminal rotation, in several anatomic specimens. We found that automatic rotation actually takes place about a unique axis distinct from that of voluntary rotation. This is also confirmed by Shaw and Murray [317] and by Wang et al. [376]. Voluntary rotation has its axis medial to the posterior cruciate ligament and tibial eminence in the posterior half of the tibial joint surface, while the axis of automatic rotation is located lateral and posterior to it. In the studies cited,

the axis of voluntary rotation is reported to lie farther medially and that of automatic rotation farther laterally than our calculations indicate. Shaw et al. [317] even place the latter on the medial side. Kelley (quoted in [317]) puts the axis of automatic rotation on the lateral side, "near the center of the lateral tibial condyle." According to Shaw, an incompetent anterior or posterior cruciate ligament permits a limited shift of the axis of automatic rotation.

If the cruciate ligaments and collateral ligament system are retained on a stable knee joint to provide kinematic guides, the joint can be stably manipulated and its articular surfaces adequately viewed from the front and rear.

When automatic rotation begins during the last 20° of extension, the fibers of the posterior cruciate ligament are already nearly horizontal. They behave, in fact, as radii of the annular sector of the medial condyle. The center of this rotation is posterolateral in location. Its axis in this position of "near extension" is situated such that it simultaneously passes through the femoral insertion of the anterior cruciate ligament. During the final stage of extension, the lateral femoral condyle impinges on the tibia at the terminal sulcus, while the annular sector of the medial condyle is still gliding into place, degree by degree. This process is shown graphically in Fig. 76. As a result of the "screwing home" of the sector, the medial condyle is forced into a medial oblique position on the tibia and in this way helps to check further extension.

In addition, it is mechanically significant that this femorotibial contact area moves anteriorly during final extension, for this greatly lengthens the lever arm of the tension exerted by the posterior capsule, which also inhibits extension (Fig. 77).

We can now understand why hyperextension injuries of the ligaments are rare in the stable knee. This is remarkable when we consider how long the lever arms of the tibia and femur are, and how much kinetic energy is often involved. Of course the posterior capsule is assisted in its checkrein function

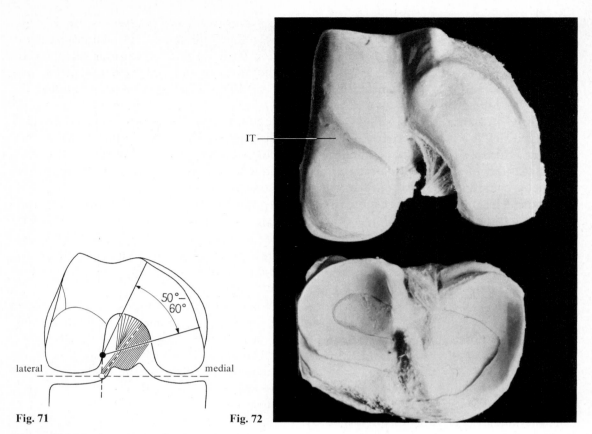

Fig. 71

Fig. 72

Fig. 71. The posterior cruciate ligament rises from the transverse plane at an angle of 50–60°. In addition, the medial femoral condyle, which (cf. Fig. 72) is significantly longer than the lateral, exhibits an extra area of articular surface that corresponds approximately to an annular sector of 50–60° (after Menschik [221])

Fig. 72. Anatomic specimen which clearly shows the different configurations of the medial and lateral femoral condyles. The angle of emergence of the posterior cruciate fibers from the femur described in Fig. 71 is also visible. The contour of the tibial plateau and difference in shape between the lateral and medial menisci conform to the differences in the femoral condyles (v. Hochstetter)

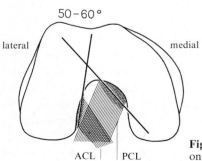

Fig. 73. The angle at which the two planes of origin of the cruciate ligaments on the femur intersect is also 50–60°

54

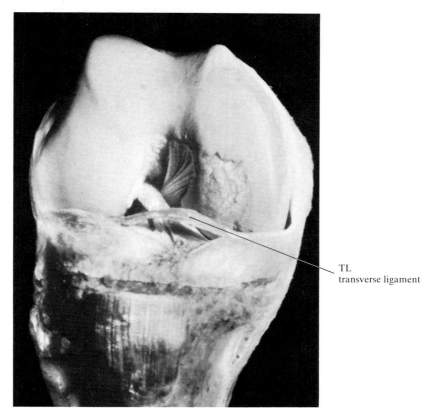

TL
transverse ligament

Fig. 74. This angle is confirmed by the examination of an anatomic specimen. In the frontal view into the flexed knee joint with cruciate ligaments, the transverse ligament of the knee is also clearly visible interconnecting the two menisci anterior to the cruciate ligaments. As it happens, cartilage damage is also evident in the stress zone opposite the eminence, which is important during rotation (v. Hochstetter)

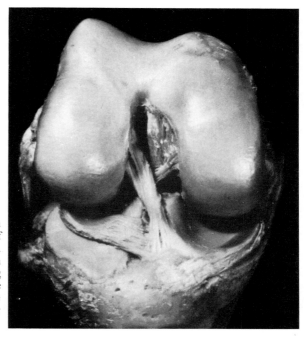

Fig. 75. These angles are visible even in maximum flexion. Also seen is the considerable posterior shift of the femorotibial contact point during normal flexion. The femoral condyles are in very close contact with both posterior meniscus horns in this position, placing a correspondingly large stress on these structures. The notch of Grant, which during extension receives the anterior cruciate ligament, is visible on the anterior roof of the intercondylar fossa (v. Hochstetter)

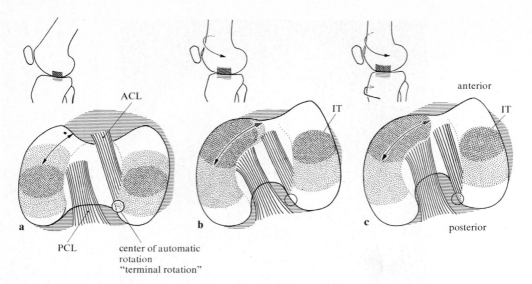

Fig. 76a–c. When the annular sector on the medial condyle is "screwed home," the tibia rotates laterally relative to the femur, producing a terminal rotation of 15°. The *darkly shaded areas* represent the contact areas; initially they are symmetrical, but with final extension the medial contact area is found to be much larger than the lateral. The center of automatic rotation during terminal extension coincides with the center of the annular sector (Fig. 71). **a** The *lightly shaded* areas represent the zones of femorotibial contact at a flexion angle of about 30°, and thus before the start of automatic rotation. **b** During further extension the annular section on the medial condyle glides posteromedially on the tibia. The lateral condyle has already finished rolling and is engaged at its "impressio terminalis." The medial condyle, on the other hand, is still able to glide in the region of its annular sector. **c** Now the gliding of the medial condyle is also complete, and the knee joint has reached full extension. The automatic rotation caused by the extra condylar bearing surface and controlled by the cruciate ligaments has led to a medial rotation of the femur on the tibial plateau, or conversely to a lateral rotation of the tibia relative to the femur

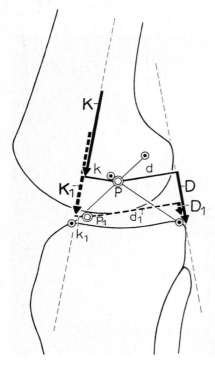

Fig. 77. During automatic rotation the center P with the instantaneous transverse axis of flexion-extension is shifted distally and anteriorly to the point P_1. This is accompanied by a substantial change in the length of the lever arms of forces acting on the joint. The extension-hyperextension force K becomes K_1 (– – –), with the very short lever arm k_1. As a result of this, the force D supplied by the posterior capsular structures is changed to D_1, which has the very short lever arm d_1. Hence the force D_1 becomes significantly smaller than the force D, their ratio being $1:6.2$ (after Menschik [221])

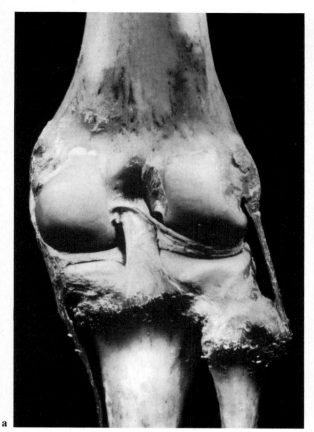
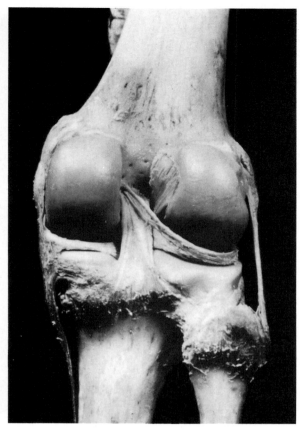

a

b

Fig. 78a, b. Representation of the position of the cruciate ligaments **a** in about 30° flexion and **b** in full extension. The terminal screwing-home of the medial femoral condyle is apparent, while the lateral condyle does not display much additional articular surface posteriorly (**b**). During final extension the posterior meniscofemoral ligament, with its fibers from the posterior cruciate ligament to the posterior meniscus horn by many strong flexor muscles. In Fig. 78 we (ligament of Wrisberg), reaches its definitive tension; its posterolateral origin corresponds approximately to the center of the annular sector on the medial femoral condyle. Note also the far posterior location of the femoral attachment of the anterior cruciate ligament (**b**), which virtually necessitates the over-the-top suturing technique described later (v. Hochstetter)

by many strong flexor muscles. In Fig. 78 we return to automatic rotation and the disparate lengths of the femoral condylar profiles. With the posterior capsule removed, the cruciate ligaments and menisci of the knee joint can be viewed. In a position of about 20° flexion, the articular surface of the medial condyle has not yet receded as far as that of the lateral condyle (Fig. 78a). After extension is reached, more medial articular surface is visible than lateral surface (Fig. 78b). The altered rotational position of the two bones with respect to each other is also visible at this time. The posterior cruciate ligament has changed its position. It is more tense and is directed more medially. The posterior meniscofemoral ligament is visibly tightened.

This screwing-home of an extra bearing surface on the medial condyle also changes the ratio of rolling to gliding over the final 20° of extension.

The mix of the movements and individual functions is shown in Fig. 79. The blending of 20° terminal extension, 15° automatic rotation and the screwing-home of the annular sector creates a situation in which gliding of the femur greatly predominates over rolling.

The profiles of the femoral condyles, like many other features, are subject to much individual variation. This may be one reason why Nietert [253] found such large deviations with regard to the size of the contact area in the stance phase, yet obtained no contradictory data on the ratio of rolling to gliding during the initial phase of flexion. Thus, according to Nietert, the claim of Braune and Fischer [36] that flexion is initiated by pure rolling can be correct only in cases where lax ligaments must first be tensed before the obligatory mechanisms of movement can become operative.

The recent studies of Girgis et al. [107] and Wang et al. [375] on the cruciate ligaments are very interesting in this regard. However, even they do not resolve the question of the degree of tension developed in the cruciate ligaments when a knee is moved under true physiologic conditions.

As stated earlier, a change in the length of the cruciate ligaments inevitably produces a change in the coupler envelope curve and thus in the shape of all articular surfaces. This may explain why Girgis et al. [107] found such great diversities in the freedom of movement resulting from the division of individual cruciate ligaments.

There was an average increase of 8° IR in extension after division of the anterior cruciate ligament, with a scatter between 0 and 15°.

There was also a pathologic hyperextension of an additional 25°, with a large scatter between 10 and 30°.

These values, of course, pertain to a knee joint with a capsule that is fully intact about its periphery. Even the capsular incision made to gain access for severing the ligament was repaired by the investigator before the stability test was performed.

Nietert [253] found in his calculations that the cruciate ligaments cannot be regarded as rigid bodies, for they are subject to displacement by other structures in the intercondylar notch. In full flexion or extension they are "wrapped around" neighboring structures (e.g., the bone) and are deformed. This is immediately reflected in a change in the shape of the pole curves.

It should be noted that there is as yet no apparatus that permits knee movements to be studied under true physiologic conditions. In the absence of the automatic rotation, valgus and varus angulations that accompany natural knee movements, the stresses that act on the ligaments are

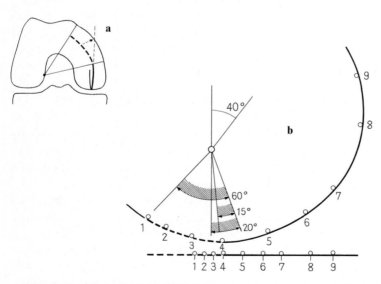

Fig. 79 a, b. Ratio of rolling to gliding during automatic rotation. If we lay out the line of femorotibial contact on the medial side in one plane (**a**), we find a new ratio of rolling to gliding during the last 20° of extension as the 50° annular sector on the medial condyle is screwed home to produce a 15° automatic rotation. On the tibia, contact points *4* through *1* are spaced closely together, while on the femur they are considerably farther apart; i.e., gliding predominates over rolling by a factor of 3–4. A similar ratio is observed during the last degrees of flexion (after Menschik [221])

unphysiologic. Frankel and Burstein [98] have recognized this difficulty. One must be wary, then, about drawing conclusions from measurements made in the absence of a rotatory component.

Automatic Rotation During Rapid Movement and During Walking on Uneven Ground

At a normal walking speed of 3.5 km/h, the leg flexes no more than 60° at the knee joint. A 7.5° downslope increases the flexion angle to about 70°. A 7.5° upslope does not increase flexion; the angle remains less than 60° [253].

A more rapid gait of 8.5 km/h increases the flexion angle to about 90° (normally 6.5 km/h is already a running pace). At no time is the knee fully extended [399]. The range of movement is then 90–20–0° (zero-passage method) for flexion-extension. Thus, automatic rotation of the knee is abolished at this pace. Obviously this is a time-saving measure, but whether it offers additional advantages, such as better cushioning of shock loads, remains unclear [253]. At a fast run of up to 30 km/h or more, the entire normal range of knee flexion is utilized. Thus, athletes treated for knee injuries must have no residual flexion loss, as this will limit their running speed.

The Cruciate Ligaments and Movement of the Knee Joint in More Than One Plane

Except for automatic rotation, we have so far discussed only the four-bar linkage in one plane. In a single plane it is easier to recognize the kinematic laws inherent in the form and function of the knee. The principle of the entire structure is clear, but its realization presents even nature with technical problems. As with the collateral ligaments, the cruciate fibers necessary for mechanical strength cannot all fit on the ideal lines of insertion.

For comparison let us return to the basic model with rigid rods representing the cruciate ligaments. These rods are attached to the femur and tibia in the sagittal plane in such a way that they trace out circular arcs when the linkage is moved. In the knee this problem is solved by the fan-shaped insertions of the cruciate ligaments, as well as by the division of each ligament into two parts [107], each of which behaves as a separate crossed four-bar linkage. This is only a well-founded hypothesis, however, and further study is needed.

The longer we deal with ligament problems, the more we come to appreciate the importance of the crossed fiber system as a structural principle. It can create conditions in which collagenous fibrous strands move at a constant length within their elastic reserve, while permitting an adequate number of fibers to attach at a given site, thereby fulfilling kinematic requirements and affording a high degree of strength.

The Three-Dimensional Four-Bar Linkage and the Central Pivot

Huson [139] described in 1974 a 3-dimensional model of a four-bar linkage and constructed a model of the knee joint consisting of a crossed linkage and two Plexiglas femoral condyles which rolled forward and backward *in one plane* between parallel guide rails. Study of this model confirmed the principles previously described. As a second model, he developed an apparatus having some freedom of rotation, i.e., a three-dimensional mobile system. The parallel rails were replaced with a circular pedestal, like a turntable, having the diameter of the intercondylar distance. This raised pivot had to recede during flexion along with the backward shift of the contact point, so that rotation remained possible.

The Central Pivot

In reality the intercondylar eminence of the tibia functions as the base of the central pivot. The fact that this pivotal base cannot move forward or backward is functionally corrected in the following way: The posterior horns of the menisci (which are particularly important in checking rotation) and the anterior horns are connected with the tibial eminence so as to form a pivotal base having a limited degree of plastic mobility. At the same time, it offers enough resistance to guarantee central guidance during flexion and rotation. Three criteria bear out this assumption:

1. The tibial eminence is covered by a very thick, tough cartilage layer that is capable of bearing loads. Equally thick cartilage is found on the opposing inner surfaces of the femoral condyles. Also, the meniscal cartilage is much harder and less deformable near its posterior junction with the eminence than in its mobile three-fifths between the attachments of the anterior and posterior horns. This fact becomes obvious when it is necessary to grasp and detach this cartilage during the course of an operation.

2. Goodfellow and O'Connor [109] have demonstrated the importance of the tibial eminence and inner aspects of the femoral condyles for absorbing compressive forces and for guiding movements under varus, valgus and rotational stress. Owing to the central position of the eminence and its anteroposterior course, it exerts optimum guidance precisely in the position of mid-flexion, and thus at a point where a high degree of rotational freedom is combined with high axial loads. In addition, the peripheral ligamentous apparatus of the knee is relatively lax at this degree of flexion, thus accentuating the need for firm central guidance.

3. Wilson [387] observed that patients with osteochondritis dissecans walk with the tibia externally rotated. This prompted him to develop his clinical test, which he performed mostly on children: With the patient supine the knee is flexed through 90° and the tibia is internally rotated. The knee is then gradually extended, and at about 30° of flexion a sharp pain is elicited. External rotation of the tibia immediately relieves this pain. Based on these findings, we no longer view osteochondritis dissecans as a lesion of the "unstressed" part of the condyle, but as a

problem of excessive stress on the growing femoral epiphysis during rotation.

Central Pivot Insufficiency and Degenerative Change

It is becoming increasingly clear that experimental cruciate ligament lesions [214] can initiate the development of degenerative change, for such measures destroy not only the function of the cruciate ligament, but also the complex function of the entire central pivot and thus the functional congruity of the knee. Kettelkamp [177] also confirms that abnormal positions of the knee components lead to incongruity and joint deterioration. He stresses, therefore, that all reconstructive measures must restore the normal instant centers of motion or at least allow the tissue to create such centers themselves by virtue of their adaptive capabilities. Kettelkamp is not alone in this view. Frankel and Burstein [98] also state that fractures and ligament ruptures dislocate the instant centers of motion, leading indirectly to an increase in stress and attrition.

The Central Pivot with Increasing Flexion

The posterior cruciate ligament is by far the most tear-resistant of all the knee ligaments. The studies of Kennedy et al. [175] indicated an average ultimate failure strength of up to 80 kg, or about twice that of the anterior cruciate ligament and medial collateral ligaments.

The measurements of Beauchamp et al. [23] showed that the posterior cruciate ligament is thicker than the anterior cruciate in 50% of cases. This is also demonstrated in the foregoing study of Girgis et al. [107] and accounts for the average greater rupture strength of the posterior cruciate ligament.

In nature, powerful structures imply correspondingly high stresses. Atrophy of disuse offers standing proof of this. Thus, the very strength of the posterior cruciate ligament is evidence that it has a particularly demanding function to perform – for during flexion, while the anterior cruciate ligament comes to lie horizontal, the posterior cruciate rears itself up, becoming practically the sole pivot point for rotation. According to Wang et al. [376], the axis of rotation then passes through the posterior part of the medial half of the joint, very close to or even through the posterior cruciate. Thus, the main responsibility for rotatory stabilization as well as the major stresses are borne by the posterior cruciate ligament.

In an important sense, then, the posterior cruciate may be considered the most important ligament of the knee. Hughston [134, 137] has made repeated reference to the predominant role of this ligament. It is significant that there are no ligamentous synergists in the flexed knee that are capable of adequately assuming its function. (The strong quadriceps muscle is an important non-ligamentous synergist that actively protects the ligament.) Although the posterior cruciate has much less protection in flexion than in more extended positions, where it is reinforced by synergists, it is relatively seldom injured.

Modern techniques of skiing pose a significant threat to this ligament, however. During the last skiing season, we had occasion to treat two unusual cases of posterior cruciate rupture. Interestingly, neither of these ruptures was the result of a fall. Both skiers described the same situation: They were skiing at high speed in a low crouch with the knees well flexed, according to modern technique. On a small rise or snow mound, each skier "caught an edge" of one ski on the side that was to be injured. Each managed to regain control of the errant ski and continue their run without falling. However, the rapid, violent twisting motion that was imparted to the knee by the ski binding and tall, rigid boot produced a tear of the posterior cruciate ligament. Because a concomitant rupture of the posteromedial corner occurred in each case, it would appear that a valgus-producing force was also present.

The specimen in Figs. 80 and 81, consisting of a proximal tibia with its cruciate and collateral ligaments, illustrates the central pivot of the knee. The posterior view in

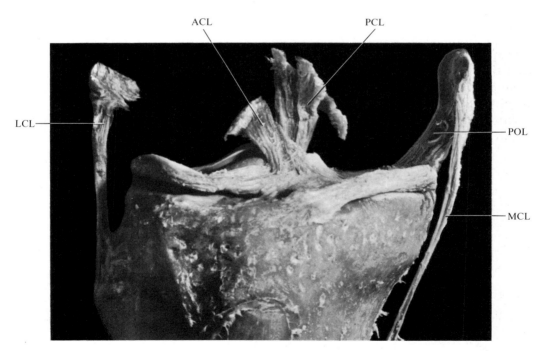

Fig. 80. The cruciate ligaments, menisci and collateral ligaments in their relation to the upper tibia as viewed from the anterior aspect (v. Hochstetter)

61

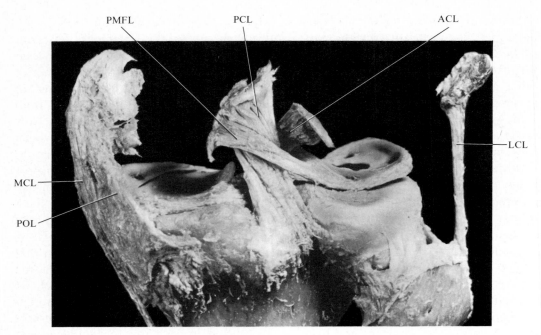

Fig. 81. The cruciate ligaments, menisci and collateral ligaments in their relation to the upper tibia as viewed from the posterior aspect. The posterior meniscofemoral ligament extends from the posterior horn of the lateral meniscus into the fan of the posterior cruciate ligament. It is Y-shaped, one arm of the Y (ligament of Wrisberg) passing posterior to the PCL, and the other arm (ligament of Humphrey) passing anteriorly between the PCL and ACL to attach to the central pivot (ligament of Wrisberg, now called the posterior meniscofemoral ligament, PMFL) (v. Hochstetter)

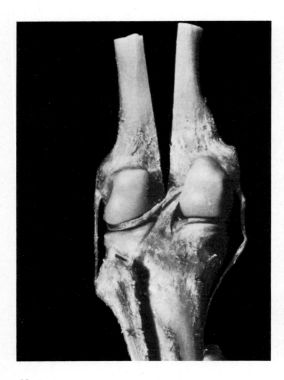

Fig. 82. If the femur is sawed in half along the sagittal plane exactly between the attachments of the cruciate ligaments and separated, these ligaments act as "medial collateral ligaments" to stabilize their respective joint half (v. Hochstetter)

62

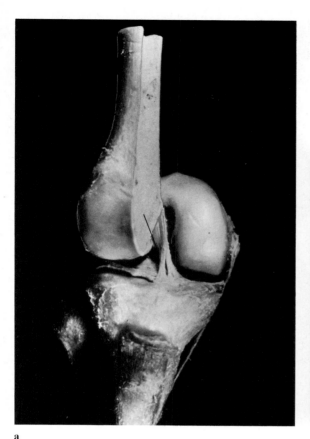

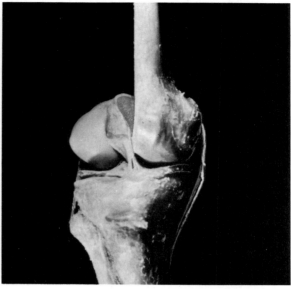

Fig. 83a, b. The lateral stability of the medial and lateral compartments thus created is surprisingly well maintained even during flexion and extension of the individual femur halves (v. Hochstetter)

Fig. 81 shows the axial orientation of the posterior cruciate ligament as well as the posterior oblique ligament with its meniscal attachment. The figure also demonstrates that the similar spatial orientation of these two ligaments is not coincidental, and that it may well account for the combined lesion of the posterior cruciate and posteromedial corner that occurred in the skiing accidents described above.

Further Functional Possibilities of the Elements of the Central Pivot

Study of an anatomic specimen in which the femur has been split longitudinally in the sagittal plane down to the central pivot, so that a cruciate ligament is retained on each half of the femur (Fig. 82), can be highly instructive. Because the medial and lateral collateral ligaments are also retained, each femoral half can be flexed and extended independently of the other (Fig. 83), with each cruciate ligament acting as a collateral ligament for its respective condyle. As Fig. 82 shows, the two femoral halves can be spread apart only a small distance in extension. Thus, if a lateral or medial ligament is incompetent because of a sprain or rupture, the cruciate ligaments can stabilize the knee against varus and valgus stresses from the center, both alone and in concert with the remaining ligaments.

A sagittal section showing the femoral half from the inside (Fig. 84) is also instructive from a physiologic standpoint because it enables the cruciate ligament insertions to be viewed from an unaccustomed angle.

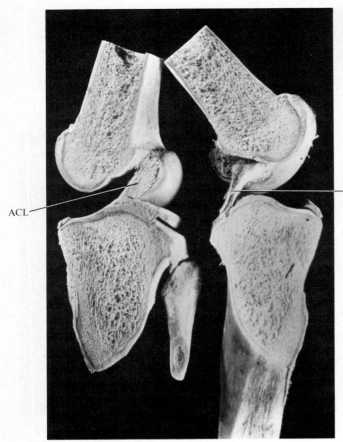

ACL

PCL

Fig. 84. In another example the sagittal cut through the femur between the cruciate ligaments has been extended through the tibia to show the course and bed of the cruciate ligaments from the median plane (v. Hochstetter)

The Posteromedial Corner (Semimembranosus Corner)

– "Posterior medial collateral ligament"
– "Posteromedial corner"
– "Posterior oblique ligament"
– "Posterior medial ligaments"
– "Posterior medial capsular corner"
– "Point d'angle postéro-interne" (PAPI)

All these terms have been applied to this functionally vital area, yet none is entirely descriptive. Some refer to specific elements, while others describe only a functional locus. One thing is certain: Despite its close topographic relation to the medial collateral ligament, the "posteromedial corner" is fundamentally different in nature and function from the tibial collateral ligament itself.

Because all its elements cannot fit on the ideal Burmester line, its posteriormost liga-

mentous components are lax during flexion. Analogous to the medial longitudinal retinaculum, which is the most anterior part of the medial stabilizers and as such must be "dynamized" by the vastus medialis muscle, the most posterior parts of the medial stabilizers are dynamically stabilized by the semimembranosus muscle. In extension the semimembranosus muscle and tendon runs parallel to the femur and is thus an active co-stabilizer of all tensed medial ligaments, while in 90° flexion, for example, it extends away from the tibia at right angles and simultaneously tenses the lax ligamentous fibers. In this position it is an active stabilizer against ER. It accomplishes this both directly as an active muscle, and indirectly by tensing the posterior portion of the medial ligament (Fig. 85). Because the semimembranosus muscle dominates the area with

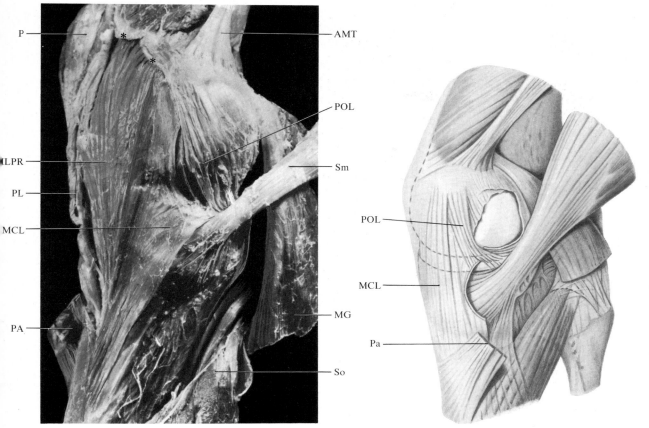

Fig. 85. The posteromedial corner (semimembranosus corner). Between the adductor magnus tendon (AMT) and semimembranosus tendon (Sm) is the posterior oblique ligament (POL). Through its connection with the Sm, the POL is a key functional element for medial stability of the knee. * the most superficial layer seperated from the vastus medialis muscle, which envelops the entire medial side and contributes to dynamic stabilization (v. Hochstetter)

Fig. 86. The posteromedial corner and its attachment to the semimembranosus tendon. Between the medial gastrocnemius tendon and POL the joint capsule is very thin. Here it has been fenestrated to show the medial condyle. This area of the capsule balloons outward when fluid is injected into the joint and so does not contribute significantly to mechanical stability at this location (Institute of Anatomy, University of Basel)

its insertions and function, we have named the posteromedial corner the *"semimembranosus corner"* (Fig. 86).

The Individual Functional Elements of the Semimembranosus Corner

From the center to the periphery, these are:

The posterior meniscus horn. As will be shown, the posterior horn of the meniscus forms a critically important site for the redirection of forces that are transmitted to it; without it the value of the semimem-

branosus corner would be seriously compromised. The very reattachment of the posterior horn to the coronary ligament during a reconstructive procedure is sufficient to reduce AP instability to a much greater degree than generally assumed.

The posterior oblique ligament, POL (Fig. 87). Hughston and Eilers [136] have emphasized the important role of the posterior oblique ligament (not to be confused with the oblique popliteal ligament). In our studies of anatomic structures and their functional relationships at the Anatomical

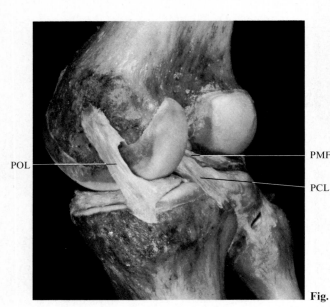

POL

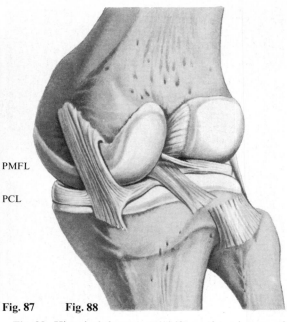

PMFL

PCL

Fig. 87   Fig. 88

Fig. 87. Drawing of an anatomic specimen of Wolf (1948) which demonstrates the POL as an isolated structure. This important femorotibial ligament is also firmly attached to the posterior horn of the medial meniscus through its femeromeniscal and meniscotibial fibers. *This is the site* at which the medial meniscus has intimate attachment with the ligament system. Anterior to this site is the MCL, which must move relative to the

Fig. 88. Historical document (1948) on the existence of the "posterior oblique ligament" of Hughston [136] or "posterior medial collateral ligament" of Meyer (1853) (Institute of Anatomy, University of Basel)

meniscus during flexion and so has no attachment with it, though such an attachment is frequently described (Institute of Anatomy, University of Basel)

Institute of the University of Basel, we have come across an interesting specimen. In 1948 (!) Wolf prepared a knee specimen (Figs. 87 and 88) on which the posterior extension of the medial collateral ligament was labeled as a separate structure. Further study revealed to our great surprise that as early as 1853, Meyer [226] had already described the "posterior medial collateral ligament" in detail. Later anatomists such as Fick [91] and Strasser [336] undertook the division of the medial ligament into the true collateral ligament (MCL) and the POL. Meyer, incidentally, also coined the term "posterior lateral collateral ligament" for the lateral side (see p. 40 and Figs. 54 and 55).

The POL is intimately attached to the medial meniscus, although about 1/2 to 2/3 of its fibers pass uninterrupted from the femur to the tibia. Thus, the POL constitutes a true femorotibial ligament. In addition, there are fibers in the deep portion that ex-

tend only from the femur to the meniscus or from the meniscus to the tibia to form the "femoromeniscal" and "meniscotibial" fibers. The latter, which connect the circumference of the meniscus with the tibial border, form a separate entity that is also called the coronary ligament.

The semimembranosus muscle. The semimembranosus is the muscle of the posteromedial corner, to which it adheres with its five arms like a rubber suction cup. Because the direction of its pull varies greatly during flexion, this mode of insertion is favorable. The five insertions are distributed as follows (Fig. 97):

1. a reflected portion (pars reflexa) passing anteriorly beneath the medial collateral ligament to insert on the tibia (direct pull in flexion);
2. a direct insertion on the posteromedial aspect of the tibia (direct pull in extension);

3. the "oblique popliteal ligament," which extends laterally and obliquely over the posterior aspect of the capsule to the site of the fabella (which may or may not be present);
4. an expansion to the posterior fibers of the POL;
5. an expansion to the aponeurosis of the popliteus muscle.

The 3rd and 4th tendon insertions connect the semimembranosus muscle with the posterior capsule, thus making it the controlling and guiding element of the semimembranosus corner.

Interaction of the Ligaments During Rotation

Having considered the two-dimensional system, we shall now return to the behavior of the ligaments during rotation (Fig. 89). The cruciate and collateral ligaments are so arranged that the cruciate ligaments are relaxed during ER, and are tightened by "coiling" during IR. In IR they develop their highest tension, causing the tibia to become pressed against the femur and checking further medial rotation.

An antagonistic mechanism is at work in the collateral ligaments: They are tightened by ER and relaxed by IR. Thus, they control and limit ER, when the cruciate ligaments are lax. Through this mechanism the cruciate and collateral ligaments alternately increase the pressure of one joint surface on the other, thereby helping to keep the joint closed in maximum IR and ER.

This stability is still present even if the ligaments are damaged and lax, although the range of rotation is increased. This increased freedom of rotation is the first stage of rotatory instability.

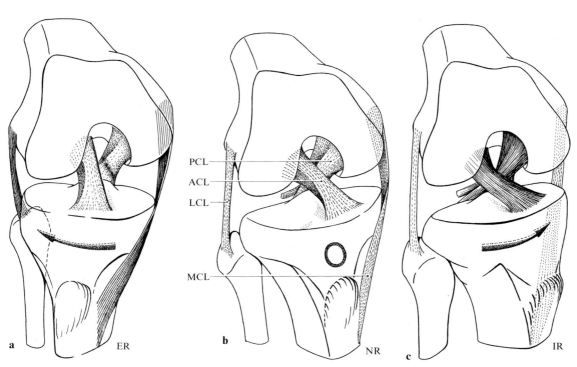

Fig. 89 a–c. Besides their synergistic functions, the cruciate and collateral ligaments also exercise a basic antagonistic function during rotation. **a** In ER it is the collateral ligaments which tighten and inhibit excessive rotation by becoming crossed in space. **b** In NR none of the four ligamentous structures is under unusual tension. **c** In IR the collateral ligaments become more vertical and so are lax, while the cruciate ligaments become coiled round each other and come under strong tension

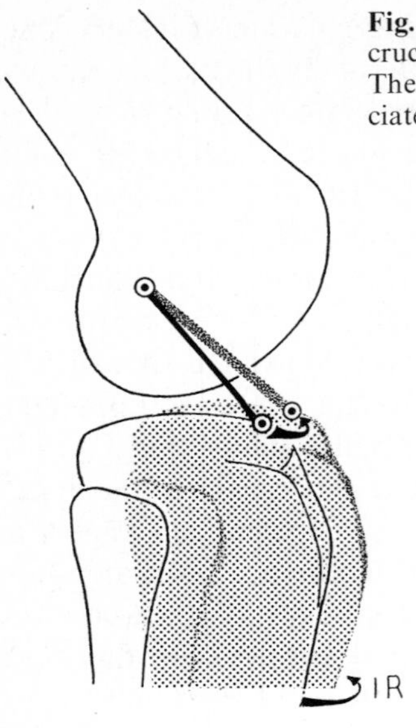

Fig. 90. The lateral tibial plateau is convex superiorly. This alone enables the tense cruciate ligaments to maintain a constant length when the knee is rotated internally. The femoral condyle glides down the slope of the plateau, providing the anterior cruciate ligament with the additional length necessary for IR

Internal Rotation, Coiling Mechanism of the Cruciate Ligaments, and Shape of the Lateral Tibial Plateau

If Menschik is correct in theorizing that the cruciate ligaments are already taut in neutral rotation (NR), then further coiling of the ligaments would no longer be possible, for the necessary length reserves would be lacking. Nevertheless, IR is possible, states Huson [139], because of the posterior downslope of the lateral tibial plateau. When the lateral tibial plateau moves forward during IR, the femur glides backward and downward. This relaxes the cruciate ligaments sufficiently to allow the normal 15–20° of IR (Fig. 90).

Voluntary Rotation, its Range and Axis

Several authors have measured rotatory movements by clamping the foot in a special apparatus and then rotating the limb at the knee. The results display a sizable individual and author-dependent range of variation. Lanz and Wachsmuth [192] report 10° IR and 42° ER, while Ross [304] found a 17° range of IR and 18° range of ER. In general, rotation of the knee was greatest in 45° flexion. Ruetsch and Morscher [306] measured 15° IR and 21° ER with the knee flexed 90°.

Since the axis of rotation does not pass through the center of the joint but is shifted toward the medial side, the extent of rotatory movements and associated excursion of the femur relative to the tibia are different on the medial and lateral sides. For this reason the cartilaginous surfaces provided solely for meniscal gliding during rotation have different lengths on the medial and lateral sides (Fig. 91). On the medial side, only short additional gliding surfaces are present for the anterior horn during IR and for the posterior horn during ER. On the lateral side, by contrast, considerably longer gliding surfaces are provided for the greater excursions of the lateral meniscus during rotations. Especially on the anterior side, the lateral meniscus can extend quite far over the tibial plateau during ER as it moves out of the way of the femoral condyle. The gliding path is shorter posteriorly in accordance with the smaller average excursion of the meniscus during IR.

Active and Passive Stabilization by the Semimembranosus Corner During Rotation and Under an Anteroposterior Stress

The knee joint is surrounded by a number of triangular structures (Fig. 100). Often the involved ligamentous and tendinous expan-

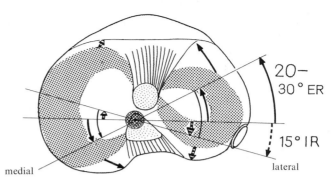

medial · lateral

Fig. 91. Right tibial plateau with the paths of meniscus movements during voluntary rotations of the flexed knee. Because the axis of rotation is located more on the medial side, somewhere in the area of the small circle, during ER the femoral condyle moves the menisci posteriorly on the medial side and a much greater distance anteriorly on the lateral side, as represented by the *solid black arrows.* Conversely, during IR the menisci are moved forward on the medial side and a considerably greater distance backward on the lateral side, as indicated by the *striped arrows*

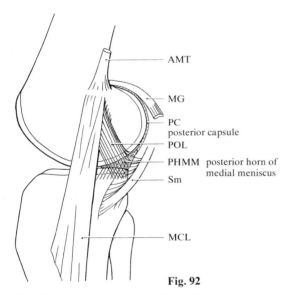

AMT

MG

PC
posterior capsule
POL
PHMM posterior horn of
medial meniscus
Sm

MCL

Fig. 92

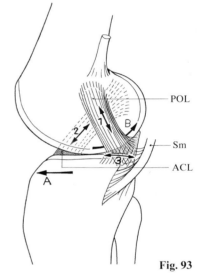

POL

Sm

ACL

A

Fig. 93

Fig. 92. Schematic representation of the semimembranosus corner

Fig. 93. The POL is a synergist of the ACL (*2*). When the tibia is displaced anteriorally (*arrow A*) relative to the femur, the ACL comes under tension. But at the same time, the femoral condyle must push the meniscus backward or ride up upon it (*arrow B*). Because the meniscus is firmly attached to the tibia via the meniscotibial fibers of the POL (*3*), its backward displacement is checked by these fibers. Thus, it functions together with the femoromeniscal portion of the POL (*1*), which also comes under strong tension, as a wedge brake against anterior tibial displacement. This structurally important system functions properly only if the POL, posterior meniscus horn and semimembranosus attachment form an intact unit. Even a small lesion leads to the first stage of anteromedial rotatory instability

sions create the appearance of simple V-shaped structures, because one side of the triangle is formed by bone.

The fiber systems connecting the tibia-MCL-femur and femur-POL-tibia are also triangular. This principle is discussed in Physiology of Rotation, p. 98. Here we are concerned with the functional details of the semimembranosus corner (Fig. 92). For simplicity, the drawings in Figs. 93–95 pertain only to stresses that displace the tibia forward or backward.

69

When the tibia is pushed forward, there must be a corresponding backward movement of the femur on the tibia. This would cause the femur to mount the posterior horn, were it not for ligamentous restraint. A particularly great stress is placed on the meniscotibial fibers of the POL that form part of the coronary ligament.

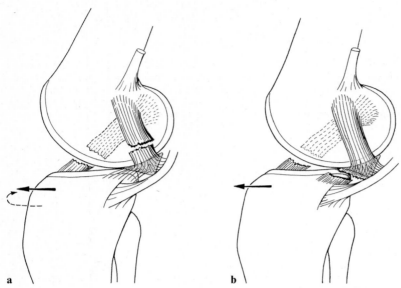

Fig. 94a, b. An anterior drawer-type displacement of the tibia (*heavy arrow*) combined with external rotation (*dashed arrow*) causes tearing of the ACL and POL (**a**). The POL may be torn proximal or distal to the posterior meniscus horn (**b**). Occasionally both portions of the ligament, the proximal and distal, may become detached from the meniscus horn. The clinical picture in such cases is that of a meniscal injury. However, the lesion is located not in the cartilaginous meniscus, but farther peripherally in the region of its capsuloligamentous attachment. Thus, the injury involves a ligamentous lesion that must be sutured, rather than a meniscus lesion; a meniscectomy in such cases is both unjustified and contraindicated

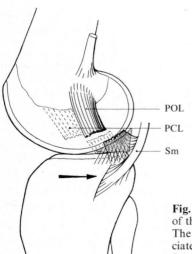

POL
PCL
Sm

Fig. 95. Posterior displacement of the tibia (*arrow*), if extensive, causes a rupture of the PCL and POL. This demonstrates the synergism of these two ligaments. The fact that the POL can be a synergist of both the anterior and posterior cruciate ligaments derives from the ability of the meniscus to transmit and redirect forces from both directions

70

In the course of reconstructive operations for fresh injuries, we have repeatedly shown how accurate repair of the semimembranosus corner with due regard for fiber isometry is in itself sufficient to correct any anterior drawer sign and anteromedial rotational drawer sign, long before the first cruciate ligament suture is in place. The importance of these fibers is particularly well demonstrated by the rare rupture of a meniscotibial ligament, in which the complex of the semimembranosus corner remains essentially intact, but the tibia is no longer restrained (see also Fig. 218g). Only 2 or 3 interrupted sutures need be placed in such a situation to repair the meniscotibial connection of the semimembranosus corner and thus restore complete anteroposterior stability to the medial joint half. The stabilizing effect of these initial sutures is so great that besides preventing the anterior drawer sign, they also abolish any valgus laxity in the extended knee, long before the MCL and anterior cruciate ligament have been sutured.

> Therefore, the semimembranosus corner is the synergist of the anterior cruciate ligament on the medial side.

It is presumed in this context that the femorotibial band of the iliotibial tract is present as a lateral synergist to form the third element of anterior stabilization [165].

In most cases these synergistic structures are conjointly injured. But while an anterior cruciate injury is almost invariably associated with a lesion of the semimembranosus corner, the femorotibial band of the iliotibial tract possesses an intrinsic dynamic mobility reserve that often enables it to escape concomitant injury. Figure 94b illustrates a rare, special form of the combined anterior cruciate/semimembranosus corner injury. This type of posteromedial lesion is apt to be overlooked or inadequately repaired and can be a source of very serious anterior instabilities.

The Functional Synergism of the Semimembranosus Corner and Posterior Cruciate Ligament

The POL runs parallel to the posterior cruciate ligament (Fig. 95), which accounts for their common function. This raises the possibility of a common lesion from forces acting in a posteromedial direction.

The Functional Synergism of the Semimembranosus Corner and Anterior Cruciate Ligament, and the Function of the Medial Meniscus

The fact that the POL and anterior cruciate ligament cross each other in space would not suggest a common function. It is only the posterior horn of the medial meniscus that makes this paradoxical function possible. The meniscus acts as a "redirector" of applied forces, as the wedge of its posterior horn checks anterior displacement of the tibia, even though the POL runs in the other direction. Thus, it is an important component of the semimembranosus corner and itself exerts a stabilizing effect against anteromedial tibial displacement. As a result, every medial meniscectomy inevitably leads to anteromedial rotatory instability. The more radical the meniscectomy, the greater the instability. Complete extirpation of the meniscus after Mandl (quoted in [397]) means a resection in the capsule, i.e., outside or peripheral to the meniscal cartilage, with a consequent severe disruption of fibers belonging to the POL (Fig. 96).

The Semimembranosus Corner and Popliteus Corner

It is no coincidence that the fifth tendinous expansion of the semimembranosus merges with the aponeurosis of the popliteus muscle. The popliteus and semimembranosus muscles form a functional pair. Both are interconnected by the fiber system. Just as the semimembranosus muscle is an active stabilizer and checkrein of the medial side, the popliteus muscle, with its pencil-thick tendon, is the corresponding stabilizer

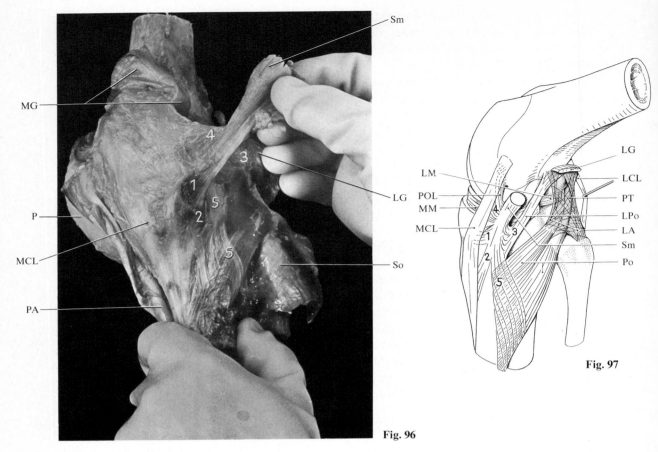

Fig. 96

Fig. 97

Fig. 96. The semimembranosus muscle is the active controlling and stabilizing muscle of the posteromedial corner. It sends tendinous expansions to the posterior meniscus horn and the POL. As a result, it tenses the posteromedial corner in various flexion angles and in IR, even when the POL is relatively lax. In extension its direction of pull runs roughly parallel to the femoral shaft to the posteromedial corner of the tibia. The semimembranosus acts as a powerful stabilizer against medial opening; in 90° flexion it exerts an approximately right-angle pull on the upper tibia and posteromedial corner. It actively limits ER and prevents excessive rotation in this direction. Anteriorly its most superficial layer blends with that of the MCL. Accordingly, this MCL fiber layer is "dynamized" from a proximal direction by the vastus medialis (see p. 35) and from a posterior direction by the semimembranosus. Parts of these tendinous expansions of the semimembranosus indirectly connect the tibia with the femur; these correspond to the "superficial arm" of the POL described by Hughston and Eilers [136] and are more tendinous in their composition than ligamentous. It is important that this connecting layer be accurately repaired in both recent and old injuries

Fig. 97. Diagram of the five sites of insertion of the semimembranosus in the posteromedial corner. *1* Pars reflexa, which passes anteriorly below the long bundle of the collateral ligament fibers, almost parallel to the tibial articular surface, and fills the semimembranosus sulcus, a bony furrow often visible in x-ray. *2* The direct insertion on the tibial margin, which blends longitudinally with the periosteum. *3* Insertion which passes as the oblique popliteal ligament into the tendon of the lateral head of the gastrocnemius to the fabella. *4* Insertion which blends with the POL (see also Fig. 96). *5* Insertion which blends with the fascia of the popliteus and thus establishes a functional connection with this muscle. This connection enables a common reception of tension changes that are indispensable for active rotational control via reflex mechanisms. The popliteus muscle with its various attachments to the posteromedial corner forms a kind of active counterpart to the lateral side. Both structures act jointly as internal rotators of the tibia when the foot is not fixed and the tibia is free to move

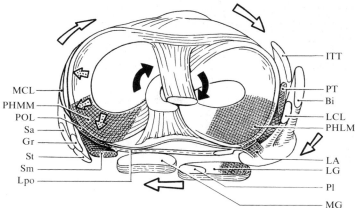

Fig. 98. The semimembranosus corner and popliteus corner each consist of a functionally-integrated triple complex. The medial complex is composed of the posterior horn of the medial meniscus, the attached POL and the semimembranosus muscle; the lateral complex consists of the posterior horn of the lateral meniscus, the popliteus tendon, the arcuate popliteal ligament as well as the lateral gastrocnemius tendon. *Black arrows:* torsional stress in the central pivot; *white arrows:* simultaneous rotational stress of the peripheral ligaments; *spotted arrows:* stress on the medial side and semimembranosus corner (adapted from Nicholas [252])

and checkrein of the lateral side. With its main tendon and its expansions to the posterior capsule, lateral meniscal posterior horn and arcuate ligament, it is a prime example of a stabilizer which 1. restrains the femur laterally on the tibia with its free tendon and 2. "dynamizes" the arcuate ligament complex, thereby contributing to stability even in flexion (Figs. 97 and 98).

The Posterolateral Corner (Popliteus Corner)

- "Arcuate popliteal ligament complex"
- "Posterolateral corner"
- "Posterior lateral capsular corner"
- "Point d'angle postéro-externe" (PAPE)

As on the medial side, none of these terms is comprehensive enough to express the functional value of this joint region.

Because the active control element is the popliteus muscle, we call this area the *popliteus corner*.

The Individual Functional Elements of the Popliteus Corner

Four components form this functional complex, which is essential for lateral stability:

1. the lateral meniscus with its posterior horn;
2. the arcuate ligament complex, consisting of:
   - the fabellofibular ligament (of Vallois)
   - deep portions of the capsule
   - a meniscotibial linkage
3. the popliteus muscle
4. the gastrocnemius muscle.

The ligamentous elements of the lateral side, while relatively inconspicuous, are nevertheless crucial for stability and may, in fact, be even more important than the ligaments of the medial side. Because the ligaments act as tension receptors, any abnormality in their length will prevent the dynamic stabilizers from functioning properly. As a result, late changes of the lateral ligaments secondary to injuries are much more debilitating than on the medial side, even though an important active stabilizing force is provided by the biceps, iliotibial tract and popliteus muscle.

The importance of these ligaments as feedback elements should not be underestimated. If they are torn or even lax, they are no longer tensed at the correct moment and so can no longer furnish the proprioceptive input necessary for active auxiliary stabilization; the motor system of the knee loses its

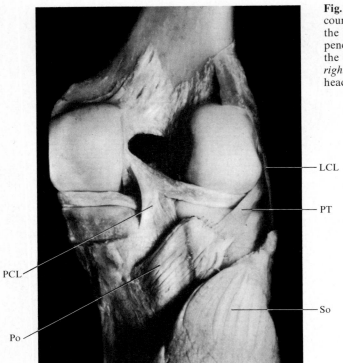

- LCL
- PT
- PCL
- Po
- So

Fig. 99. Posterior aspect of the knee joint showing the course of the popliteus muscle and its tendon running past the posterior horn of the lateral meniscus; as a rule this pencil-thick tendon passes below the LCL and attaches to the femur anterior to it. The greater muscle mass (*bottom right*) belongs to the soleus muscle attaching to the fibular head (v. Hochstetter)

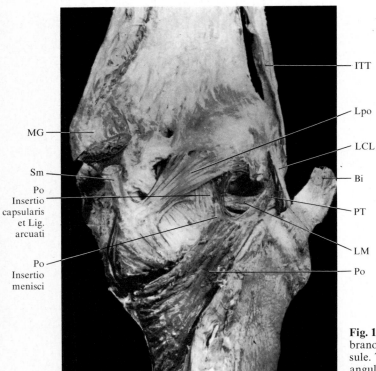

- MG
- Sm
- Po
- Insertio capsularis et Lig. arcuati
- Po Insertio menisci
- ITT
- Lpo
- LCL
- Bi
- PT
- LM
- Po

Fig. 100. The tendinous expansions of the semimembranosus and popliteus muscles to the posterior joint capsule. This specimen documents the typical V-shaped or triangular arrangement of the fiber bundles, which is very important for passive rotatory stability (v. Hochstetter)

feedback and reference points, and active-passive coordination can no longer function in a controlled, orderly way.

The popliteus muscle (Figs. 99 and 100) is perhaps the major controlling element of the lateral side, acting both as a sensor and a moderator through its many tedinous extensions and tension receptors.

According to Basmajian and Lovejoy [21], the Y-shaped origin of the popliteus also gives it the important function of pulling the lateral meniscus backward during flexion and IR, out of the way of the rapidly receding lateral femoral condyle. Its position also makes it a synergist of the posterior cruciate ligament.

Because the most proximal portion of the arcuate ligament from the site of the fabella to the femur blends with the tendinous plate of the gastrocnemius muscle, the gastrocnemius also belongs to the popliteus corner in the broadest sense.

Active Stabilization Under Proprioceptive Control

According to Hochstetter (personal communication and unpublished documents), the tendon spindles that function as tension receptors are most concentrated in the fan-shaped ends of the tendons, which, as in the semimembranosus muscle, have connections with ligaments, the joint capsule and other tendons. A comparative count of these receptors would be highly interesting and instructive.

In the same context, it is noteworthy that there is a larger-than-average area of the cerebral cortex devoted to the reception of sensory input from the lower limb. Its processing must be of special importance for the cybernetics of balance and the manifold sequences of movement. The corresponding area for the upper limb is significantly smaller.

Freeman and Wyke [100] have studied the innervation of the knee joint in cats and have found a rich supply in the region of the posterior capsule as a whole, the POL, the posterior cruciate ligament, and the coronary ligaments of both menisci. They described a "posterior articular nerve," a "medial articular nerve" (located on the anteromedial side), and a "lateral articular nerve." The medial and lateral nerves supplied rather small areas compared to the posterior nerve. Freeman and Wyke identified four types of nerve endings. They called types I, II and III mechanoreceptors, characterizing type I as low-threshold, slowly adapting; type II as low-threshold, rapidly adapting; and type III as high-threshold, very slowly adapting. They assigned type IV endings to pain perception and vasomotor functions. The different types were not evenly distributed in all tissues. Type III was found in all ligaments, including the cruciates, as Kennedy et al. [174] have confirmed.

Stilwell [333, 334] has also described the innervation of fibers, aponeuroses and tendons in detail. He found three kinds of structures apparently involved in the proprioceptive control system, noting that "facilitating and inhibiting influences emanate from stretch afferents in the knee joint capsule."

Many nerve endings occur at the musculotendinous junctions, and the fasciae are also richly supplied with nerve branches arising from both the muscles and the skin.

The phenomenon of postpoliomyelitic flail joint provides a clear illustration of the importance of active auxiliary stabilization by the muscles. Passive ligamentous support alone cannot withstand long-term stress unless supplemented by active protection.

A study by Palmer [280] merits special attention in this context. He stimulated the deep portions of the medial collateral ligament and noted a contraction of the vastus medialis muscle in response.

In patients with anteromedial instabilities of the knee, Schmitt and Mittelmeier [311] found longstanding vastus medialis atrophies which had their cause not in a lack of training but probably in reflex-kinematic factors like those described by Ségal et al. [314].

Rotation

Physiology and Pathophysiology of Free and Active Rotation

Active Rotation by the Extensors

All muscles that bridge the knee joint are found to exert some degree of rotatory effect during careful functional testing. Even the two bellies of the gastrocnemius, whose function in the knee is still somewhat obscure, contribute to this action.

The Quadriceps Muscle

This muscle is comprised of various extensors and shows an axial deviation of about 10–15° in its course across the patella and patellar ligament (Fig. 101). This angle, whose vertex lies on the patella, is called the Q angle (Fig. 102a; cf. schematic diagrams in Dejour [63] and Insall et al. [144]). Disregarding for the moment the vastus medialis and vastus lateralis, the rectus femoris and vastus intermedius rotate the tibia internally on the femur due to their angled direction of pull (Fig. 102a). This IR of the tibia occurs if the tibia is freely mobile; if it is fixed, the patella pushes the lateral femoral condyle backward causing ER of the femur.

But the Q angle is not the only mechanism underlying rotation of the knee by the quadriceps apparatus. The arrangement of the vastus medialis and vastus lateralis is at least equally important for the active control of rotation by the quadriceps muscle. The distal transverse part of the vastus medialis, the vastus medialis obliquus, directly counteracts the rotatory force K resulting from the Q angle (Fig. 102a). It also rotates the tibia

medially via the patellar ligament, with a simultaneous relief of compression in the lateral patellofemoral area. The vastus lateralis can act as an antagonist to counteract this tension: In strong IR or with a large varus stress, it pulls the patella laterally toward the lateral femoral condyle and checks further medial rotation of the tibia. The Q angle also lateralizes the quadriceps force that presses the femur and tibia together. This antagonism is especially important when pressure transmission is shifted medialward by a dynamic varus stress, as during sprinting (Fig. 116).

Observations in athletes have revealed interesting aspects of these mechanisms. Weight lifters, who perform their feats with the knee internally rotated, display a relative hypertrophy of the vastus lateralis. The vastus medialis, by contrast, is relatively poorly developed in these athletes. According to the studies of Cadilhac et al. [43], the two muscles show differences in the quantitative distribution of type-I (slow-twitch) and type-II (fast-twitch) muscle fibers. The vastus lateralis contains a predominance of type-I fibers, which are suited for a sustained, static retention function, while the vastus medialis contains many type-II fibers better suited for rapidly changing, phasic actions.

Our clinical experience indicates that the tone of the vastus muscles alters in response to a varus or valgus stress applied to the knee (see also Palmer [279, 280]). If a varus or valgus force is applied to the knee joint of a thin patient with good reflexes and a well-defined patella, with the knee flexed about 15°, varus pressure is seen to cause a lateral deviation of the patella, and valgus pressure a medial deviation. Though the extent of this displacement is slight, it nevertheless constitutes a separate and distinct movement.

It was once thought that the vastus medialis became active only in the final 20° of extension, and thus during automatic rotation. However, an analysis of sports photos (Fig. 102 b–d) reveals that the vastus medialis can be powerfully active in all degrees of flexion.

As Fig. 103 shows, moreover, the activity of the vastus medialis is also dependent on the rotational position of the knee joint (cf. Kapandji [164]). The ER in Fig. 103 c increases the activity of the vastus medialis, while the IR in Fig. 103 a does not provoke marked vastus medialis contraction.

The changing actions of the vastus medialis and lateralis muscles are associated with varying degrees of compression between the patellar halves and the femur.

In neutral rotation (NR) (Fig. 103 b), there is no great disparity in the forces of muscular tension. In strong IR the patella is passively compressed against the medial femoral condyle, while the active tension of the vastus lateralis increases and counteracts this compression. Conversely, in strong ER of the tibia the patella is spontaneously pressed against the lateral femoral condyle, while the active muscular tension in the vastus medialis increases (Fig. 104). The ligaments extending between the patella and menisci play an important role in this control mechanism (Fig. 103). They have been described by Pauzat [221] after Kaplan [170] as the patellomeniscal ligaments. We believe that these ligamentous attachments, which do not occur with equal prominence in all individuals, also explain why the clinical picture of medial patellar chondromalacia is often so difficult to distinguish from that of a medial meniscus lesion. These ligaments place both lesion sites on a single functional axis, so to speak, and may cause pain to radiate from one site to the other.

The *patellofemoral articulation* is entirely dependent on the function of the quadriceps muscle and displays certain peculiarities. It is surprising, for example, that the entire articular surface of the patella is never in full contact with the femur at any one time. Several authors, such as Grant [113], Maquet [205], Henche et al. [401] and Goodfellow [110, 111], have confirmed that while patel-

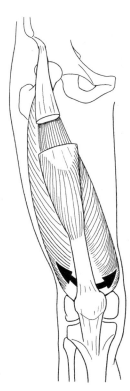

Fig. 101. The quadriceps extensor apparatus acts with the vastus medialis obliquus (*right arrow*) and vastus lateralis (*left arrow*) as an active rotator and rotational stabilizer

Fig. 102. a Even in the frontal plane, the quadriceps muscle does not pull vertically over the patella to the tibial tuberosity, but exerts an oblique pull that forms a laterally obtuse angle called the quadriceps or *Q* angle. In accordance with the parallelogram of forces, this *Q* angle causes a laterally-directed force *K* to act on the patella. The lateral portion of the femoral condyle is pushed posteriorly by this force, while the tibia is rotated medially relative to the femur. The distal transverse portion of the vastus medialis (the vastus medialis obliquus) acts as an antagonist to this force *K*. It can pull the patella medially, thereby restraining the medial femoral condyle. **b–d** This vastus medialis is active not just in full extension, but also in 30, 60 and 100° flexion (102 b from *Schweizer Illustrierte*, 1974; 102 c, d from *World Cup*, 1974)

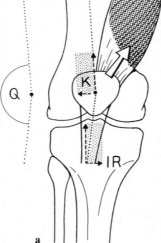

a

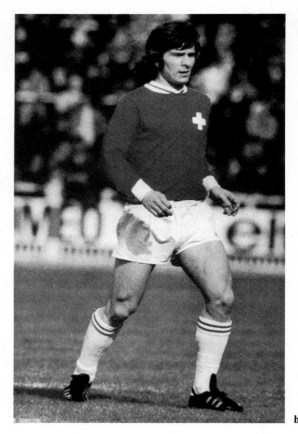

b

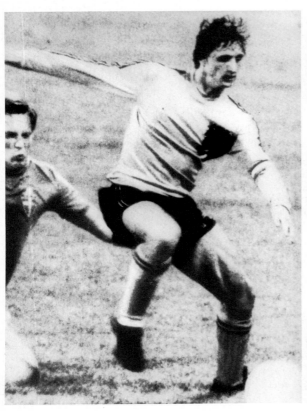

c

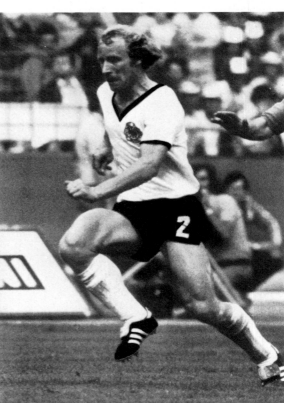

d

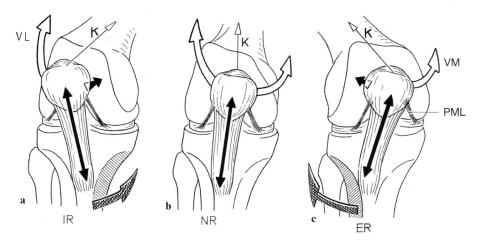

Fig. 103a–c. The quadriceps extensor apparatus with its patellofemoral component in various positions of rotation. **a** The angulation in IR causes pressure to be exerted against the medial femoral condyle (*short arrow*) under the pull of a central force *K*; the vastus lateralis muscle contracts antagonistically to compensate. **b** In NR the vastus medialis and lateralis can function equally as agonists and antagonists. **c** In ER the patella is pressed against the lateral femoral condyle (*short arrow*) under the action of the force *K*, and the vastus medialis reflexly contracts to compensate

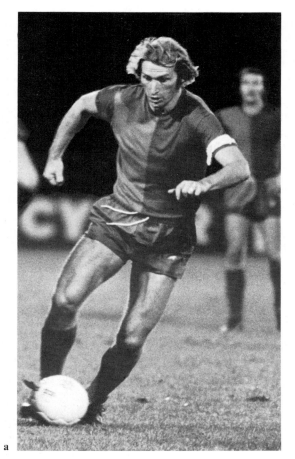
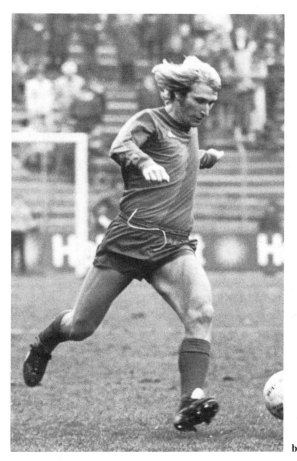

Fig. 104a, b. A soccer player controls the ball with a combination of internal and external tibial rotation. **a** ER is stabilized by a powerful contraction of the vastus medialis; **b** in IR the vastus medialis is under very little tension (photo Baumli)

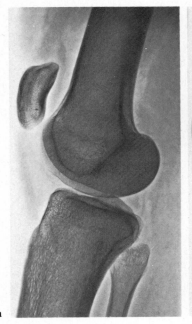
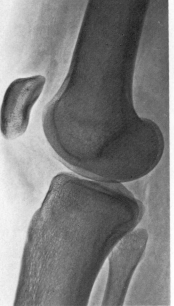
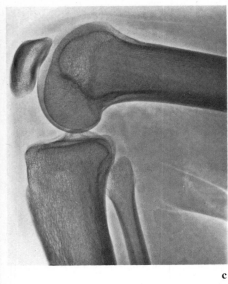

a

b

c

Fig. 105a–c. The relation of the patella to the femur. **a** In extension with the quadriceps *tensed,* only the distal part of the patella articulates with the femur. The similarly tensed patellar ligament (*shadow*) is stretched to its full length. **b** In extension with the quadriceps *relaxed,* the patella descends, articulating with the femur in its central portion. The patellar ligament is also relaxed. **c** In 90° flexion the proximal articular surface of the patella rides on the trochlea just above the intercondylar notch

lo-femoral contact may indeed obey certain rules during flexion-extension, the patella is never in complete contact with the femur. The distal portion, the wedge-shaped patellar apex, has no articular surface and can never come in contact with the femur, because it is completely ensheathed by the patellar tendon. With the knee in extension, the patella contacts the femur at a point just proximal to its apex (see Fig. 105). As the knee is flexed, this contact area migrates toward the proximal pole of the patella. If flexion is continued past 90° to the normal limit of 135°, the patella comes to lie in front of the intercondylar fossa of the femur, and its contact area encompasses only the lateral facet and the medial "odd facet" (Fig. 106). As in the femorotibial joint, there is a rolling-gliding mechanism at work in the femoropatellar articulation, except that in the latter, the direction of patellar gliding is opposite to its direction of rolling.

The presence of a particularly thick layer of articular cartilage on the medial facet of the patella should also be mentioned in this context. As Bandi [17] and Morscher [231] point out, the thickness of this layer makes it prone to nutritional disturbances, since the exchange of materials by diffusion is slowed as the diffusion path lengthens. As a result, there is a fine line between sufficiency and insufficiency, and even minor functional disturbances, according to Ficat [86, 88], can cause this finely balanced system to become decompensated. Little is known as yet about the relationship between rotational physiology, cartilage nutrition and patellar chondromalacia in the patellofemoral joint. Clearly, the physiology and pathophysiology of rotation as well as ligamentous instability must play an important role, as Ségal [314] has emphasized. The changing pressures on the various patellar contact surfaces – medial, lateral, proximal and distal – together with the transverse movements of the patella by medial and lateral quadriceps tension have a crucial bearing on the health of the tissues in the femoropatellar joint.

80

In operations on fresh injuries, even in athletes, we frequently find various forms of cartilage pathology such as edema, fibrillation and ulceration for which the patient has voiced no previous complaints. Typical chrondropathic symptoms may arise postoperatively, however (see also Rehabilitation, p. 267).

The Patellofemoral Joint and Dislocation of the Patella

The phenomenon of patellar dislocation, as a pathophysiologic product of active rotation, is ranked among the physiologic processes in the region of the quadriceps muscle and femoropatellar joint.

Case example: An adolescent girl of mature bone growth presented with a patellar dislocation from pulling on a boot. To learn the mechanism of the injury, we asked the patient to demonstrate with the healthy limb. What we observed deepened our understanding of the functional relationships in the femoropatellar articulation: With the tibia internally rotated (!) and toes pointed, the patient slipped her foot and lower leg into the very narrow, knee-high boot. At the moment her heel passed the ankle of the boot, and resistance increased, the patient countered by forcibly extending the leg at the knee joint, which was still internally rotated. At this point there was a snapping subluxation of the patella of the healthy leg. At a flexion angle of about 30°, it could be seen how the vastus lateralis pulled the patella up onto the lateral femoral condyle until, with increasing extension, the patella was able to slip back to its central position.

This observation also demonstrated that the patella does not dislocate over the lateral femoral condyle at just any point, but only in the area of the terminal sulcus, and thus at the junction of the femoropatellar and femorotibial articular surfaces. Obviously lateral guidance is lacking in the area of this depression (see Mechanics, p. 15), and the path is cleared for patellar dislocation in the truest sense of the word. In addition, the clinical experience of Eriksson [80] and the work of Scheller and Martensen [309] show that flake fractures are occasioned not by the patellar dislocation itself, but by its reduction. This confirms our observation that the patella dislocates along a least-resistance path having no obstructions that could cause an osteochondral fracture. This occurs only when the dislocation is reduced in subsequent extension by pulling the patella back over the high lateral lip of the femoral patellar surface (Fig. 107). Based on these facts, we do not believe that the "lateral patellofemoral angle" of Laurin et al. [196] is significant in the causation of patellar dislocation. This angle exists only momentarily in a specific patellar position relative to the femur and is inadequate for a tridimensional assessment of the dynamic processes involved (Fig. 108 a–d).

Osteochondral fragments from the patella and femur have also been described by Morscher [231], who notes further that the literature contains no account of meniscal injuries occurring in association with patellar dislocation, even though a valgus flexion-ER mechanism was the presumed cause of the lesion. We, too, have encountered no combined injury of this type in our patient material.

At this point it is important to consider the question of whether patellar dislocation takes place with the knee in ER or IR. The case described above involving dislocation from the pulling on of a boot with the leg extended and internally rotated is supplemented by more recent observations.

One case involved a young skier who was running a practice slalom course laid out on level ground. As he was leaving a gate to the right, he caught his right ski tip on the gate pole. His leg was rotated internally, and his patella dislocated when he attempted to force the ski on past the pole with his right leg. As in the previous case, active extension in forced IR caused the dislocation to occur.

The assumption that we are dealing with an active dislocation mechanism driven by the pull of the vastus lateralis is strengthened by the fact that no meniscal injury has ever been observed in association with a dislocated patella, for sooner or later such a combination would have been observed if an ER mechanism were involved. It may be that such dislocations can occur in either position of rotation, with the quadriceps muscle playing different roles in each of the two mechanisms. It is conceivable that in the valgus-ER mechanism, the quadriceps could move the patella laterally in its entirety because of the

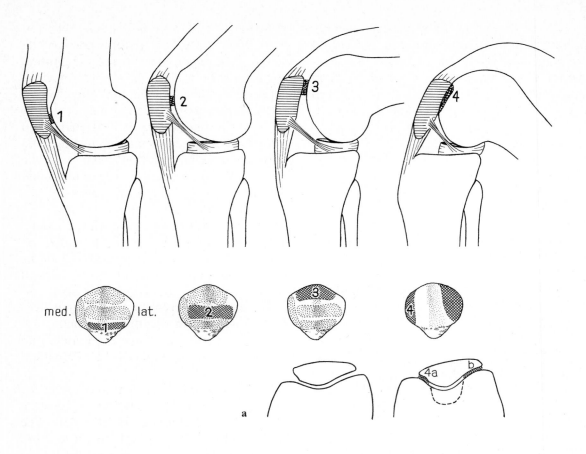

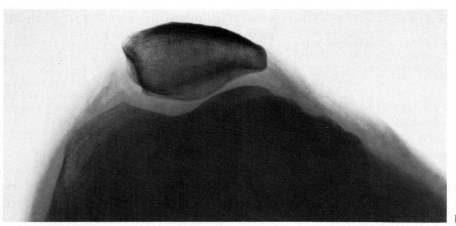

Fig. 106. a Schematic representation of patellofemoral contact after Grant and Basmajian [113] and Goodfellow et al. [110, 111]. Each joint position from full extension (*1*) to intermediate flexion (*2* and *3*) to full flexion (*4*) is characterized by a different area of patellofemoral contact. Note that it is not until phase *4* that the true medial patellar edge facet, or "odd facet" (*4a*), articulates with the femur. In the femoropatellar joint, as in the femorotibial, there is a rolling-gliding mechanism, except that the direction of gliding is opposite to that of rolling. **b** Axial roentgenogram of a patella demonstrating the medial "odd facet," which exhibits a conspicuous subchondral layer of osteosclerosis as a sign of stress

Fig. 107. Patellar dislocation and reduction. Spontaneous dislocation occurs in the flexed knee when the patella slips laterally in the area of the terminal sulcus (*arrow A*). Reduction occurs when the patella snaps back during extension; in the process, it passes the high lateral lip of the trochlea in the area of *arrow B*, causing osteochondral flake fractures to occur (see also Fig. 108a). The patella may sustain two types of fracture, one involving the central margin or patellar crest (fragment *1a* in the drawing), and one involving the odd facet (fragment *1b*)

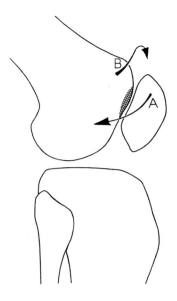

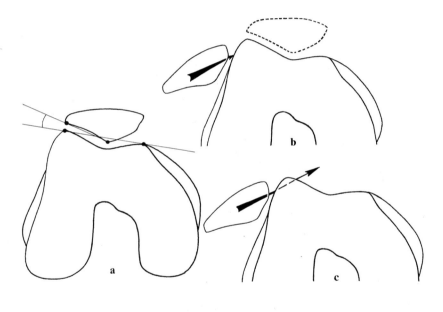

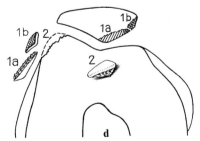

Fig. 108a–d. These flake fractures occur only when the dislocation is reduced. **a** The angle indicated by Laurin exists in only one plane and so is of limited use in describing the dynamic phenomenon of patellar dislocation. **b, c** Stages of dislocation, unaccompanied by flake fractures. **d** The reduced patella with osteochondral fragments. The condylar edge fragment *2* is displaced into the anterior half of the joint, while the sheared-off patellar fragments (*1a* and *1b*) tend to remain on the lateral side of the condyle

83

greater Q angle, without the need for the vastus lateralis to exert any special action.

Whatever the details of the process of patellar dislocation may be, the finely-tuned function performed by the quadriceps in the control of rotational and varus-valgus stresses remains undisputed.

Active Rotation by the Flexors

Monoarticular Flexor-Rotators

For too long the *popliteus muscle* has been given little attention in functional considerations of the knee joint, as Southmaid and Quigley [330] point out. Its juxta-articular location and oblique course make it almost a pure rotator. But its location behind the flexion axis also makes it a flexor, although this action is slightly due to the short lever arms.

The popliteus mucle has several functions:

1. With the tibia hanging free and its proximal attachment fixed, it acts as an internal rotator of the tibia.

2. With the tibia fixed, it exerts an external rotating action on the femur and serves as a general rotatory stabilizer. This mechanism also corresponds to internal rotation, though this time the femoral condyle is the moving member.

3. The popliteus reinforces the biceps muscle and iliotibial tract as a general stabilizer of the lateral side (Figs. 109 and 110) when the knee approaches extension.

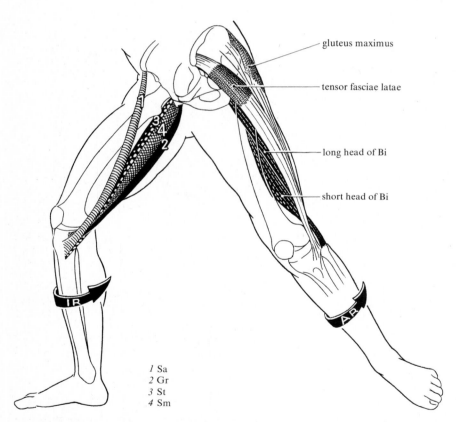

gluteus maximus

tensor fasciae latae

long head of Bi

short head of Bi

1 Sa
2 Gr
3 St
4 Sm

Fig. 109. The active voluntary rotators of the knee joint. The *right* leg shows the active internal rotators: the muscles of the pes anserinus group, the sartorius, gracilis and semitendinosus, supported by the powerful semimembranosus which inserts farther posteriorly. The active external rotators are shown in the *left* leg. The short head of the biceps, with its purely fibulo-femoral course, is a monoarticular external rotator, while the long, ischiofibular head of the biceps is a biarticular external rotator of the knee and extensor of the hip. The two active muscles whose forces are transmitted to the tibia via the iliotibial tract are the biarticular tensor fasciae latae and gluteus maximus

84

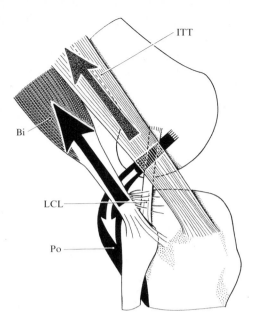

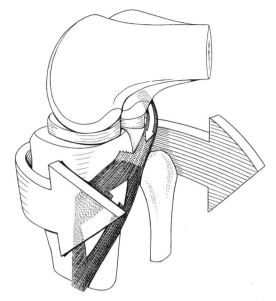

Fig. 110. The active-passive stabilizing mechanisms of the lateral side. The purely passive stabilizing structures are poorly developed on the lateral side compared to the medial. They consist of the LCL with its relatively small cross-section and the passive elements of the popliteus corner and ALFTL. Active stabilization is provided by the dynamic portion of the iliotibial tract and by the popliteus and biceps muscles. As on the medial side, the lateral active elements act in extension to check varus opening; as flexion increases their rotatory action becomes more powerful

Fig. 111. Schematic representation of the popliteus muscle. The course of the popliteus, with its distal muscle belly and tendon passing below the LCL to the femur, can act in two directions as a pure rotator of the knee: With the tibia fixed and the foot planted on the ground, it exerts a posterolateral tension on the femur and thus stabilizes the lateral side and popliteus corner. With the femur fixed and the tibia hanging free, it rotates the tibia internally relative to the femur

Its pull then protects the anatomically weak capsulo-ligamentous elements of the posterolateral side of the knee.

4. It contributes somewhat to flexion owing to its location in the posterior region of the joint. But its main function is stabilization, as indicated by its tendinous attachments with the arcuate ligament and posterior horn of the lateral meniscus (Fig. 111).

The Short Head of the Biceps. The short head of the biceps is another monoarticular muscle of the flexor group. It is an external rotator and thus an antagonist of the popliteus. It is also a flexor, owing to its attachment behind the flexion axis. It is a more efficient flexor than the popliteus, because its anatomic position gives it a greater mechanical advantage for this action (Fig. 112).

Biarticular Internal Rotators

With the exception of the popliteus, all active internal rotators of the flexor group are biarticular, attaching to both the knee and hip. The fan-shaped pelvic origin of the muscles, from the anterior iliac spine for the sartorius to the ischial tuberosity for the semimembranosus, enable the internal rotators to exert a smooth, continuous action in a variety of positions.

As Meyer writes in his *Mechanics of the Knee Joint* [226], the Weber brothers were among the first to recognize the important role of the flexor-rotators. They collected interesting comparative data by systematically weighing these muscles in cadavers. They used these data as a measure of the importance of particular muscles in flexion-rotation, applying the simple but valid rule

Table 1. Proportionality data on weight differences of the internal and external rotators

Flexion with IR		*Flexion with ER*	
Sartorius muscle	125.7	Biceps femoris muscle	274.4
Gracilis muscle	82.2		
Semitendinosus muscle	128.2		
Popliteus muscle	24.0		
Semimembranosus muscle	206.5		
Internal rotation	566.6	External rotation	274.4

that the size of a structure is proportional to its functional importance. Their findings, expressed as proportions, are given in the table above (Meyer and Weber).

The Weber brothers (quoted in [226]) did not mention the tensor fasciae latae or gluteus maximus as external rotators. Both muscles exert an active force on the knee joint through the iliotibial tract. The fact that the gluteus maximus sends a powerful muscular extension into the tract from the posterior side is not widely known. Because the Weber brothers neglected these two important external rotators, their results are biased in favor of the internal rotators.

A particularly interesting finding of this early study is the significantly greater weight of the semimembranosus compared to the other internal rotators. This underscores the importance of this muscle, which is now generally recognized.

Kapandji [164] presents a drawing that shows the course of the rotators in relation to the moving limbs. In Fig. 109 we have

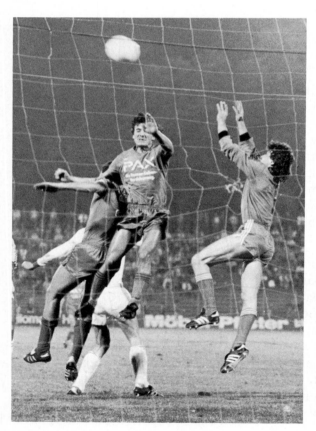

Fig. 112. The short head of the biceps acts as a pure external rotator of the tibia. The active external rotation by both heads of the biceps is clearly seen in the high-jumping goalkeeper. The short head passes to the distal half of the femur and like the popliteus is a monoarticular rotator and flexor. A situation equivalent to an acute semimembranosus injury can occur on the lateral side when the fibular head dislocates as a result of excessive biceps traction with the knee strongly flexed and the foot planted (see also Fig. 120) (photo Baumli)

adopted his basic scheme, supplementing it with greater detail.

Biarticular External Rotators

Besides the biceps femoris, which, according to the Weber brothers (quoted in [226]), weighs half as much as all the internal rotators, there are the external rotators which act on the knee via the iliotibial tract.

The Iliotibial Tract

Functionally the iliotibial tract is a multifaceted structure. Its distal posterior portions, which we call the anterolateral femorotibial ligament (ALFTL), extend from the linea aspera of the femur to the tubercle of Gerdy, as previously described. Just as these deep portions produce passive stabilization of the knee joint, the more anterior, superficial parts of the tract actively stabilize the lateral side as the tendon of the tensor fasciae latae and gluteus maximus. This active stabilizer is peculiar (see also p. 27) in that it crosses the flexion axis during knee movement. As a result, it acts as an extensor beyond about 30° extension, and as a flexor beyond 30° flexion. From this angle on it can exert its external rotating action on the upper tibia. The active force which acts via the iliotibial tract to stabilize the knee laterally against varus stress, extend it between 0 and 30° and rotate it at greater angles of flexion is provided by the tensor fasciae latae and gluteus maximus muscles. Their Y-shaped arrangement, in which the gluteus medius may also be actively involved, shows that this lateral stabilizing and rotating force is present both when the hip is in an extension phase via the gluteus maximus and when the tensor fasciae latae is active in a flexion phase.

These references to the biarticular function of these rotators further illustrate how active and passive elements work together over the entire length of the limb to produce stability.

Varus-Flexion-IR and Valgus-Flexion-ER

The normal knee has a full range of motion between the position of varus-flexion-IR and valgus-flexion-ER. The soccer players in Fig. 113 illustrate both positions, which are more extreme in the player on the left and about average in the player on the right. The player on the left has practically exhausted the available range, but as yet he runs no risk of injury because the stress is still entirely within physiologic limits. A lesion will occur only if an additional valgus-producing force acts upon on his left leg, which is in valgus-flexion-ER. Conversely, an additional varus-producing force would have to act on the right limb, which is in varus-flexion-IR, for an injury to occur, as Noesberger and Paillot [256] have demonstrated with films. The majority of knee injuries occur when stress limits are exceeded in these extreme positions. This is why some 80% of ligamentous knee injuries take the form of a medial or lateral "unhappy triad," with excessive stress in ER causing a lesion of the *medial collateral ligament, anterior cruciate ligament* and *semimembranosus corner,* and excessive stress in varus causing injury of the *lateral collateral ligament, posterior cruciate ligament* and *popliteus corner.*

These extreme positions can be assumed voluntarily, as in the case of hurdlers (Fig. 114), who place their trailing leg in valgus-flexion-ER when clearing a hurdle.

The weight lifter chooses the other extreme of varus-flexion-IR in order to achieve maximum performance (Fig. 115).

Interestingly, varus-flexion-IR is a position favored by all running athletes (Fig. 116). We are so accustomed to this pattern that we do not notice it. Only by watching an untrained individual run in valgus-flexion-ER are we reminded of the link between style and performance.

Differences of Stabilizing Potential in Varus-Flexion-IR and Valgus-Flexion-ER

Experience has shown that combined injuries are 10–20 times more frequent on the

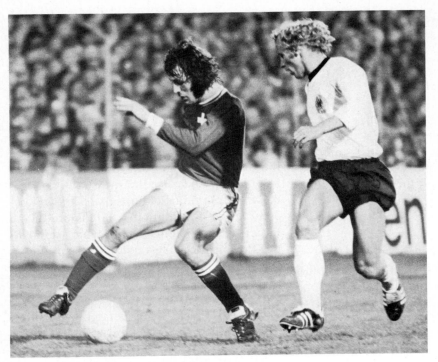

Fig. 113. Possible extreme positions of the knee joint. In each case the right leg is in varus-flexion-IR and the left leg is in valgus-flexion-ER. Within these two physiologic extremes is a wide range in which the knee joint can be actively moved with no danger of injury. If an additional valgus-producing force is applied to the left leg, a complex injury of the medial triad type will result; an additional varus force applied to the right leg will produce a lateral triad injury (photo Baumli)

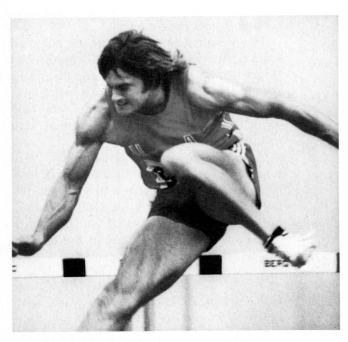

Fig. 114. The hurdler demonstrates the extreme degree of active external rotation needed to clear a hurdle (Montreal, 1976)

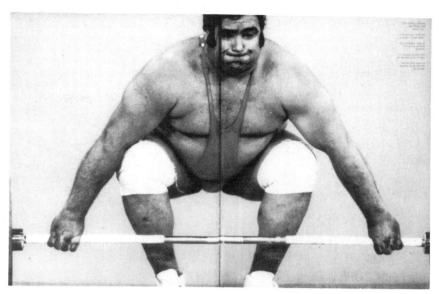

Fig. 115. The weightlifter places his legs in the typical varus-flexion-IR position. These athletes develop hypertrophy of the vastus lateralis as a result of working in IR and due to the primarily static exercise of the type-II muscle fibers. These men contrast with dynamic athletes, who work rapidly in all rotational positions and thus develop hypertrophy of the vastus medialis (Montreal, 1976)

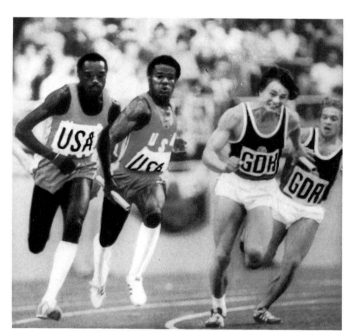

Fig. 116. Runners also exhibit a typical rotational position of the knee. During the actual performance phase of the race, the position of varus-flexion-IR can always be observed. When running the cool-down lap after the finish line, the runner reassumes a position of valgus-flexion-ER (Montreal, 1976)

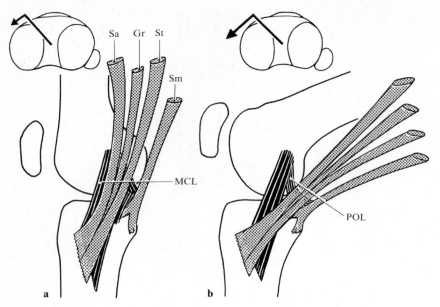

Fig. 117a, b. The pes anserinus group and semimembranosus exert considerably more rotational force in flexion, when they pull almost at right angles to the tibia, than in extension, when their lever arm for rotation is shorter. **a** Parallel course of the pes anserinus tendons to the MCL. Their attachment, too, obeys the Burmester Curve. When a valgus-producing stress is exerted on the MCL in extension, the parallel pes anserinus tendons also come under tension and can reflexly augment passive stabilization by their active protection. This protective reaction can increase several-fold the purely passive medial stability provided by the MCL. **b** In flexion the rotators afford active protection by counteracting excessive ER. The pes anserinus group can act with the semimembranosus to check ER, and the biceps with the iliotibial tract and vastus lateralis (!) to check IR

medial side of the knee than on the *lateral* side. This fact suggests that the varus-IR so often seen in trained athletes is no coincidence. When walking on a steep or slippery surface, we instinctively place the leg in varus-IR, for it is easiest to keep the knee under control in this position.

Active Synergistic Protection of Ligament Function by the Rotators of the Knee

Dejour [63] has shown that the rotational force of the internal rotators increases with the degree of flexion, owing to the corresponding lengthening of the available lever arm. The muscles of the pes anserinus group insert just anterior to the tibial insertion of the MCL (cf. Kinematics, p. 36). In extension the three tendons of the pes are parallel to the MCL and closely overlie it. In this position the pes anserinus muscles provide an active protective restraint which greatly augments the passive restraint of the MCL. Every good soccer player knows this intuitively and keeps his leg straight and internally rotated when cutting off a hard-kicked ball. Kaplan [167] quotes Duchenne, who refers to the biceps, semimembranosus and semitendinosus as "active ligaments" that are of fundamental importance in the knee joint.

As Fig. 117 shows, this active restraint protecting the MCL diminishes with increasing flexion. As the rotatory force increases, some protection against valgus stress is lost, and the knee joint is at greater risk for injury. But by the same token, the greater freedom of rotation in flexion enables the knee to evade a varus or valgus stress to a large degree. Now the main task of the rotators is to protect the knee joint from excessive ER or IR. As long as this is successfully done under reflex control, injury can be avoided.

The observations of Slocum and Larson [325] in patients who have undergone a pes anserinus transfer are of interest in this context. While such patients may exhibit stronger IR with training, the knee joint shows an elastic valgus laxity in extension and especially in 30° flexion. In many patients this instability increases over the years, and they become unable to stabilize the knee actively against a valgus stress. Thus, while pes anserinus transplantation increases the force of IR by lengthening the lever arm for this movement, it simultaneously decreases the leverage for active valgus stabilization by the pes anserinus group.

The Rupture Strength of the Ligaments of the Knee and Active Protection

Kennedy et al. [175], who conducted comprehensive experiments on the rupture strength of the cruciate and collateral ligaments, report that the medial collateral and anterior cruciate ligaments have similar ultimate failure strengths of 35–40 kg, while that of the posterior cruciate ligament is approximately 80 kg. When we consider these values, we are struck by the apparent disproportion between potential stress and rupture strength. When ski racers fall or pole vaulters land, the forces that are neutralized must far exceed 40–80 kg. Yet trained athletes suffer relatively few injuries. Thus, the forces acting on the joints must be actively transformed and redistributed. According to Kennedy and Fowler [172] and Freeman and Wyke [100], widely ramified nerve branches are present in both the cruciate and the collateral ligaments. It can be concluded from the study of Freeman and Wyke that, based on the nerve endings described, tension reception takes precedence over pain sensation and vasoregulation. This would strongly suggest that the registered tensions are promptly utilized as feedback for the control of muscular actions, which in turn serve to counteract excessive strain of the purely passive structures and thus guard against injury. Only in this way could the often massive discharges of force (see Fig. 118, for example) be neutralized within the elas-

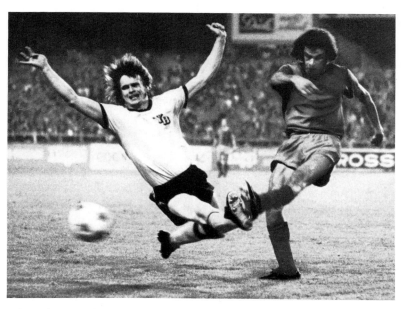

Fig. 118. Extreme dynamic forces such as these can be tolerated without ligamentous injury only when well-conditioned muscles act in concert to exercise their full stabilizing and protective function. Note the violent collision of the extended legs and the momentary recurvation. Stresses are still within elastic reserves, however, and so no injuries are incurred (photo Grossenbacher)

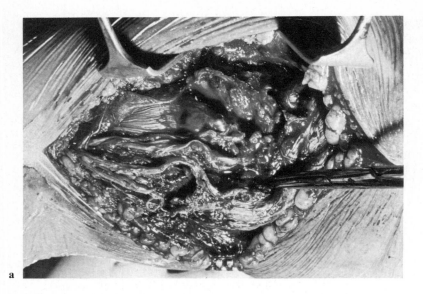

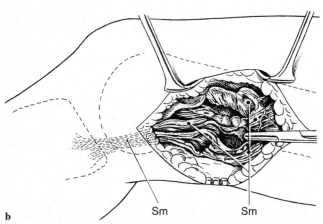

Sm   Sm

b

Fig. 119 a, b. Clinical example of an active rotational injury with spontaneous rupture of the semimembranosus tendon at its junction with the muscle belly. The soccer player had planted his right leg and rotated his upper body counterclockwise, causing extreme pas-sive ER of the right knee joint. When he attempted to correct for this, spontaneous rupture of the muscle oc-curred; the injury was at once perceived and recognized by the player (**a** operative photo for documentation; **b** positional drawing)

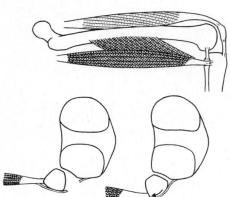

Fig. 120. Schematic representation of the mechanism underlying dislocation of the fibular head

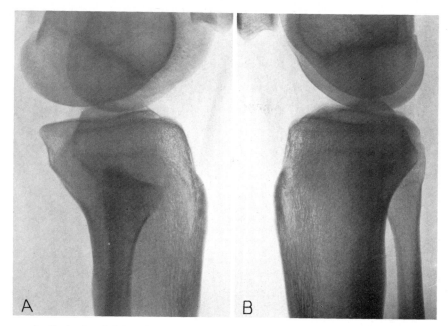

Fig. 121 a, b. Roentgenograms of a fibular head dislocation. **a** Injured side; **b** healthy side

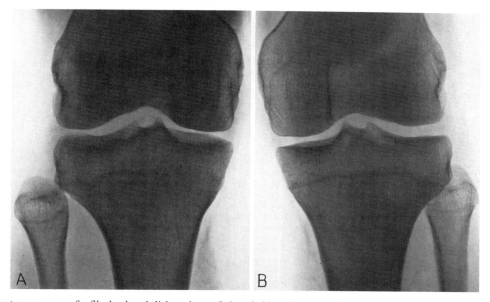

Fig. 122 a, b. Roentgenograms of a fibular head dislocation. **a** Injured side; **b** healthy side

tic reserve of the individual ligaments. The ligaments can, in fact, withstand an extreme force that acts for only a short time in the same direction. The direction and duration of the deforming force are key variables in the occurrence of injury.

Injuries of the Active Rotational System

Semimembranosus Rupture

Besides tendinitis and bursitis-type irritations, we have come across only three

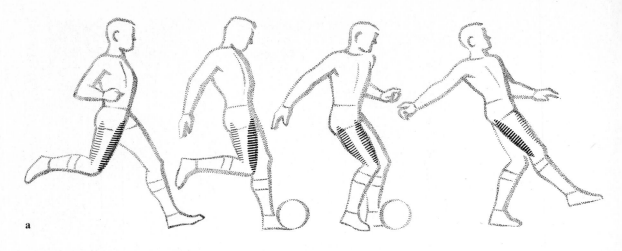

a

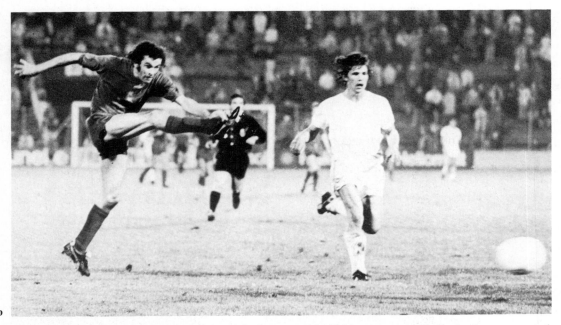

b

Fig. 123. a The "paradox of Tschaidse," which shows that the antagonists are utilized even during extremely powerful extension movements like those associated with kicking a soccer ball; b they are rotational stabilizers which simultaneously act to check hyperextension (photo Baumli)

cases of severe spontaneous injury of the internal rotators. One case involved a complete rupture at the musculotendinous junction of the semimembranosus muscle, as shown in Fig. 119. The rupture occurred in the supporting leg of a soccer player as he tried reflexly to rotate the knee back from extreme ER with the foot planted on the ground. He immediately felt the tear and was able himself to diagnose the mechanism of its occurrence. The wavy collagenous fibers of the aponeurotic layer are visible distal to the rupture site. Two later cases involved a smooth avulsion of the semimembranosus muscle from its origin on the ischial tuberosity.

Dislocation of the Fibular Head

On the lateral side of the knee, we have observed ten cases of a dislocated fibular head,

94

a condition analogous to the semimembranosus rupture on the medial side. When the biceps muscle rotates the tibia externally with the knee flexed and the foot planted, the weakest point in the system is at the proximal tibiofibular attachment. In the presence of a sufficient trauma, a rotatory dislocation will occur in the proximal tibiofibular articulation, accompanied by tearing of the biceps tendon fibers that extend across the fibular head to the tubercle of Gerdy. Figs. 120–122 illustrate this mechanism and show the radiographic result.

Agonism and Antagonism Between Extensor-Flexors and Rotators

Donskoi [71] cites "Tschaidse's paradox," which states that flexors and extensors act simultaneously. The greater the extension, the greater the countertension exerted by the flexors (Fig. 123 a). Presumably this represents a reflexly-based safeguard against active overextension (cf. Fig. 118). In addition, these flexors also act as rotatory stabilizers and so are not only antagonists to the extensors, but are also rotators in their own right. This is illustrated in Fig. 123 b, which shows active rotation during extension as a soccer player makes a shot.

Passive Rotatory Stabilization

To enable the active structures to check rotatory movements in an orderly fashion, passive elements are needed to provide guidance for the rotational system of the knee. The active forces alone are incapable of maintaining stability in a situation of extreme rotational stress like that shown in Fig. 124, where the knee joint serves as a pivot point for the total rotational momentum of the body.

The passive rotatory stabilizers are, from the center to the periphery, the two cruciate ligaments, the menisci, and the surrounding capsuloligamentous structures (Fig. 125).

When the knee is flexed, the powerful posterior cruciate ligament runs parallel to the longitudinal axis of rotation [137] and has few synergists in this position. This may account in part for its great rupture strength, which is twice that of the anterior cruciate.

The peripheral portions of the menisci surrounding the posterior cruciate ligament are of special importance, as will be shown in the following chapter.

The Principle of the Triangular Structure in Passive Rotatory Stabilization

The drawing in Fig. 126 b explains the anatomic specimen in Fig. 126 a. The posterior capsule offers an excellent illustration of how the collagenous fibers interconnect through V-shaped expansions while displaying typical triangular patterns of attachment. There is the oblique popliteal ligament, which blends with the bulk of the semimembranosus tendon (e.g., its 4th insertion) to form a three-dimensional triangle linking the medial proximal femur, posteromedial tibia and posterolateral femur. On the lateral side, the individual elements of the arcuate ligament also form complex triangular structures. Besides the femorofibular attachment formed by the lateral collateral ligament, there is a linkage between the fibular head and fabella or posterior femur called the fabellofibular ligament or ligament of Vallois. These two elements are accompanied by a more transverse portion of the arcuate ligament. This blends with the V-shaped expansion of the popliteus muscle, which can thus exert a dynamizing action on the arcuate ligament complex.

Also interesing is the fact that two ligaments, the oblique popliteal and the fabellofibular, both attach to the fabella. Kaplan [169] also uses the term "short lateral collateral ligament" for the fabellofibular ligament.

The manner in which these V-shaped or triangular structures act as rotatory stabilizers is explained below, taking as examples the MCL and the POL (see p. 98).

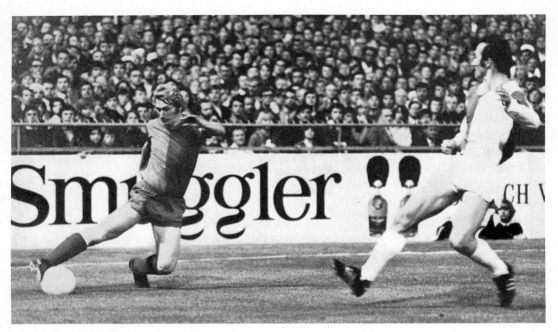

Fig. 124. The knee joint, as a pivot point, is often subjected to violent forces (as illustrated by the soccer player on the left). The theoretical rupture strength of the ligaments alone is insufficient to stabilize the knee passively against kinetic forces of this magnitude (photo Baumli)

The Role of the Fabella

A fabella is present in only about one-fifth of the population. Nevertheless, the site at which it occurs is significant. In the same way that the patella on the anterior side of the knee is located at an intersection of collagenous structures that exert tension in various directions, the fabella lies at a point on the posterolateral side of the knee where multidirectional collagenous tensile stresses intersect. Besides the oblique popliteal ligament and fabellofibular ligament mentioned above, the tendon of the lateral gastrocnemius also contributes to these stresses.

We made the following interesting observation concerning the origin of the fabella: An 18-year-old girl sustained a complex knee injury, and x-rays were taken. The injury was treated conservatively. Ten years later the patient presented with residual complaints in the same knee, and x-rays were again ordered. Suddenly a fabella was present, despite the fact that the closest scrutiny had revealed none on the original films. This suggests that the fabella may form in response to an appropriate stress, providing a structure which, by way of analogy with the patella, can come under tension from all directions.

The patella, too, lies at a point of intersecting tensile stresses. It acts like a mobile pulley to redirect tensile forces from the quadriceps tendon and patellar ligament longitudinally, from the transverse retinacula transversely, and from the meniscopatellar ligaments, longitudinal retinacula and tendons of the vastus lateralis and medialis muscles, transmitting them to the femur in the form of compression. Thus, the patella provides a mobile yet firm site for the attachment of ligaments and tendons on the extensor side, while the fabella assumes this role on the flexor side. We might mention in this context the localized "fabellar arthrosis" described by Taillard [400]; it may also be the product of a special stress configuration.

Having performed a variety of ligament reconstructions in an attempt to eliminate the pivot-shift phenomenon, we have found time and again that these new ligaments are unable to follow flexion and extension movements without becoming either stretched or wrinkled. There is a line extending from the tubercle of Gerdy to the fabella

96

Fig. 125. The active extensor, rotator and flexor apparatus contributes to the synergistic interaction of the passive elements. Important parts of this containment system are the lateral and medial menisci, which play a major role in the modification and neutralization of rotational forces

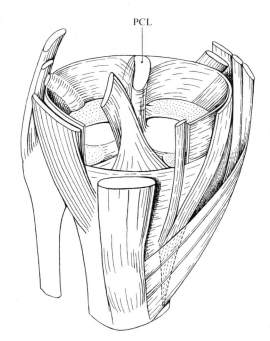

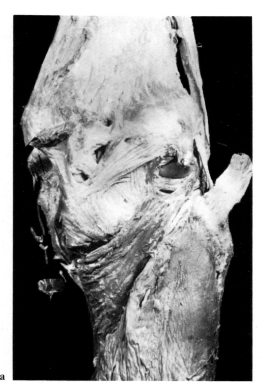

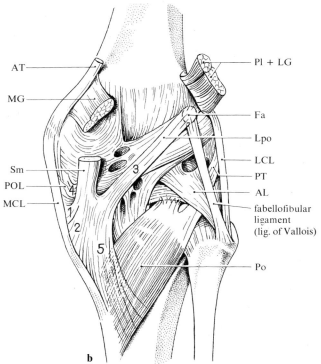

Fig. 126. a Anatomic specimen (v. Hochstetter) and **b** positional drawing showing the triangular passive elements in the posterior capsule of the knee that are crucial for rotatory stability. The oblique popliteal ligament (*3*) is dynamically stabilized by the semimem- branosus muscle, and the arcuate ligament by the popliteus muscle. (**a** shows the biceps tendon emerging to the right, which is not drawn in **b**) (numbers explained in Fig. 97)

97

which undergoes little or no length change during flexion-extension. Knowledge of this line is important when performing lateral stabilizing operations to correct a pivot shift. In contrast to reconstruction of the anterolateral femorotibial ligament (ALFTL), which exerts only an anterolateral stabilizing action, a connection with the fabella can also stabilize the posterolateral side. Kaplan [169] touches on this problem, pointing to the connection between the existence of a strong "short lateral ligament" (fabellofibular ligament) and the presence of a fabella. In all other cases the components of the popliteus corner must be correspondingly stronger in order to compensate.

The Triangular Arrangement of the MCL and POL as an Aid to Passive Rotatory Stabilization

Figs. 127 and 128 show how these structures, with their schematically triangular arrangement, can limit rotation. Two sides of the triangle are formed by ligaments and the third

by the upper tibia. If the vertex of the triangle is fixed and the tibia is moved backward or rotated internally, the POL tightens while the MCL becomes lax (Fig. 128 b).

In neutral rotation the ligamentous sides of the triangle are under only a basic tension.

In ER the tibia moves forward with respect to the femur, while the femur glides backward and upward on the posterior meniscus horn, thus tightening both ligamentous sides of the triangle. As shown in Fig. 93, the posterior side is tightened by its attachment to the posterior meniscus horn, and the anterior side by virtue of its orientation in the triangle.

Due to the shortness of the posterior side (POL), its fibers are more quickly stretched beyond their elastic reserve and so tear more quickly during excessive ER than the long fibers of the triangle's anterior side (MCL).

The triangle is only a schematic concept, of course, for a rigid triangle is immobile. In reality the MCL and POL form the familiar crossed four-bar linkage, since the sides of the triangle do not meet at a point on the

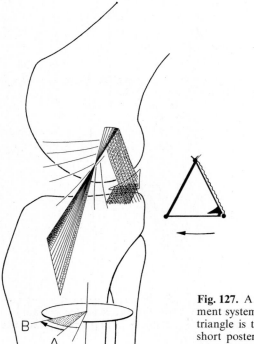

Fig. 127. A triangular structure is also present in the medial collateral ligament system: During ER of the tibia from *A* to *B*, the anterior side of the triangle is tense. But owing to the intervening meniscus (cf. Fig. 93), the short posterior side also comes under tension, so that both ligamentous sides of the triangle are tense in ER

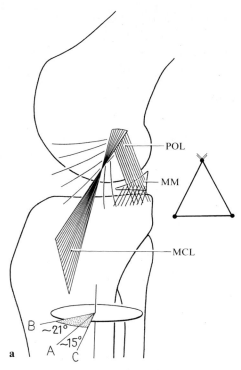

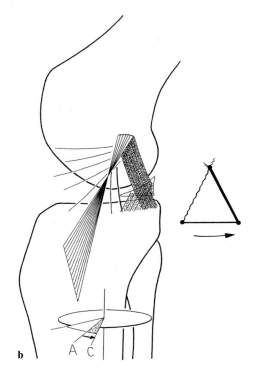

Fig. 128. a In NR neither the anterior nor posterior side of the triangle is under much tension, **b** while in IR from *A* to *C*, the posterior side of the triangle is tensed while the anterior side is lax

femur, but cross each other just before inserting. Unlike the triangle, which would have a constant flexion axis at its vertex, the crossed linkage can follow the axis as it changes position.

Physiology and Pathophysiology of the Menisci During Rotation

Figure 129 again shows the extended "dynamic socket" of the knee joint, reiterating the principle in Fig. 125. In this view we see only a small part of the tibial cartilage that forms the base of the socket. The concavity of the medial tibial plateau and convexity of the lateral plateau are visible within the encircling menisci. The adjacent soft tissues that project anteriorly and posteriorly form an important part of this "dynamic socket." The various muscular and tendinous extensions are the elements of active adaptation, which influence even the internal pressure of the joint. In the lower half of the picture are the "condylar plates," which cover the posterior portions of the femoral condyles and line the deep surface of the overlying muscles. It is also apparent that, with the exception of the iliotibial tract and the patellar and parapatellar extensor apparatus, the elements of active and passive stabilization are concentrated in the posterior half of the joint.

Physiologic Movements of the Menisci During Rotation

As stated under Kinematics, the menisci have to move backward during flexion as they follow the contact point of the femur, their radius of curvature decreasing in conformance with the diminishing radius of the femoral condyles (Fig. 130). Similarly, during rotation of the flexed knee, the menisci move back and forth and become highly distorted. We showed in Kinematics that there is a considerably greater rotational excursion

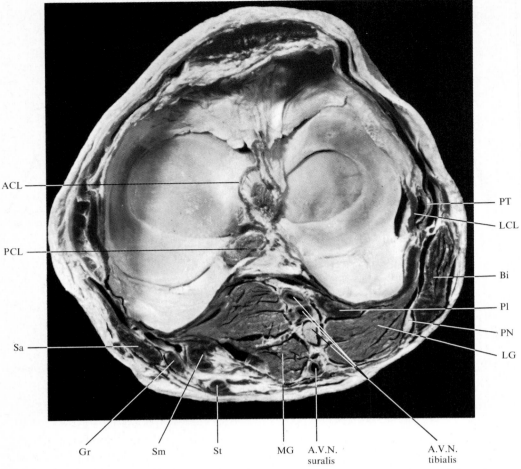

ACL —
PCL —
Sa —

PT
LCL
Bi
Pl
PN
LG

Gr   Sm   St   MG   A.V.N.   A.V.N.
                            suralis   tibialis

Fig. 129. View of the expanded socket of the knee joint from above. The menisci are an important component of this socket. Anterior to them are the fat pads held by the patellar ligament and longitudinal retinacula, and posterior to them are the condylar plates, which are supported from the popliteal side by the gastrocnemii and the rest of the flexors (v. Hochstetter)

in the lateral half of the joint than on the medial side, due to the medial location of the axis of voluntary rotation.

It is not easy to measure accurately the range of IR and ER at 90° of flexion. All who have made such measurements have found sizable differences with regard to the individual range of total rotation. The average range of 36° measured by Ruetsch and Morscher [306] is similar to the value of 37° found by Ross [364]. Of this 36° range, ER accounts for 21° and IR for 15° (Fig. 131). The scatter for 42 knees was considerable, varying between 27 and 54° for total rotation, between 14 and 29° for ER, and between 9 and 29° for IR. We know of no spe-cific correlations between the range of knee rotation and the incidence of meniscal injuries, but such a connection would not surprise us.

The two semilunar cartilages are in any case strongly displaced by these rotations, the lateral meniscus far more than the medial. The medial meniscus is firmly anchored at the site where it is subject to the least displacement (Fig. 132). It has a firm peripheral attachment with the POL, for it must not move relative to this ligament when the knee is flexed or rotated. The lateral meniscus, by contrast, requires a much greater mobility and could not have a similar attachment in the area of the popliteus corner.

100

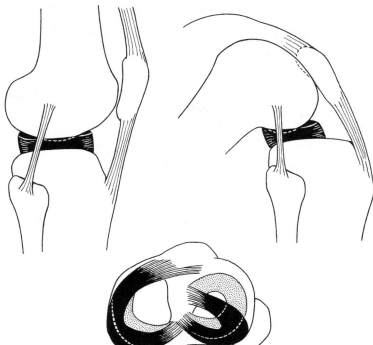

Fig. 130. The posterior displacement and distortion of the menisci on the tibial plateau during normal flexion

Because the lateral popliteus corner is far more dynamic than the semimembranosus corner and is stabilized by muscular action, the meniscus is allowed, by virtue of the popliteal hiatus, a free mobility that is to some extent independent of the accompanying action of the popliteus tendon. This is the main reason why tears of the lateral meniscus are at least ten times less frequent than tears of the medial meniscus. As will be shown, tears in the medial meniscus tend to occur within the circular sector belonging to the POL.

The Importance of the Menisci for the Knee Joint

Most authors today agree that a knee joint with two healthy menisci has a far better long-term prognosis than a knee joint after meniscectomy. Fairen et al. [82] from

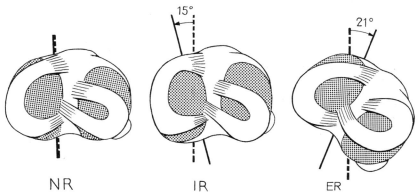

Fig. 131. Range of IR and ER with the associated movements of the menisci on the plateau. The average range of 15° for IR and 21° for ER corresponds to measurements of Ruetsch and Morscher [306]

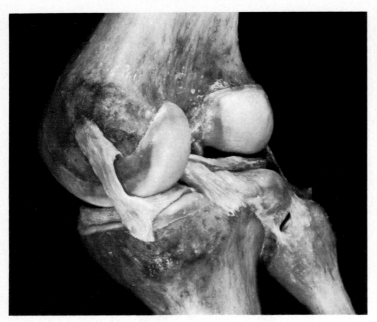

Fig. 132. The medial meniscus is fused to the collateral ligament apparatus only in the region of the POL. In other areas it must be mobile to follow all movements of flexion, extension and rotation. Anterior to the POL the MCL lies in a second, more peripheral layer that is freely mobile. In this area the meniscus is attached only to the deep capsular structures; between these and the MCL there is usually a bursa-like space (Institute of Anatomy, University of Basel)

Cabot's group are typical of many other authors who emphasize that a knee joint after meniscectomy is on its way to degenerative change. This change is dependent upon many, often obscure factors. One factor is sex, for joint deterioration is significantly more rapid and prevalent among women than men. Concomitant instability is another key factor. Individual factors, perhaps even the individual range of rotation, can also predispose to degenerative change.

While there is wide agreement as to the negative consequence of meniscectomy, little is known about the specific mechanisms by which the menisci act to reduce cartilage stress. For the purpose of our discussion, it is irrelevant whether the menisci improve joint congruity and thus enlarge the load-bearing surface (Fairen et al. [82]); whether they improve joint lubrication by spreading the synovial fluid; whether they act like a circular wheel brake to check rotation (Trillat et al. [359]); or whether they function as a kind of elastic shock absorber. Presumably all these factors work together as the menisci reduce peak loads by transforming the forces in such a way that the stresses imposed on the involved tissues remain tolerable. What we wish to emphasize here is that removal of the menisci is justified only if there is an overriding indication for it.

True Traumatic Meniscal Injuries

Only rarely have we seen a true, fresh avulsion of a meniscus caused by a single trauma. Usually this injury is combined with a ligamentous lesion of the knee. Fig. 216 f shows how these *traumatic* detachments of the meniscus occur in its ligamentous periphery, rather than in the actual cartilaginous substance of the meniscus. In such cases the avulsed meniscus is suitably exposed and reattached when the ligamentous lesion is repaired (Fig. 214–216 g).

In the overwhelming majority of meniscal lesions, two elements must be present: First and foremost, there must be attrition of the meniscal cartilage with associated incipient

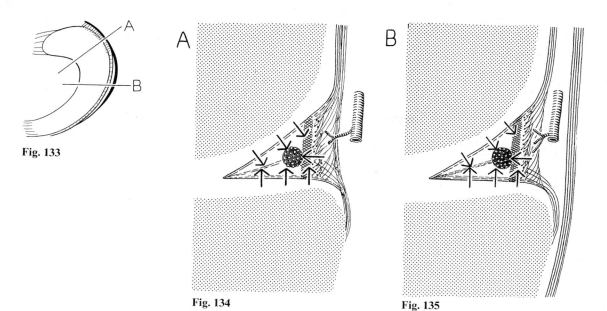

Fig. 133

Fig. 134

Fig. 135

Fig. 133. Relation of the medial meniscus to the medial collateral ligament system. *A* Situation in the region of close attachment with the POL. *B* Situation in the region of the MCL, where there are no ligamentous attachments with the meniscus

Fig. 134. Cross-section through ligament and meniscus in the region of *A* (Fig. 133). The medial meniscus itself shows three zones of collagenous fiber attachment with the ligament: *1.* a superficial zone made up of femoromeniscal fibers; *2.* a basal zone made up of tibiomeniscal fibers; and *3* a central fiber layer that approximately bisects the meniscus wedge. In addition, the meniscus displays a vascularized peripheral zone with a dense network of interwoven ligamentous fibers. At the center of the meniscal cross-section there is a usually circular zone of poor nutrition, owing to the long diffusion path from the upper and lower surfaces and from

Fig. 135. Cross-section through ligaments and meniscus in the region of *B* (Fig. 133). The situation in the deep layer is fundamentally the same. In this case, however, the MCL runs freely past the deep layer with the meniscus

the vascular periphery. This zone is drawn as a vesicular structure due to the mucoid degeneration that occurs there. Just peripheral to it is the optimum zone for meniscectomy (*cross-hatched area*), for a resection here will remove the degenerative, tear-prone areas while sparing the perfused portions and the ligamentous portions important for stability. The zone of degeneration runs like a curved cylinder throughout the meniscus. The diameter of the cylinder is correspondingly greater in the thicker posterior horn than in the thinner anterior portion; hence it may be more accurate to describe the degenerative zone as a curved cone-shaped region

tears; and second, there must be an acute trauma which enlarges these primary tears. These attrition tears tend to occur in the thinner central portion of the meniscus rather than in its thicker periphery.

The firm attachment of the medial meniscus with the POL is an important factor both in true traumatic detachments of the meniscus at its periphery and in the development of attrition tears. This follows the well-known principle that structures are torn or avulsed at sites where they are fixed, but can escape injury in areas where they are mobile.

The Structure of the Menisci and Their Integration into the Capsular Ligament System, with Implications for the Technique of Meniscectomy

1. In the area of the posterior horn (Situation A): Figs. 133 and 134 show the course of the fibers from the capsule to the meniscus according to studies by Wagner [370]. Some fibers pass directly from the femur to the tibia as the deep capsular ligament, while others pass from the femur to the meniscus and from the upper tibia to the meniscus (see Ligamentous Injuries, General, p. 148).

103

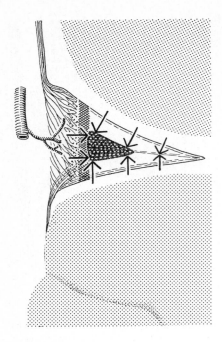

Fig. 136. The cross-section through the posterior portion of the lateral meniscus is somewhat different from the medial in that the posterior horn is clearly more voluminous. As a result, the central poorly-nourished zone is also more voluminous than on the medial side. This larger zone of mucoid degeneration accounts for the greater frequency of ganglia of the lateral meniscus

These fibers interlace in the peripheral third of the meniscus. The nutrient blood vessels also ramify in this area. The fibers extend into the cartilaginous substance of the meniscus in three parts: The femoromeniscal fibers entering the superficial surface of the meniscus, the tibiomeniscal fibers entering the inferior surface of the meniscus, and a third layer formed by fibers which pass with the blood vessels toward the center of the meniscus. They form a plane that approximately bisects the angle of the meniscal wedge.

2. The situation is different at the level of the MCL (Figs. 133 and 135, Situation B). The MCL fibers run external to the deep fibers, entirely separate from the meniscus and the capsular layer; in between are the blood vessels that supply the meniscus. The femoromeniscal and tibiomensical fibers are distributed as in Fig. 134 but are somewhat more numerous. As before, there is a third, intermediate fiber layer entering the meniscal border.

3. The attachments of the lateral meniscus (Fig. 136) are similar to those described in 1., the main difference being that the lateral meniscus is considerably more bulky than the medial meniscus, especially in its posterior half. This has an important bearing on the considerations that follow.

Nutrition of the Menisci

The cartilaginous substance of the meniscus is nourished by three different pathways: from the border of the meniscus, via the blood vessels present in the peripheral third, and from the superior and inferior surface of the meniscus by diffusion from the synovia (Figs. 134–136). Thus, the central portion of the meniscus is located farthest from the nutrient sources and is a site of predilection for early degenerative change. Even the slightest disproportion will lead to initial disturbances and, histologically, to mucoid degeneration. Therefore, this zone is represented schematically as a round vesicular structure in the drawings. In reality the zone is cylindrical or even conical, for it is more voluminous in the posterior horn than in the thinner anterior horn. This conical cylinder is not straight, of course, but follows the curved contour of the meniscus.

Slany [321] has sectioned and stained menisci in his serial autopsy studies of knee joints, and has clearly demonstrated these

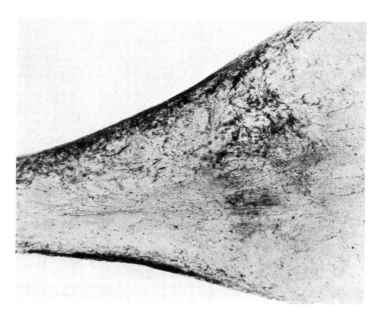

Fig. 137. This section, prepared by Slany [321] in 1941, shows both the mucoid degeneration (*colored zone*) and the fiber architecture of the middle layer of the meniscus attached to the peripheral ligaments

degenerative zones of circular cross-section with his stains of mucoid substances (Figs. 137 and 138). We shall not delve into the countless papers that have been published on this subject. Both Ficat [85] and Zippel [397] present detailed discussion of the literature and of various theories. We should mention, however, that Mittelmeyer [228] also described a longitudinal zone of degeneration in the meniscus. His drawings also place this zone in the boundary area be-

tween the central two-thirds and the peripheral third of the meniscus. This location is of clinical importance, for it allows us to define the most suitable zone for the excision of torn or pathologically altered menisci. This zone is indicated by the grid lines in Figs. 134–136. In removing the damaged meniscus, the line of resection should be just peripheral to the degenerative zone. This leaves a rim of intact meniscus that will aid stability, yet removes damaged portions that

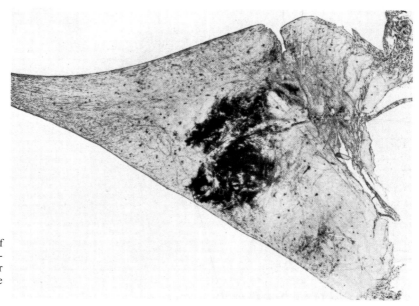

Fig. 138. Another section of Slany [321] shows a primary attrition tear from the inferior surface to the degenerative zone

might tear and form flaps if left in the joint. Peripheral tears in the *outer, ligamentous, vascular portion* should be sutured to avoid further instability. Old peripheral tears can generally be freshened without difficulty. A careful intraoperative examination is essential, for it is not uncommon for two concentric longitudinal tears to occur: one in the ligamentous periphery and the other in the area of the more centrally located degenerative zone. These dual or multiple tears are almost always associated with anterior cruciate ligament insufficiency. Multiple tears of the posterior horn are often found in such cases.

We have already mentioned these relationships in Physiology and Pathophysiology of the Cruciate Ligaments, p. 22. It is left to the operator's judgment whether all free parts of the meniscus should be resected, or whether at least *one* portion may be retained by a suture at the ligamentous periphery. Such a suture is useless, however, unless the causative anterior instability is also corrected.

Cysts of the Menisci

Meniscal cysts, called also meniscal ganglia, are often found incidentally during the course of a meniscectomy or ligament operation. They may be pin-head- to walnut-sized and are associated with the degenerative zone described above. Jaffrès [152] showed that these ganglia arise in the substance of the meniscus and extend peripheralward. This prompted us to puncture the ganglia and fill them with contrast material. We were not surprised to find that the material flowed from the ganglion into the central portion of the meniscus (cf. also Fig. 139). Based on this experience, we have in some cases carefully dissected the ganglion free outside the joint until the pedicle was identified in order to preserve the meniscus and ganglion as a unit during the resection (Figs. 140–142). In two cases the menisci were bulky, which was probably significant. The pedicle of the ganglion with its lumen could be traced into the degenerative zone, where, as expected, attrition tears were also

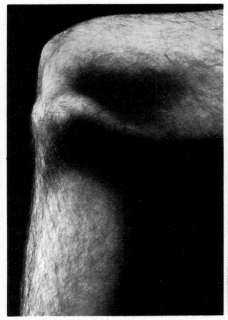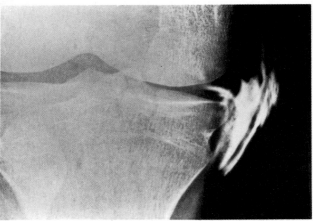

a
b

Fig. 139. a Clinical photo showing prominent ganglion of the medial meniscus. **b** This contrast film is from the same patient after the ganglion was punctured and filled with contrast medium. Note the flow of contrast material from the ganglion through a channel through the capsule wall and into the degenerative zone of the meniscus. In addition, the sulcus semimembranosi is clearly visible on the medial side of the upper tibia between it and the contrast material

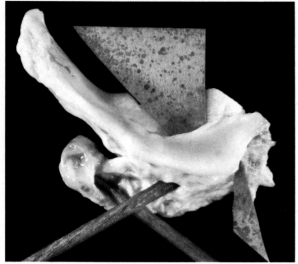

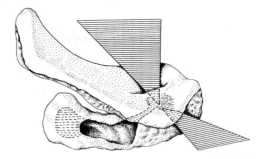

Fig. 140

Fig. 140. In this lateral meniscus, pathologic changes have caused ganglion development as well as primary tears. The ganglion and its follicle are clearly visible at the *lower left* of the excised meniscus. The *wooden rod* has been inserted into the zone of degeneration, and the *triangles* into the attrition tears. The fortuitous drainage of ganglion by such a tear may explain the occasional spontaneous disappearance of a ganglion

Fig. 141. Positional drawing for Fig. 140 showing the intercommunication of the channels and cavities

present. These observations suggest that the ganglia develop as long as there is no communication between the degenerative focus and the joint cavity, i.e., as long as the mucoid substance is not drained into the joint interior by a meniscal tear. Spontaneous cures of meniscal cysts may be attributable to such drainage. If the tear remains small, it may cause the patient no complaints. Even if a cyst is present, we attempt to preserve the peripheral portion of the ring wherever possible and limit the resection to the cyst and the central focus of mucoid degeneration.

Fiber Architecture and the Shapes of Meniscal Tears

Meniscal tears are generally classified according to their morphology (e.g., Trillat's system [374]). Wagner [370] deepened our understanding of meniscal tears by his in-

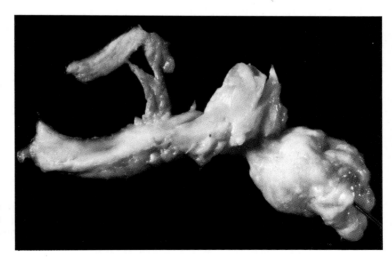

Fig. 142. Another meniscus specimen with a ganglion confirms the fact that such ganglia can occur even in combination with multiple tears

vestigations of the architecture of the collagenous fiber system in the menisci. On the one hand, he showed us how the minisci are actually integrated into the capsuloligamentous system; on the other, he explained why meniscal tears follow certain lines of predilection. The arcade shape of the individual fibrous strands, combined with the large number of such strands in the meniscus, results in a high fiber density in the peripheral third. The result is a tension-resistant ring about the periphery of the meniscus. As other authors confirm, this tension-resistant ring is important for it enables the meniscus to absorb compressive forces between the femur and tibia. If the meniscal ring offered no resistance to deformation, it could have no effect on pressure distribution between the two bones. It also resists the deforming forces associated with flexion, extension and rotation of the knee.

In the central two-thirds of the meniscus are the more radially oriented limbs of the fiber arcades (Fig. 143), creating a less dense fiber architecture.

Attrition tears develop at sites where zones of varying strength adjoin, i.e., at the junction between the peripheral fiber ring and the central zone with its more radial fibers. The initial tear at the level of the POL can subsequently enlarge in either of two ways, as shown in Fig. 144.

Figures 145 and 146 show the three-layered structure of the meniscus and illustrate how a tear need not pass vertically through the whole meniscus, but may deviate along its central fiber plane to form a flap. Thus, the classification of meniscal tears according to Trillat [347], derived from clinical features, finds a morphological correlate in the fiber architecture of the meniscus (Fig. 147).

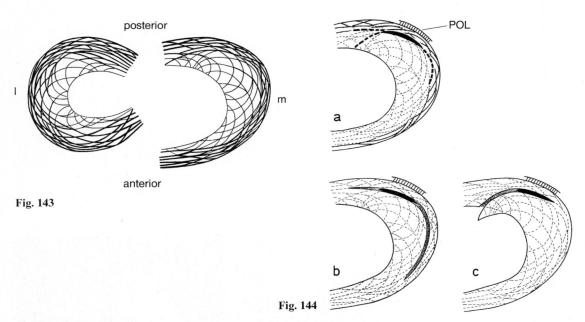

Fig. 143

Fig. 144

Fig. 143. Collagenous fiber architecture of the menisci according to Wagner. It accounts for the various types of tear that are observed

Fig. 144a–c. The most frequent types of meniscal tears and their relation to the fiber architecture of the menisci. The zone between the peripheral third and the central two-thirds of the meniscus where the collagenous fibers arc toward the center is a line of predilection for tears. Here there is a relatively abrupt transition between a self-contained, tear-resistant peripheral zone of dense, circumferentially oriented fibers and the central zone of more radially oriented fibers. The area where

the meniscus is anchored to the POL is a classic site of primary tear formation (**a**). This longitudinal tear may lengthen anteriorly or posteriorly to form a "bucket handle" that may ultimately dislocate into the intercondylar notch (**b**), or it may follow a curved fiber bundle inward and emerge through the inner free edge of the meniscus (**c**), forming a tab or "parrot beak" tear of the posterior horn

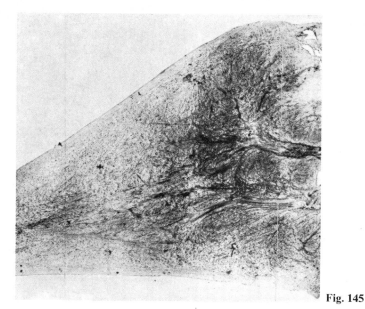

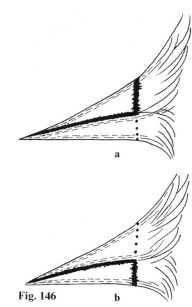

Fig. 145   **Fig. 146**

Fig. 145. Meniscal section from the study of Slany [321] showing a supply vessel and its ramification in the peripheral third of the meniscus. Just below, the central fiber layer is seen running horizontally into the meniscus from the periphery

Fig. 146a, b. Not all tears pass vertically through the substance of the meniscus; many run through the center, roughly parallel to the upper tibial surface. Again, the explanation lies in the fiber architecture, this time in cross-section: The tear follows a horizontal course just above or just below the central fiber layer, forming a tab that opens toward the femur, as in **a**, or toward the tibia, as in **b**

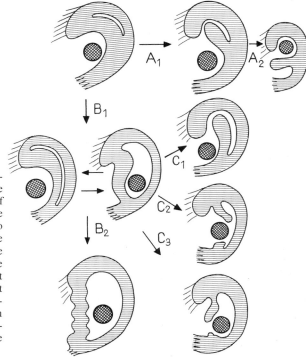

Fig. 147. Development of the main types of meniscus tear according to Trillat [347]. Starting from the stage at *upper left* with a primary longitudinal tear of the posterior horn, the tear may progress along line *A* to form the parrot-beak tear A_2, or along *B* to form a complete longitudinal tear which leads to the bucket-handle tear B_1 with consequent locking. The bucket handle may remain displaced, in which case the tear will enlarge as in B_2, perhaps to the point where it no longer prevents extension. If the bucket handle continually slips in and out of the intercondylar notch, it may become secondarily torn or ruptured in its posterior (C_1), middle (C_2) or anterior portion (C_3). The *dark circle* represents the area of femorotibial contact

109

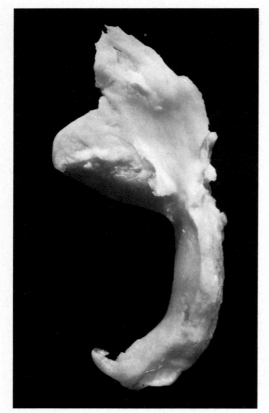

Fig. 148

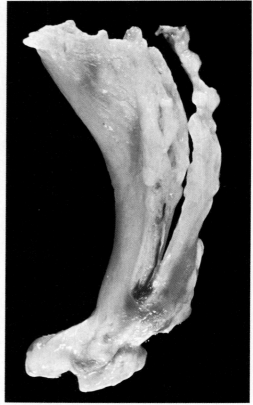

Fig. 149

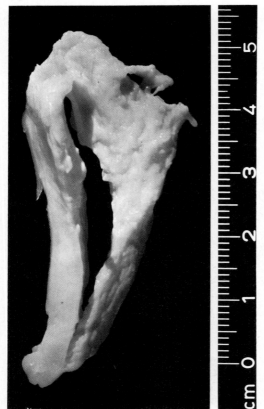

Fig. 150

110

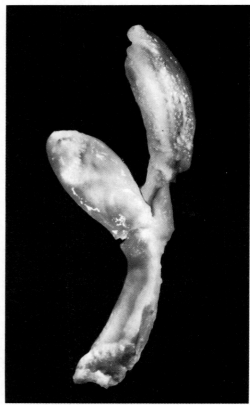

Fig. 151

The tear of the posterior horn found by Trillat in 22% of cases (top left drawing) can develop into a tab tear or "parrot beak" tear of the posterior horn (arrows A_1 and A_2). Far more often, however (see arrow B_1), the primary lesion progresses to a bucket-handle tear (41%). If this bucket handle remains displaced in the intercondylar notch for a long enough time, the tear may enlarge (as in B_2) to a point where typical clinical symptoms disappear (6%).

If the bucket handle snaps in and out of the intercondylar notch for a prolonged period of time, it may tear secondarily, forming various types of flap (C_1, C_2 and C_3). Eighty-three percent of these secondary tears occur in the posterior part or the bucket handle (C_1), 11% in the central part (C_2), and only 6% in the anterior part (C_3). These latter tears are often mistaken for tears of the anterior horn. It is difficult in such cases to identify the origin of the lesion as a tear of the posterior horn.

Figures 148 and 149 show examples of these various types of tear. A typical tab tear of the posterior horn is shown in Fig. 148. In this case the tab has been formed in part by a horizontal shearing force.

Figure 149 shows a fresh bucket-handle tear as seen at operation. In this case the tear ran perpendicular to the tibial plateau and left only a little meniscus tissue with mucoid swelling in the periphery. Figure 150 shows a bucket-handle tear with horizontal displacement. If the bucket handle alone had

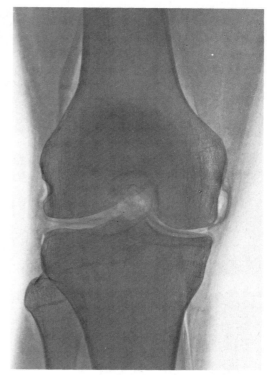

Fig. 152. Arthrogram of the knee joint before removal of the meniscus in Fig. 151. The upright, club-shaped flap is seen on the medial side, and the short meniscus stump is visible in the joint space. Note also the conspicuous indentation of the popliteal sulcus on the lateral femoral condyle; this groove receives the often pencil-thick popliteus tendon

been resected in this case, the degenerative zone in the critical posterior horn region would have been left in the joint, predisposing to recurrent tearing and flap formation. These resections were carried quite far pe-

---

Fig. 148. Typical example of a parrot-beak tear of the posterior meniscus horn, here with displacement

Fig. 149. Typical complete longitudinal tear at the classic location in the region of the older posterior horn tear. Irregularities associated with older tears are seen in the plane of the longitudinal tear, and the smooth track left by the most recent bucket-handle incarceration is visible (*lower half of photo*). Traces of fresh bleeding are also seen at the bottom of the tear

Fig. 150. Bucket-handle tear in a meniscus with marked degenerative changes peripheral to the tear zone. If only the bucket handle had been removed in this case, new tab tears would have formed in the dissociated remnant. Therefore, it is necessary that the resection also include any peripheral portions of the cartilage showing degenerative change. Firm peripheral portions should be left in place, for they contribute importantly to stability, lubrication and load distribution in the joint

Fig. 151. Torn bucket handle corresponding to type C_1 in Fig. 147. The torn handle became incarcerated between the femoral condyle and medial collateral ligament, caused occasional locking and acquired a rounded clublike shape while in its pathologic position

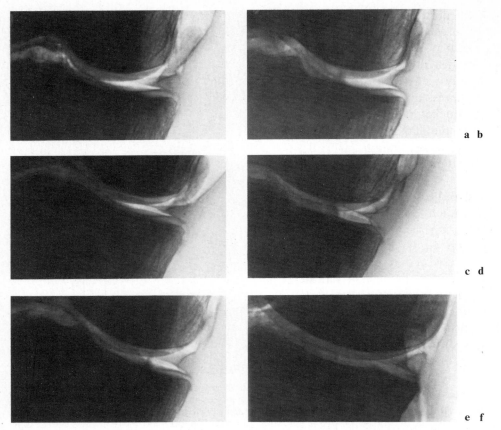

Fig. 153a–f. Closeup arthrograms of the knee (Fig. 152) bring out additional details of the club-shaped flap

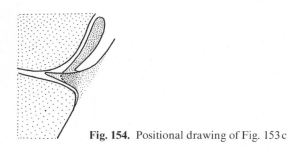

Fig. 154. Positional drawing of Fig. 153c

ripherally and each could have been done more sparingly.

Figure 151 shows a torn bucket handle of the C_1 type. The patient's history showed a single episode of locking, followed thereafter by a sensation of something "loose" on the medial side of the knee. The arthrographic findings for this meniscus are given in Figs. 152–154. The club-shaped flap rears itself up next to the medial femoral condyle, entrapped between it and the collateral ligament. In exceptional cases such an upright flap located farther back in the capsular plate could cause an unusual form of locking in which flexion is prevented.

Figure 155 shows a special phenomenon involving the incarceration of a hypermobile posterior horn. During examination for anterior drawer sign, the femoral condyle rides up onto the posterior horn and then snaps back into its normal position. This "jumping" of the femur may be audible and was called the "signo del salto" by Finochietto [92]. We have found that this phenomenon is usually associated with anterior cruciate insufficiency. A knee with normal ligamentous stability will not allow such an interposition to occur.

Discoid Meniscus

For completeness, this special defect should also be mentioned in connection with menis-

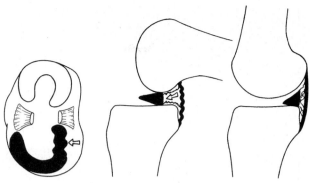

Fig. 155. A hypermobile posterior meniscus horn on the medial side, with or without a tissue bridge, can become incarcerated between the femoral condyle and tibia during flexion, leading to a snapping mechanism that is often audible (the "jump" of Finocchietto [92]). This form of instability is the result of anterior cruciate ligament insufficiency with pronounced hypermobility of the meniscus

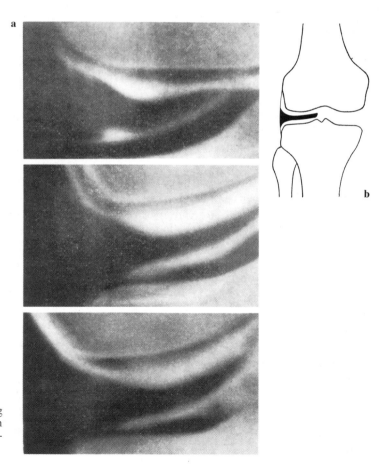

Fig. 156. a Arthrogram and **b** drawing of a rare discoid meniscus, which can develop special tears and cause corresponding symptoms (see Fig. 157)

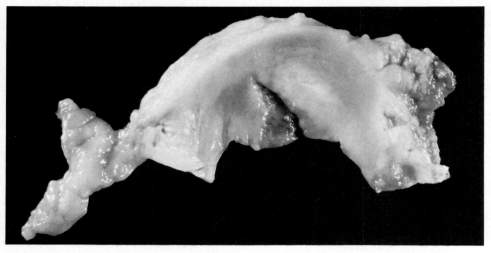

Fig. 157. The transverse tear is more or less typical in the discoid meniscus, while it is a definite rarity in the normal-shaped meniscus and is usually caused by shearing mechanisms associated with upper tibial fractures. In the discoid meniscus, on the other hand, this type of tear can result from a pure "soft tissue trauma," because the meniscus is not elastic enough to tolerate much displacement without tearing

cal lesions. As shown by Fig. 20 in Kinematics, p. 18, the menisci are initially discs that are fused with the upper tibia. Only later do spaces appear, first between the menisci and femur and then between the menisci and tibia. Further maturation with development of the characteristic crescent shape is not always complete and may become arrested at various stages. Thus, three different types of discoid meniscus can occur:

1. the primitive disc with its early-embryonic oval shape;
2. the intermediate disc with a thin interposed segment between the horns;
3. the infantile disc with a broadened middle segment [328, 363].

These menisci can be well demonstrated by means of arthrography (cf. also Fig. 156a). Figure 156b explains the arthrographic picture.

The mechanical behavior of discoid menisci is different from that of semilunar menisci. On sudden deformation the short free border will tear from the center toward the periphery, due to a lack of central tension resistance. Thus, even a simple fall onto the knee without twisting can cause a discoid meniscus to tear (Fig. 157). The case depicted clearly involves a traumatic rupture of the meniscus, for from the moment after the fall there were effusion, complaints, and an audible clicking of the knee with each movement. Understandably, the classic meniscus symptoms were absent, which caused the patient to consult several doctors before surgery was prescribed.

In conclusion, and with reference to the latter specimen photo, which is several years old, we wish to emphasize once again that we have adopted a less radical approach to meniscectomies, combining these procedures with a greater number of stabilizing ligament operations than in the past. In the present case we would today leave a larger rim of meniscus in the joint. It is difficult to give specific guidelines, for the momentary situation has much bearing on the necessary extent of the resection. As a rule, damaged tissue must be thoroughly removed to avoid a recurrence, but at the same time the meniscus should retain at least part of its function if at all possible.

Concluding Remarks on Meniscectomy

If the meniscus problem is a *chronic* one, then a coexisting problem is usually present. Hence, a meniscectomy alone in the pres-

114

ence of associated anterior cruciate insufficiency can hardly represent a definitive treatment. Too often we have seen patients who first underwent a medial meniscectomy and then had to undergo a lateral meniscectomy a few months or years later. Even then, the patients were not free of complaints, because the preexisting anterior cruciate insufficiency was too severe and continued to cause problems. These cases will almost certainly progress to degenerative joint disease due to the functional incongruity left in the wake of the meniscectomies.

Because, for the reasons cited, a substantial number of meniscectomies require reoperation at a later date, the selection of the primary incision is important. For years we have favored the straight, medial parapatellar approach even for simple meniscectomies (see Approaches, p. 160). Preexisting oblique incisions from earlier operations limit the surgeon in his choice of approaches and incisions at reoperation. The medial parapatellar approach is suitable for practically all knee operations.

Examination of the Injured Knee Joint

At the Heidelberg Symposium of 1977 [312], various experts such as O'Donoghue, Trillat, Blazina, Kennedy and James independently examined knee joints in a selected patient group and made diagnoses. Their techniques differed, but their results were very similar.

Roaas and Nilsson [301]: "A correct diagnosis depends upon a knowledge of functional anatomy, accurate history taking, and a painstakingly thorough examination. Often repeated examinations must be made over a period of several days before a final diagnosis can be reached." According to Hughston et al. [in 140], the classic clinical findings in knee injuries, such as spontaneous pain, swelling, effusion, localized tenderness and disability, are of no absolute diagnostic value, but do have an important relative value. They evaluated the significance of these symptoms in recent knee injuries as follows:

General Symptoms

Spontaneous Pain

Nearly three-fourths of the patients with medial ligament tears walked into the clinic unaided, without a cane or crutches, and had little pain.

Swelling

Two-thirds of the patients had localized swelling over the site of the rupture on the medial side.

Effusion

Joint effusion was absent in most cases. None of the 18 patients with tears of the pos-terior cruciate showed intraarticular effusion. This absence of effusion was explained by the extent of the tears, which allowed the fluid to extravasate into surrounding tissues.

Localized Tenderness

In 76% of the patients, tenderness was maximal just over the site of the lesion on the medial side. Of 28 patients with a tear of the medial collateral ligament at its tibial attachment, 21 had marked tenderness at that site. In 10 patients with a tear of the ligament at its femoral attachment, 8 had the greatest tenderness there. The more complex the tear, the poorer the site of tenderness as an index of the location and extent of the lesion. Nevertheless, the information obtained was still adequate to indicate the correct operative procedure.

Disability

Although 38 of the 50 patients could walk unaided, none could sprint or "cut" or go up and down stairs and slopes, because the sense of giving-way was too great.

Testing the Stability of the Knee

General Considerations and Methods

The articular surfaces of the knee are not congruent. On the medial side the femur meets the tibia like a wheel on a plate, and on the lateral side like a wheel on a dome. Only the ligaments, acting in concert with the remaining soft tissues, provide the knee with the necessary stability.

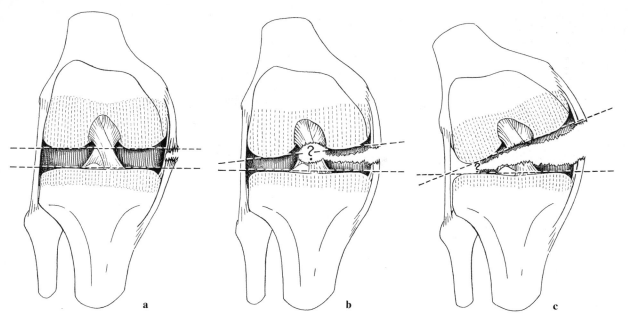

Fig. 158a–c. The ligamentous lesion and associated passive instability. **a** If the tear is confined to the MCL and the posterior "corner" and posterior capsule (*shaded*) are intact, then a valgus stress applied to the extended knee will not cause medial opening of the joint. This is possible only when the knee is flexed about 30° to relax the posterior capsule, thereby eliminating its lateral stabilizing action. **b** If the knee shows medial opening in extension, involvement of the cruciate ligaments is a possibility, even if no significant drawer sign can be elicited. **c** If the valgus instability extends across to the lateral side in both flexion and extension, there is no question that both cruciate ligaments are torn. The only question that remains is the degree of involvement of the posteromedial corner and femorotibial iliotibial tract fibers

Hence, ligamentous injuries of the knee, more than of any other joint, are essentially a problem of motion guidance.

Ligamentous stability is not an end in itself but is a prerequisite for achieving apposition, stability and integral function of the joint members – a situation we call "functional congruity."

Instabilities occur in a variety of forms. Broadly speaking, instabilities may be classified as straight, rotatory or combined.

The classic example of a straight instability is the isolated medial collateral ligament instability, characterized by an abnormal medial opening of the joint space under a valgus stress. The comparison with an opening book is appropriate.

Referring to Fig. 158a and considering the effects of a simple tear of the medial collateral ligament, we can see that valgus laxity will be minimal unless portions of the posterior capsule are also involved in the injury. Moreover, the findings will vary de-

pending on whether the knee is tested in flexion or extension. Because extension tightens the posterior capsule, there will be little or no medial opening in this position even with a torn collateral ligament. When the knee is flexed, however, the posterior capsule is relaxed, and the same ligamentous lesion will result in a much greater degree of valgus laxity (Fig. 160).

If the tear extends to the middle of the posterior capsule, it must be asked whether the cruciate ligaments could withstand such a severe valgus trauma without injury (Fig. 158b).

If the tear extends through the posterior capsule to the lateral collateral ligament (Fig. 158c), there can be no doubt that both cruciate ligaments are torn (Fig. 158).

Thus, the degree of opening of the joint space, when compared to the uninjured side, is a direct measure of the overall extent of the lesion. Volkov [367] has shown with stress roentgenograms of the knee that a val-

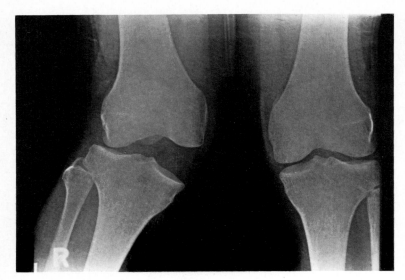

Fig. 159. Stress roentgenogram of a knee injured in a fall from a moped, with ruptures of both cruciate ligaments and extreme valgus instability

gus opening of 5–6 mm (sic) in extension denotes a rupture of the collateral ligament, and that an opening of 12–15° (sic) must signify an associated injury of the posterior cruciate ligament.

An anterior drawer sign of 8 mm is a sure indication of an anterior cruciate ligament tear.

On the one hand, this confirms our experience that the posterior cruciate ligament is involved far more frequently in combined injuries than is generally assumed. In many cases we have found a residual posterior drawer sign, where only an anterior drawer had been diagnosed prior to surgical repair.

On the other hand, it is clear that the posterior drawer sign is very often mistaken for a positive anterior drawer sign. This is due to the paradox that an abnormal anterior displacement of the tibia may represent a posterior drawer.

Testing Lateral Stability

Any effusion-filled knee will appear unstable relative to a "dry" knee during testing. In a "floating knee" of this type it is even difficult to recognize neutral rotation or hold the knee in that position.

Examination in Extension

This functional test (Fig. 160a) provides information on the state of the semimembranosus or popliteus corner. If these corner structures are intact, there will be no varus or valgus instability. A mild instability signifies a tear in one of these structures. A severe instability denotes an associated tear of the posterior cruciate ligament or even of both cruciates (see also Fig. 158).

An intact semimembranosus corner allows no medial opening, even if a complete tear of the MCL is found at operation.

Examination in 30° Flexion

The posterior capsule is relaxed (Fig. 160b) and so cannot mask tears of the MCL. As the degree of instability increases, it becomes increasingly likely that the semimembranosus corner is torn. Lateral stability must always be tested with the leg rotated externally due to the anatomic course of the ligament (Fig. 89).

Individual differences are more pronounced in flexion than in extension. Most knees will show complete ligamentous stability when extended, whereas the flexed knee shows instabilities, which can often be consid-

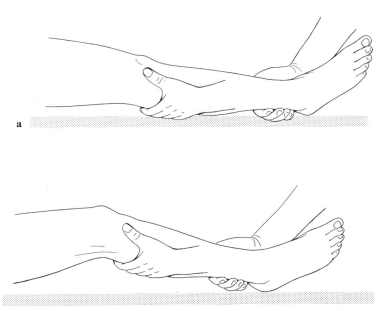

Fig. 160 a, b. Example of stability testing under a varus and valgus stress with the knee extended (**a**) and flexed 30° (**b**). The examination should be performed in both positions. Lateral stability in flexion should always be tested in ER

ered normal, however. Experience has taught us that these individual, physiologic instabilities correlate with the shape of the condyles. The greater the "average condylar radius" (a term useful for descriptive purposes), the more stable the knee in all degrees of flexion. Knee joints with a small "average radius" of femorotibial condylar curvature are often quite lax in flexion. This unfavorable circumstance hampers reconstructive surgery both in recent injuries and in chronic instabilities. Small condylar radii are more common in women than in men. Although we have not yet evaluated therapeutic results in terms of these criteria, it is our impression that results are generally better in large knee joints.

These differences make evaluation correspondingly more difficult. It is *imperative* that the injured limb be compared with the opposite, uninjured side.

Measurement of Instability

An instability of 5 mm or less is described as a "1+ instability" (mild); between 5 and 10 mm as 2+ (moderate); and 10 mm or more as 3+ (severe). Noesberger (personal communication) uses 3–5 mm as the 1+ range. This interpretation seems to be more practical, for values of 0–3 mm (relative to the healthy side) are not pathologic in the majority of cases. An equivocal or borderline result is indicated by (1+).

The more experience one gains with regular examinations, the more one will be inclined to test lateral stability in all flexion angles up to 90° and beyond. The difference in ligamentous closure between the medial and lateral sides should be mentioned at this point. Generally speaking, the lateral side is more lax than the medial side, presumably by virtue of its greater rotational freedom. Any loosening of the ligaments will accentuate the rotatory laxity. We consider this to be one reason for the more frequent detection of instability on the lateral side of the knee, where even a slight rotational displacement greatly increases the distance between the femoral condyle and tibial plateau due to the convexity of the tibial articular surface. Thus, an objective assessment is especially difficult on the lateral side.

119

In both anterior and posterior instability, the examiner will note an abnormal anterior displacement of the tibia when a pull is exerted. In the case of anterior instability, the femur retains its normal central position on the tibia. In the case of posterior instability, gravity will cause the tibia to sag posteriorly at the start of the test, and a pull will restore the tibia to its normal central position. Hence, it is wise to follow this important rule:

> A positive anterior drawer sign is present only if it has been proved that the posterior drawer sign is negative.

Examination in Extension

There are anterior and posterior drawer instabilities that can be clearly demonstrated even in extension. They signify a recent injury or chronic instability of extreme severity. Trillat [359] was one of the first to stress the functional importance of the *drawer sign in extension* ("le tiroir en extension"). Mild drawer signs in extension often cause the patient considerably more discomfort than more severe drawer signs in 90° flexion.

Examination in Flexion

Every examiner has his own routine. Nevertheless, the anterior drawer test must be performed in several angles of flexion, because the drawer sign is more conspicuous in some positions than in others.

This anterior drawer test is performed up to about 30° of flexion. It is an important test because if positive, it is virtually a sure sign of an anterior cruciate ligament rupture.

Anterior stability is particularly well demonstrated at 20–30° of flexion, for the iliotibial tract crosses the transverse flexion axis and thus contributes little to active stabilization in this phase – a fact also exploited by Slocum's test, among others. Moreover, the MCL is not very tight in 20–30° flexion.

For the test the examiner grasps the upper tibia with one hand and the lower femur with the other and tests anterior stability at the flexion angle indicated.

Isolated anterior cruciate ligament tears can also be demonstrated in this manner, while anterior instabilities at a flexion angle of 90° denote an associated injury of the semimembranosus corner.

Another important position for testing anteroposterior stability is 60–90° flexion. The patient is placed supine with the knee flexed and the foot resting on the table top. First the leg is examined from the side to detect any posterior sag of the tibia (Fig. 161). This is the best way of determining whether a posterior, anterior, or anterior and posterior instability is present. The patient must be fully relaxed so that the tibia can sag under the weight of the lower leg. Sometimes this is possible only after repeated examinations.

If the patient is now told to lift the foot slowly from the table without moving the upper leg, the tibial plateau will be seen to move forward under the pull of the patellar ligament before the foot entirely leaves the table and extension is commenced. The examiner can manually reproduce this anterior shift of the tibia by pulling the lower leg forward. If a posterior drawer is present, this pull will reduce the tibia from its abnormal sagging position into the normal neutral position (Fig. 161e). If there is no anterior drawer, the tibia will come to rest firmly in this neutral position as soon as the anterior cruciate ligament is tense (Fig. 163c).

On the other hand, if an anterior drawer is present and there is no posterior drawer, then the tibia can be pulled out of the neutral position into a true anterior drawer position (Fig. 162). When the tibia is pushed back out of the anterior drawer position, its posterior movement will be noticeably checked by tightening of the posterior cruciate ligament (Fig. 163 b).

If both cruciate ligaments are intact, this checking will occur in both the anterior and posterior direction (Fig. 163 a). An anteroposterior displacement of 2–3 mm may be normal if a similar displacement is found on the unaffected side. If both cruciate ligaments are torn (Fig. 163 d), this checking will be absent in both directions. Movement of the tibia by the examiner is then checked exponentially by the increasing resistance of the peripheral capsuloligamentous structures.

To evaluate rotatory stability, all the drawer tests must be performed in ER, NR and IR.

Assessment is difficult in cases where anterior and posterior instability coexist, for then there is no longer a zero point in the system. Stress roentgenograms should be made in doubtful cases.

Roentgenographic Examination

General

Because every unstable knee may have accompanying bone lesions, a roentgenographic study is an essential part of the examination (Fig. 164).

> Three films are taken under an anterior drawer stress in NR, IR and ER, and then under a posterior drawer stress in the same rotational positions.

Besides the standard a.p. and lateral views, the p.a. "tunnel" view of the knee and the axial or "sunrise" view of the patella are necessary.

The tunnel view permits an accurate assessment of the tibial and intercondylar attachments of the cruciate ligaments, while the sunrise view will demonstrate any osteochondral flake fractures in the area of the femoropatellar articulation.

Problems of Stress Roentgenograms

A stability examination without anesthesia is of only relative value. Most patients unconsciously counteract a pathologic laxity with their active stabilizers, often creating a false impression of normal ligamentous stability. A positive drawer test is obtained only by catching the patient "off guard." But if the same patient is tested under anesthesia, the drawer test will be unmistakably positive. Moreover, an anterior drawer sign may now be accompanied by a posterior drawer, or vice-versa. Only a roentgenographic examination under anesthesia can yield truly objective results. For practical reasons, however, this cannot be done routinely.

Stress films must be taken with the tibia held in both the anterior and posterior positions. Even then the examiner can be deceived, for the abnormal rotatory laxity of the unstable knee can still alter the results. Only when the drawer sign is demonstrated by x-ray in all three rotational positions (NR, IR and ER) can the examination be called truly objective. The examiner must decide how many views are needed, according to the difficulty of the case to be assessed. Even with fixation devices, it is difficult to take standard, reproducible films in all rotational positions. Ideally up to six views should be taken; this number is doubled if the healthy knee is used for comparison, and is multiplied several times if drawer signs in extension (Trillat-Lachmann) are also to be demonstrated.

We have not yet employed this systematic routine. The cost is prohibitive as long as the films cannot be routinely and reproducibly compared, even under anesthesia, although this would be of great interest from a scientific standpoint.

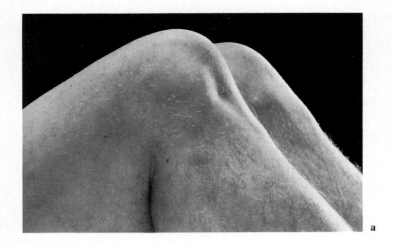

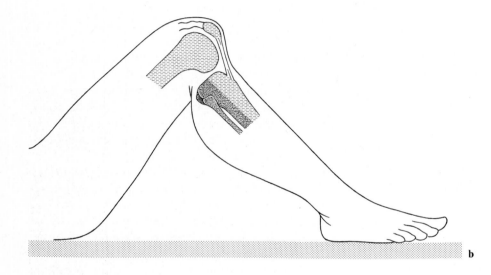

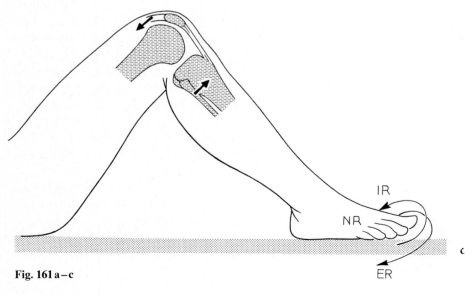

Fig. 161 a–c

122

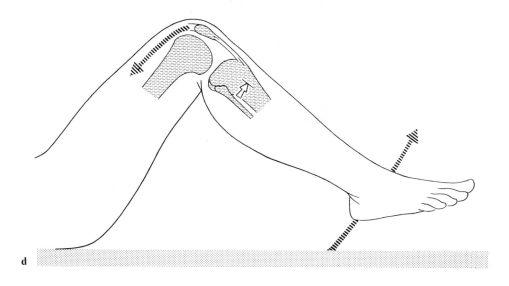

d

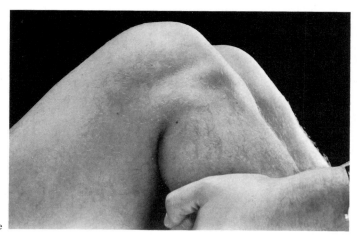

e

Fig. 161 a–e. The "posterior drawer" is very often mistaken for an "anterior drawer," because the tibia sags posteriorly and appears to move an abnormal distance forward when the examiner tests for an anterior drawer phenomenon. **a** The "posterior sag" of the right tibia is obvious compared to the normal silhouette of the healthy knee joint. **b** The tibial sag in the resting position. If the patient starts to raise his foot from this position, the pull of the quadriceps first displaces the tibia anteriorly into the neutral resting position, until the anterior cruciate ligament is tight (**c**). Only then is the foot raised from the table (**d**). **e** The same knee joint as in **a**, now manually restored to its normal position. Both silhouettes are again equal. As a rule, all examinations for drawer signs should be performed with the tibia in IR, ER and NR. However, the test should not be done in extreme IR or ER, for even a highly unstable knee joint can be passively stabilized by ligamentous coiling when subjected to maximal rotation

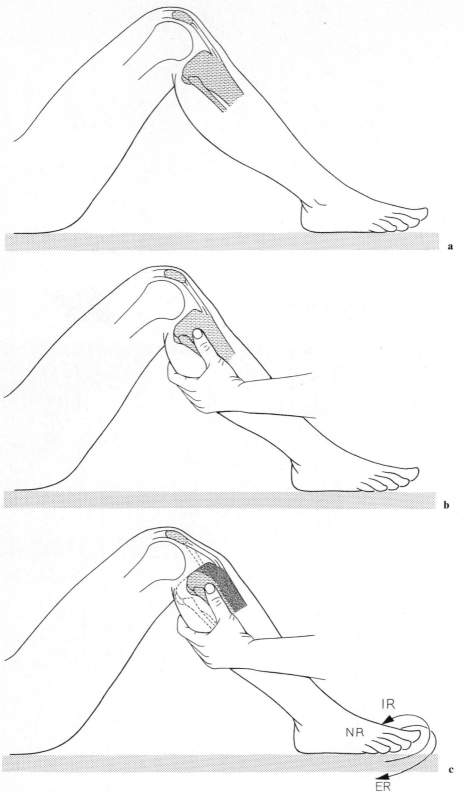

Fig. 162a–c. The anterior drawer test. **a** In the resting position the tibial plateau is held in its normal position by the intact posterior cruciate ligament. **b, c** With an- terior cruciate insufficiency the tibia can be pulled for- ward against the force of gravity and the tone of the flexors

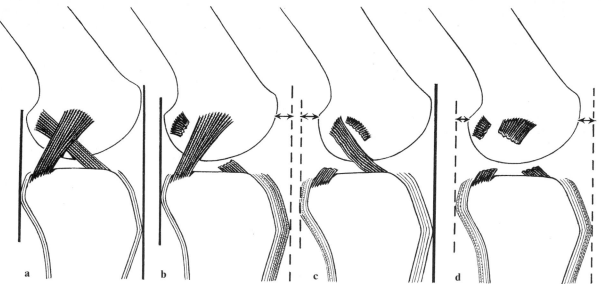

Fig. 163a–d. Testing for anterior, posterior and combined anteroposterior instability in the healthy and injured knee. **a** Even in the healthy knee with intact ligaments the tibia can be displaced forward and backward a small degree relative to the femur; this is due to the elastic reserve of the system and of the individual collagen fibers. In the normal knee, however, there is a distinct limit (*vertical lines*) beyond which relative motion is prohibited by tightening of the fibers in the synergistic ligamentous complexes. **b** With rupture of the anterior cruciate ligament, the tibia can be displaced pos-

teriorly to a slight degree, but a definite stop is felt; however, anterior displacement of the tibia is opposed not by an abrupt stop, but by a steady rise of resistance. The degree of displacement varies with the amount of force applied. **c** With rupture of the posterior cruciate ligament, the opposite is observed: a definite limit anteriorly and an ill-defined limit posteriorly. **d** With rupture of both ligaments, no abrupt stop is felt in either direction, and the anterior and posterior drawer displacements are opposed only by increasing resistance

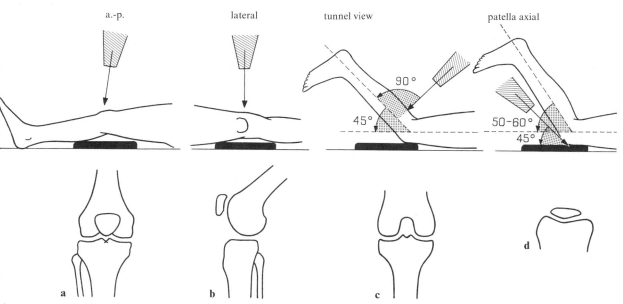

Fig. 164a–d. Every clinical examination of an acutely injured knee should include a roentgenographic evaluation. Besides the standard *a.-p.* **a** and lateral **b** views, it is important that the intercondylar fossa also be visualized **c**. This will demonstrate minimal bony lesions or other signs that can help to localize cruciate ligament tears, while lesions in the periphery often provide evidence of collateral and capsular ligamentous tears. Such findings

can have great bearing on the choice of operative tactics. **d** The axial "sunrise" view of the patella is also important for the demonstration of osteochondral flake fractures of the patella and femoral condyle. Bone fragments dislodged by patellar dislocation are most frequently found in front of the intercondylar fossa and next to the lateral femoral condyle or in the suprapatellar pouch. Illustration from Morscher [198]

Individual Variability of Normal Values

The studies of Jacobsen [146] have documented the empirical observation that knee joint stability varies from one individual to the next. Hence, an injured knee should be examined only after the healthy knee has first been tested to establish an individual baseline.

Jacobsen (1976) reports the following normal ranges of variation:

Medial laxity in 30° flexion: 5.8–12.1 mm (women 5.2–9.8 mm)
Lateral laxity in 30° flexion: 9.2–16.9 mm (both sexes)
Anterior drawer sign in 90° flexion: 0–5 mm (both sexes)
Posterior drawer sign in 90° flexion: 0–5 mm (Both sexes).

Jacobsen states that a positive should be declared only if there is an instability of 3 mm or more relative to the normal side. In any case a clear difference must be demonstrated before therapeutic implications may be drawn.

Reference Lines as an Aid to Stress Roentgenogram Interpretation

In the lateral view of the knee in 90° flexion and NR, a line tangent to the posterior part of the femoral condyle and posterior edge of the tibial plateau will normally be parallel to the posterior border of the tibial shaft.

If an anterior drawer sign is present, we can measure (in mm) the distance of the posterior tibial plateau from the vertical tangent to the femoral condyle.

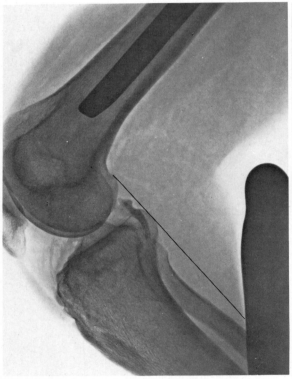
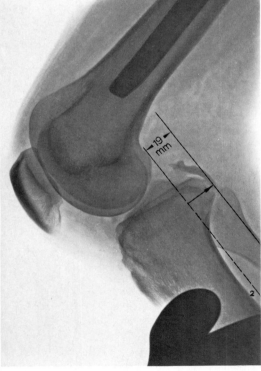

a
b

Fig. 165a, b. Normal and stress roentgenogram to demonstrate the posterior drawer. The stress film **b** is especially important if anterior and posterior instabilities coexist. Due to individual differences, findings should always be compared to the uninjured side. To measure anterior and posterior instability, the knee is flexed 90°, and a line is dropped from the posterior edge of the femoral condyle parallel to the posterior margin of the tibial shaft and tangential to the posterior tibial plateau. The posterior drawer sign is elicited, and then a second line is drawn parallel to the first and also tangential to the posterior tibial plateau. The distance between the lines can be measured in mm

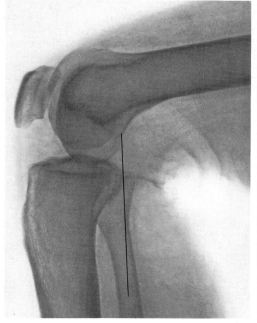 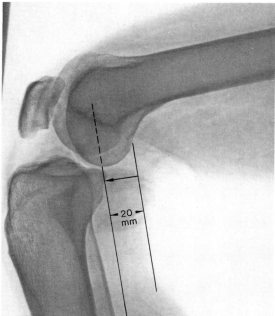

a b

Fig. 166a, b. Normal and stress film to demonstrate the anterior drawer. Again, with the knee in the drawer position, a second parallel line is drawn tangential to the posterior tibial plateau, and the drawer distance is measured in mm

With a posterior drawer sign, the tibial plateau projects beyond the vertical line, and we can again measure this distance in mm (Figs. 165 and 166).

Testing Rotational Stability

Slocum and Larson [324] were the first to show that besides medial, lateral, anterior and posterior instabilities, the knee is also subject to rotatory instabilities.

In principle the rotatory stability tests are performed like the drawer tests, with the knee in flexion. This can be done with the foot resting on the table, as shown in Figs. 161 and 162 for the drawer test, or with the knee flexed 90° over the side of the table (Fig. 167). We use the latter position for testing rotatory stability as well as for the anterior and posterior drawer tests, because many patients are better able to relax with the lower leg hanging free. If the patient has learned to relax sufficiently, the examination should be concluded by also testing rotatory stability with the knee *extended.*

The basis of these rotation tests is the systematic examination of anteroposterior drawer mobility in three rotational positions:

Neutral rotation (NR), external rotation (ER), internal rotation (IR)

This enables the instability to be categorized in more precise terms.

An anterior drawer test that is 2+ in NR, 3+ in ER and 0 in IR signifies a rotatory instability in the *anteromedial* quadrant.

An anterior drawer test that is 1+ in NR, 0 in ER and 2+ in IR indicates instability in the *anterolateral* quadrant.

In both cases an anterior cruciate ligament insufficiency is the central finding.

The two anterior rotatory instabilities – anteromedial and anterolateral – are much

127

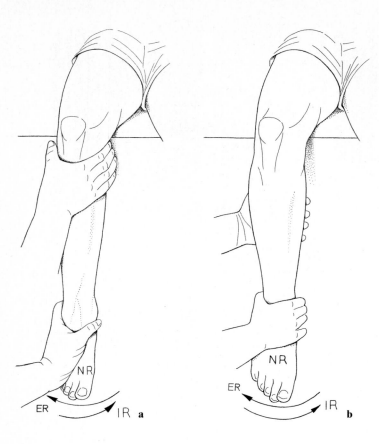

Fig. 167a, b. The clinical drawer test is meaningful only if the patient is relaxed and does not exert active countertension against the instability. This is best achieved by having the patient sit on the examining table with his lower leg hanging freely over the side

easier to demonstrate than the corresponding posterior instabilities. Posteromedial and posterolateral instabilities are usually subtle and are detected by appropriate testing in NR, ER and IR with the tibia resting on the table and hanging free.

Pathophysiology of Rotatory Instabilities

The discussions that follow are based on the scheme of Castaing et al. [47] and Bousquet [32] published in 1972. We have supplemented this scheme with more recent findings on the physiology of the ligaments.

The basis for all assessments is a knowledge of functional synergisms. That is, it must be understood the ligaments act *in concert,* rather than individually, to carry out a given function, as we have shown in our discussion of the semimembranosus corner (Fig. 168).

The modified scheme of Bousquet illustrates such a synergism between the anterior cruciate ligament and the POL and posterior meniscus horn. Normal stability can be expected only as long as both structures act together.

Ligamentous Stability of the Knee in Extension

If we examine the *extended knee* (Fig. 169[2]) to learn which ligaments are responsible for stability in this position, we find on the medial side that both the MCL and POL are taut. On the lateral side the taut structures are, from the front backward, the ALFTL, LCL and popliteus corner.

The entire posterior capsule is tense, as are both cruciate ligaments.

---

2 Figs. 169–176 modified from Castaing et al. [47]

Fig. 168. The instabilities that have been demonstrated are analyzed in terms of lost ligamentous functions, based upon a knowledge of the actions of the ligaments and their synergistic relationships. Thus, for example, a significant anterior drawer sign in NR and ER signifies not only a rupture of the anterior cruciate ligament, but also a tear in the region of the semimembranosus corner

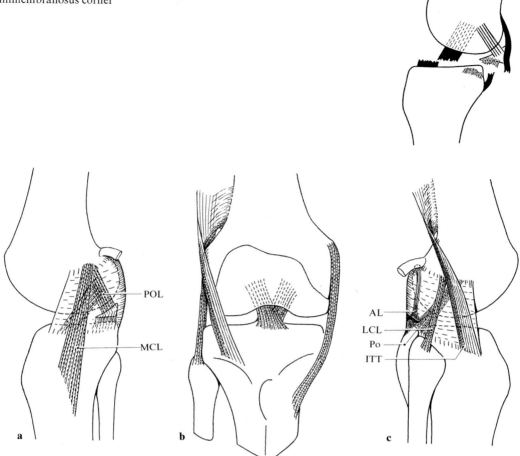

Fig. 169a–c. Semischematic representation of ligamentous stability in the extended knee. The MCL, POL, ALFTL, LCL, popliteus corner, capsule, ACL and PCL are all taut

Ligamentous Stability at 30° Flexion in NR

In this situation (Fig. 170) the passive stabilizing elements of the posterior capsule are relaxed. The MCL and LCL are less tense than in extension but are not lax. The anterior cruciate ligament is under very little tension, while the posterior cruciate is tight.

Ligamentous Stability at 30° Flexion in ER

At 30° flexion in ER (Fig. 171) the medial and lateral peripheral ligaments are taut, while both cruciate ligaments are relaxed.

Ligamentous Stability at 30° Flexion in IR

In this position (Fig. 172) the semimembranosus corner, both cruciate ligaments, the ALFTL, the arcuate ligament are taut; the popliteus tendon may also be reflexly tensed. The MCL and LCL are lax.

Ligamentous Stability at 30° Flexion on Anterior Displacement of the Tibia (Fig. 173)

In NR the anterior cruciate ligament is tense, as are the semimembranosus corner and ALFTL to some degree.

129

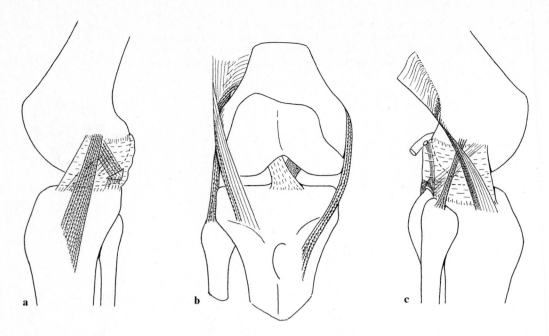

Fig. 170a–c. Ligamentous stability at 30° flexion in NR. The MCL, semimembranosus corner, ALFTL, LCL and PCL are less tense, while the ACL is lax

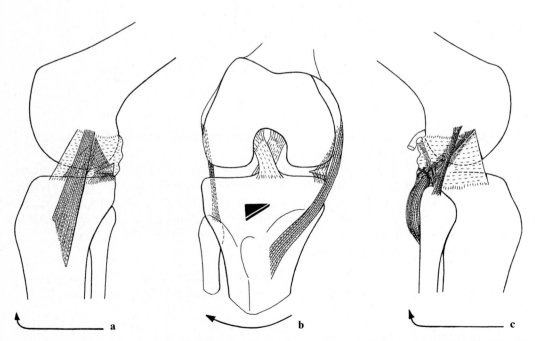

Fig. 171a–c. Ligamentous stability at 30° flexion in ER. The MCL, semimembranosus corner, LCL and popliteus corner are taut; the ACL is lax, and the PCL is under only slight tension

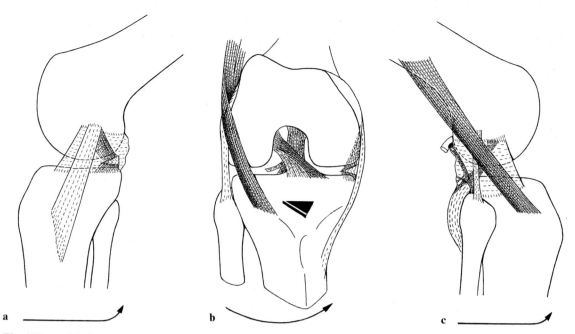

Fig. 172 a–c. Ligamentous stability at 30° flexion in IR. The semimembranosus corner, ALFTL, arcuate ligament, ACL and PCL are taut; the MCL and LCL are lax

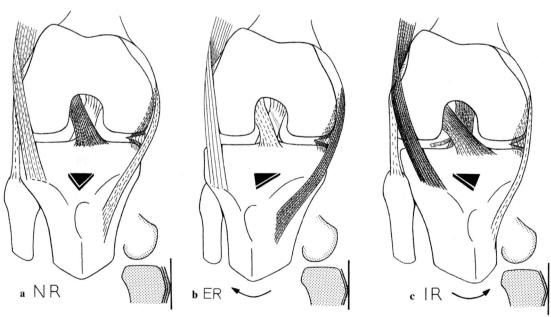

Fig. 173 a–c. Ligamentous stability at 30° flexion with anterior displacement of the tibia (anterior drawer test). **a** In NR the ACL is taut, and the semimembranosus corner and ALFTL are under slight tension. **b** In ER the MCL, semimembranosus corner and LCL are taut, while the ACL, PCL and ALFTL are relaxed. **c** IR tightens the ACL, PCL and ALFTL and slightly tenses the semimembranosus corner. In the normal knee, anterior displacement is greatest in NR. In ER and IR, the anterior stability of the tibia is enhanced by twisting of the peripheral capsular and ligamentous structures, and so there is less anterior displacement; this displacement is nil in extreme ER and IR

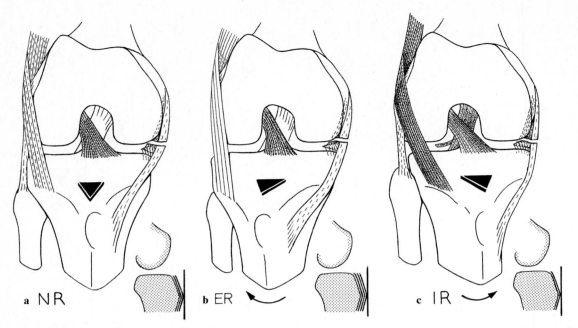

Fig. 174a–c. Ligamentous stability at 30° flexion with anterior displacement of the tibia and division of the medial ligaments. **a** Following division of the MCL and POL, the anterior drawer in NR is the same as in the intact knee (Fig. 173). **b** In ER, on the other hand, failure of restraint by the MCL and semimembranosus corner allows an abnormal degree of ER, which continues until checked by the ACL. Anterior drawer displacement is greater in this ER than in NR. **c** In IR anterior stability is again normal due to tightening of the cruciate ligaments and the ALFTL. Hence, there is little or no anterior drawer displacement in IR, as in the normal knee

In ER the MCL and POL are very tense, while the anterior cruciate ligament and ALFTL are lax.

In IR the iliotibial tract with its ALFTL is the most tense, followed by the cruciate ligaments and semimembranosus corner (cf. Fig. 95).

Thus, in the healthy knee the normal anterior drawer mobility is greatest in NR, where it is about 2 mm. In ER and IR there is little or no anterior drawer sign due to the twisting of the peripheral ligaments.

Ligamentous Stability at 30° Flexion on Anterior Displacement of the Tibia with the MCL and POL Severed (Fig. 174)

In NR, as before, the anterior cruciate ligament is the most tense, and there is still an anterior drawer sign of about 2 mm.

In IR the situation is likewise unchanged, and the drawer sign is reduced practically to 0 mm.

In ER, on the other hand, the stabilizing action of the MCL and POL is lost, and all the tension is placed on the ACL. The latter cannot prevent an anterior drawer sign of up to 5 mm. Therefore, *anteromedial rotatory instability results.*

Ligamentous Stability at 30° Flexion on Anterior Displacement of the Tibia with the Anterior Cruciate Ligament Severed (Fig. 175)

In NR, with the loss of stabilization by the anterior cruciate ligament, all the tension is placed on the MCL, POL and ALFTL. But these medial and lateral peripheral bands are incapable of producing anterior stability by themselves, and the anterior drawer sign is increased by 2–3 mm.

In ER stability is again normal with no anterior drawer, and all tension is borne by the MCL and POL.

In IR stability is also normal with no anterior drawer, and all tension is borne by the ALFTL and semimembranosus corner.

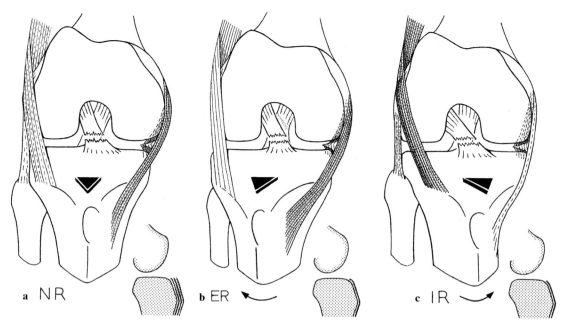

Fig. 175 a–c. Ligamentous stability at 30° flexion with anterior displacement of the tibia and division of the anterior cruciate ligament. **a** With isolated division of the ACL, we find a greater drawer displacement in NR than in the intact knee. Anterior displacement is finally checked by tightening of the semimembranosus corner, MCL and ALFTL. **b** In ER the situation does not differ from that in the normal knee, for in this position the ACL is lax and exerts no restraining action. **c** Stability is similarly unchanged in IR owing to a "coiling" of the ALFTL and semimembranosus corner

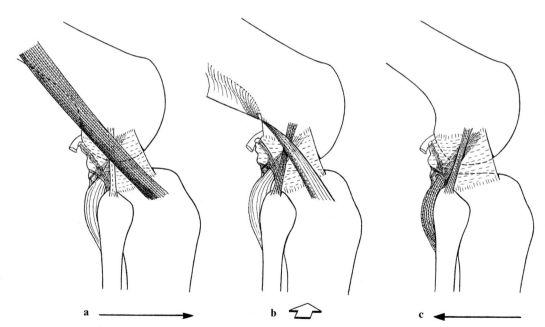

Fig. 176 a–c. The ligamentous structures of the lateral side as stabilizers in 30° flexion under stress in various directions. **a** On anterior displacement of the tibia, the ALFTL and portions of the arcuate ligament are tense. **b** Under a varus stress the ALFTL, LCL and portions of the arcuate ligament and popliteus tendon are taut. **c** On posterior displacement of the tibia, the LCL, popliteus tendon and portions of the arcuate ligament are taut

133

Thus, *there is a simple anterior instability in NR with no rotatory instability.*

Lateral Ligamentous Structures as Stabilizers at 30° Flexion in Various Stress Directions (Fig. 176)

On anterior displacement of the tibia, the iliotibial tract with its ALFTL bears most of the tension, with some assistance from the popliteus corner.

Under a varus stress the ALFTL, LCL and popliteus corner are under tension.

On posterior displacement of the tibia, the LCL and popliteus corner absorb all the tension, while the ALFTL remains tension-free.

Cruciate Ligament Insufficiency and Lateral Subluxation Phenomena with the Corresponding Clinical Tests

Subluxation in Anterior Cruciate Insufficiency

Anterior cruciate insufficiency leads to a disintegration of the rolling-gliding mechanism, which is especially obvious on the lateral side and was pointed out by us in 1976 [241]. Because the axis of rotation in the normal knee is shifted toward the medial side (Fig. 91), the lateral plateau normally has a greater anterior and posterior excursion during rotation than the medial plateau, and the posterior convexity of the lateral plateau predisposes to subluxation phenomena on that side.

The lateral pivot shift test of McIntosh. The examiner lifts the foot of the extended, internally rotated leg with one hand, forces the knee into valgus with the other hand by pushing on the side of the calf, and slowly flexes the knee while maintaining the valgus stress. In a positive test a "subluxation snap" (Figs. 34 b–39 b) will occur at about 30–40° flexion. The test is positive in the presence of anterior cruciate insufficiency. Associated insufficiency of the ALFTL and semimembranosus corner accentuates the sign, while a severe valgus instability makes it difficult to elicit for lack of medial support [153, 371].

The "jerk" test of Hughston. In this test the examiner flexes the knee to about 60°, grasps and internally rotates the distal tibia, and with his other hand applies a valgus stress to the knee. He then gradually extends the knee, maintaining the IR and valgus pressure. The femoral condyle remains behind the summit of the plateau until, at about 20–30° flexion, the tightening posterior structures of the popliteus corner pull the tibial plateau back, and the subluxation relocates with a jerk.

This test is positive in essentially the same injuries as the lateral pivot shift test of McIntosh (see above), but the jerk cannot be elicited as regularly as the pivot shift, even when the corresponding ligamentous lesions are present.

Slocum's test. The patient is positioned laterally with the healthy side down. The leg with the injured knee rests only on the medial side of the foot; the knee is unsupported. The examiner grasps the distal femur with one hand and the proximal tibia with the other and slowly flexes the knee. Again, a subluxation sign can be observed at about 30° flexion if anterior cruciate insufficiency is present.

In this position the iliotibial tract lies above the flexion axis and so is excluded as an active stabilizer. The collateral ligaments are relatively lax, as in the Lachmann test (see p. 120), thus making it easier to demonstrate the cruciate insufficiency. The test may be used like the Lachmann test, therefore.

Severe valgus instability often makes the subluxation snap more difficult to demonstrate.

The main advantage of Slocum's test is patient relaxation, which is more easily achieved in lateral recumbency than in the other tests.

Losee's test. This is similar to the jerk test, in that the limb is moved from flexion to extension.

If the left knee is being tested, the examiner stands to the left of the patient, grasps the foot with his left hand, flexes the knee to about 40° and uses his abdomen as a fulcrum to apply a valgus stress to the knee. With his right hand he increases the valgus pressure, placing the fingers on the patella and the thumb behind the fibular head (taking care to avoid peroneal nerve compression), while simultaneously pulling the upper tibia forward. On subsequent extension, during which the lower leg may rotate inward, a lateral snapping will occur between the femur and tibia at about 20° if there is an anterior cruciate insufficiency with anterolateral rotatory instability (McIntosh and Darby [215], Hughston [in 140], Slocum et al. [327], Losee et al. [201]).

Subluxations in Posterior Cruciate Insufficiency

External rotation-recurvatum test of Hughston. The feet are lifted with the legs relaxed. If there is a tear of the posterior cruciate ligament, popliteus corner and LCL in one knee, then the affected knee will fall into recurvatum with ER and increased tibia vara.

"Reverse posterior pivot shift" test of Jakob. If the posterior cruciate ligament, popliteus corner and LCL are torn, the tibial plateau can be pushed backward in flexion, so that the lateral femoral condyle is in front of the summit of the plateau and glides there during subsequent extension until the lateral gastrocnemius muscle and capsule are tightened, causing the femur to return to its normal position in extension with a snap (Hughston [in 140], Jakob [153]). There are anterior as well as posterior subluxation signs, and so care must be taken to differentiate a posterior instability from an anterior one.

Thus, there is not just *one* pivot shift but several kindred phenomena that all have their origin in the pathophysiology of the cruciate ligaments.

Classification of Instabilities

Hughston et al. [137], Kennedy [in 312], Nicholas [252], Slocum and Larson [324] and Trillat [359] are the names most often associated with the classification of instabilities. Nicholas published his "4-quadrant" classification scheme in 1973 [252], and Hughston published comprehensive papers in 1974 [136a] and 1976 [137]. Recently Kennedy [in 312] has published several summaries on current knowledge, and Trillat [359] has developed a lesion-based classification system which is based on the ligament sections of Paillot, and which in turn serves as the basis for our discussions.

Differences in nomenclature and evaluation persist (Dexel [in 233]), but progress toward standardization is being made. This enables us to present the following classification:

Instabilities in One Plane or About One Axis

Hughston [137] uses the term "straight instability," Kennedy [312] "one-plane instability," and Trillat [359] speaks of a "direct drawer." All denote stabilities that are nonrotatory in nature.

Medial Instability About One Axis

In extension. Valgus instability indicates a lesion of the MCL and POL and, if severe, an associated lesion of the medial half of the posterior capsule. A concomitant injury of the posterior cruciate ligament should always be suspected.

In 30° flexion. Mild medial opening denotes a lesion of the MCL and POL; the severity may be 1st, 2nd or perhaps 3rd degree (Fig. 192e). The posterior capsule no longer contributes to lateral stabilization in the flexed knee.

Any severe medial opening is associated with rotatory instability and suggests a cruciate ligament injury.

Lateral Instability about One Axis

In extension. Varus instability signifies a lesion of the LCL, the ALFTL (the arcuate complex and popliteus corner), all or part of the biceps tendon, the PCL and perhaps the ACL.

In 30° flexion. Mild lateral opening indicates a possible lesion of the LCL, ALFTL and popliteus corner.

Any severe lateral opening is associated with rotatory instability.

Anterior Instability in One Plane

This is demonstrated by a *positive anterior drawer sign in NR* at any flexion angle.

A severely positive drawer sign denotes injury not just of the ACL but also of the MCL, POL and ALFTL; a very severe instability further indicates that the posterior femorotibial structures and popliteus corner are torn.

Thus, *any severe anterior drawer sign in NR* is also associated with rotatory instability or even with varus or valgus instability.

Posterior Instability in One Plane

This is demonstrated by a *positive posterior drawer sign in NR* at any flexion angle.

A severe drawer sign indicates injury of the ACL and PCL, with involvement of the semimembranosus corner and popliteus corner.

Thus, *a severe posterior drawer sign in NR* is associated with additional varus, valgus and rotatory instabilities, for, like a massive anterior instability, it indicates involvement of the peripheral ligaments in the injury.

Rotatory Instabilities

The lesion of a peripheral ligament increases the range of rotational motion in the knee joint. If the lesion is complicated by a tear in the central pivot, this mobility is further increased. Because the normal axis of rotation can be maintained only by normal ligamentous stability, it, too, will be shifted by ligamentous injuries. On the one hand, such injuries enlarge the normally small area on the tibia within which the longitudinal axis of rotation intersects the tibial plateau. In other words, the longitudinal rotational axis is now free to "wander" over a larger area than is normally possible.

On the other hand, because in the flexed knee this longitudinal axis is largely defined by the posterior cruciate ligament, it can shift only a small distance as long as this ligament is intact. This is the case in instabilities of three of the four quadrants: the anteromedial, anterolateral and posterolateral. A posteromedial instability cannot exist if the posterior cruciate ligament is intact. If this ligament is ruptured, then the axis of rotation moves entirely out of the central pivot to the lateral periphery. Thus, Hughston et al. [137] do not include a "posteromedial rotatory instability" in their classification, because this no longer represents a classic rotatory instability with its axis at the joint center, but a different type of instability in which the axis of rotation is shifted to the lateral joint periphery (Fig. 177). According to Kennedy and O'Donoghue [312], however, it is possible for a posteromedial rotatory instability to exist even when the posterior cruciate ligament is intact.

It is unclear whether a partial or old lesion of the PCL with scarring was not in fact present in these cases. In any event, it is clear that the posteromedial "rotatory" instability represents a special type of rotatory instability. This is also true of posterolateral instabilities with a ruptured posterior cruciate ligament.

But because all these cases involve an instability in at least one of the four quadrants, we include all four types in our classification for didactic purposes.

For the posteromedial type, we have chosen the variant with a ruptured posterior cruciate ligament (Fig. 177b) in order to illustrate the difference.

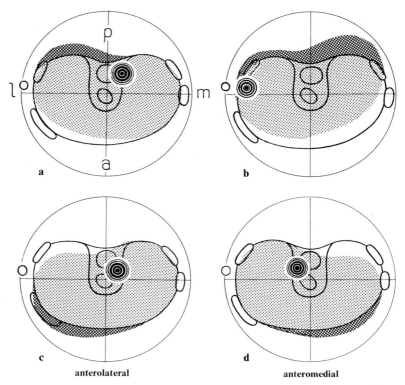

Fig. 177a–d. Schematic representation of the right tibial plateau with its 7 passive stabilizing elements as viewed from above. The possible instabilities of the knee joint occur in the four quadrants superimposed on the tibial plateau. The anteromedial instability (**d**) is the most frequent, followed by the anterolateral (**c**) and posterolateral (**a**); these are classed as "simple" rotatory instabilities, inasmuch as the intact PCL minimizes the abnormal shift of the rotational axis. In posteromedial instability (**b**), the PCL is necessarily insufficient and thus allows the rotary axis to shift entirely out of the central region of the joint to the lateral periphery. Thus, this type of instability represents a special case and is not entirely comparable to the other rotatory instabilities

Anteromedial Rotatory Instability

In this classic rotatory instability, the *medial* tibial plateau rotates too far anteriorly. There is medial opening of the joint space. The injured structures are, in order of increasing instability:
– the semimembranosus corner
– the MCL
– the ACL.

Anterolateral Rotatory Instability

This is an obvious rotatory instability in which the *lateral* tibial plateau rotates too far anteriorly. The joint space opens on the lateral side.

The injured structures are, in order of increasing instability:
– the ALFTL
– the ACL
– the popliteus corner.

Posterolateral Rotatory Instability

This is another obvious rotatory instability in which the *lateral* tibial plateau rotates too far posteriorly. There is lateral opening of the joint space. The injured structures are, in order of increasing instability:
– the popliteus corner
– the LCL
– PCL.

137

If the posterior cruciate is torn, the axis of rotation also shifts from the center, but this time to the *medial* joint periphery.

Posteromedial Rotatory Instability

If the posterior cruciate ligament is still intact, then rotatory instability with a central axis is possible. But if the ligament is ruptured, this axis shifts to the *lateral* joint periphery. The tibial plateau rotates posteromedially, and there is medial opening.

The injured structures are, in order of increasing instability:

- the semimembranosus corner
- the MCL
- the ACL (partly)
- the PCL (interstitial tear).

With a clear-cut rupture of the PCL and an intact ACL, a posteromedial instability is present (Kennedy [in 312]).

Every *severe* rotatory instability in one quadrant is associated with rotatory instability in another quadrant or with valgus or varus instability.

Combined Instabilities

General

We have intentionally limited ourselves to a simple classification. A survey of the literature (in [330]) shows that discrepancies still exist in the evaluation of these instabilities. Standards differ, depending on whether the classification is based anatomically on the PCL (Hughston) or is biomechanically oriented (Trillat).

In our opinion a clear line cannot be drawn between one instability and another in either the acutely or chronically unstable knee. Classification is not an end in itself, but is simply an aid to clarifying the nature of a complex lesion. When confronted with a recent injury, our primary task is to identify clearly all the involved ligaments in order to optimize the chance of functional recovery after surgical repair.

In chronic instabilities, we are dealing with a situation in which the former combined injury is masked by partial healing, producing changes in the clinical picture.

But the surgeon who is familiar with the connections between ligamentous lesions and instability, both from study and experience, should have little difficulty in analyzing even chronic instabilities.

For this reason we favor the classification of Trillat et al. [359], which relates instabilities to the division of individual ligaments or entire ligament systems. The combined instabilities can be subdivided into two main groups:

Combined Rotatory Instabilities in Several Quadrants

In this form anteromedial and anterolateral rotatory instabilities may coexist or one may progress to the other by the "stretch-out" mechanism of Ellison [in 12].

The longer such an abnormal rotatory laxity persists, the greater the progressive stretching of the peripheral capsular ligamentous sheath in the other quadrants, especially in young, physically active individuals. The most common mode of progression is anteromedial to anterolateral and, when this combination decompensates, even to posterolateral instability [66].

Combined rotatory instabilities of this type are commonly mistaken for valgus instability.

138

Though one might expect to find a severe degree of valgus laxity, in reality the lateral femoral condyle glides anteriorally or posteriorally off the convexity of the tibial plateau, resulting in increased valgus of the joint with an *apparent* valgus instability. This slipping of the femoral condyle with rotational displacement of the tibial plateau can be recognized by careful observation, however.

> Severe rotatory instabilities (including combined types) are always associated with varus or valgus instability.

Rotatory Instabilities with Valgus-Varus Instability

As a rule, the more severe the rotatory instability, the greater the associated medial or lateral instability. The capsular sheath is stretched and *must* allow considerable varus or valgus opening if the rotatory instability is severe. By the same token, a severe medial or lateral instability must result in considerable rotatory instability.

Ligamentous Injuries and Instabilities

It is known that the capsule does not envelop the knee like a ligament, providing passive stability at all points. It is reinforced by seven key ligaments. Besides the cruciate ligaments in the central pivot, these are, proceeding clockwise from the anterolateral quadrant (Fig. 178):

1. The ALFTL. The underlying deep capsule has no ligamentous fibers back to the level of the LCL and popliteus tendon and consists only of a highly elastic synovial investment. Only the meniscotibial fibers in the mid-lateral portion of the joint, together with the expansions of the arcuate ligament and biceps, are firm.

2. The LCL. Its stabilizing function depends strongly on the rotational position of the knee joint.

3. The popliteus corner. This is adjoined by the posterior capsule (Vidal [365]), which extends around to the semimembranosus corner on the medial side. The last tendinous strands of the popliteus and semimembranosus corner terminate in this portion of the capsule. It performs a purely *passive stabilizing function* only in extension. In flexion its ligamentous strands contribute to active rotation as extensions of the popliteus (arcuate popliteal ligament) and semimembranosus tendon (oblique popliteal ligament). They then function as active dynamic stabilizers.

4. The semimembranosus corner.

5. The MCL is the most imposing of all these true ligaments. Between it and the patellar ligament is the longitudinal patellar retinaculum, an active stabilizer.

Analysis of the Biomechanical Effects of Ligamentous Injuries on Stability in the Four Quadrants

The basic idea for this discussion was adopted from Trillat et al. [359] and embellished with some additional details. We find that more than 20 different instabilities can be qualitatively and quantitatively distinguished according to the severity and complexity of the ligamentous lesion (cf. also Fig. 178 ff.).

Anteromedial Instabilities

Moving from the simple monad to duad A, duad B, the triad and the tetrad (Fig. 180), we find a logical increase in the degree of instability as the severity of the injury worsens.

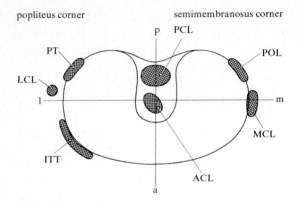

popliteus corner   semimembranosus corner

Fig. 178. Schematic representation of the right tibial plateau showing the 4 quadrants and the 7 main passive stabilizers of the knee joint. Two of these, the ACL and the PCL, are located in the central pivot. Five are in the periphery: the MCL and semimembranosus corner medially, and the iliotibial tract (ALFTL), LCL and popliteus corner laterally

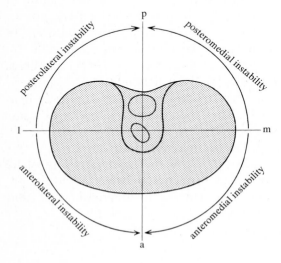

Fig. 179. Representation of the 4 quadrants and designation of the corresponding instabilities

The "unhappy triad" of O'Donoghue [265, 266] also fits into this series. The duads and tetrad represent further types of complex injury that are of differential diagnostic importance (lateral pivot shift with involvement of the ACL).

Posterolateral Instabilities

On the lateral side as well, the severity of injury increases from the simple monad to the tetrad (Fig. 181) (posterior pivot shift with involvement of the PCL and popliteus corner).

Anterolateral Instabilities

In these instabilities the complexity of injury ranges from the monad to the triad

(Fig. 182). The duad and triad are typically associated with a lateral pivot shift.

Posteromedial Instabilities

It is unclear whether a monad or duad can exist in this quadrant. On the other hand, we have personally observed the triad shown in Fig. 183 on more than one occasion.

For the reasons cited earlier (Fig. 177), we regard this simply as an instability, rather than a rotatory instability (no pivotal shift is known).

Posterior Instabilities

An isolated tear of the posterior cruciate ligament is known (Fig. 184a). Unlike the isolated anterior cruciate tear, it not only

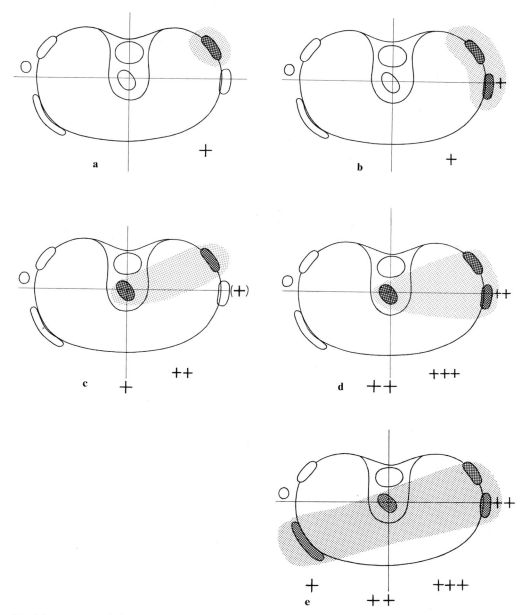

Fig. 180 a–e. Possible *anteromedial* instabilities, presented in order of complexity of the ligamentous injury. **a** The *monad* is a solitary lesion of the POL (semimembranosus corner) which causes a 1 + anteromedial rotatory instability. **b** *Duad A* is a combined injury of the POL and MCL; it causes a 1 + anteromedial rotatory instability and 1 + valgus instability. **c** *Duad B* is a combined injury of the POL and ACL; it causes a 2 + anteromedial rotatory instability, 1 + anterior drawer sign in NR and a (1 +) valgus instability. **d** The *triad* is a combined injury of the POL, ACL and MCL; it causes a 3 + anteromedial rotatory instability, 2 + anterior drawer sign in NR and a 2 + valgus instability. **e** The *tetrad* involves injury to the POL, ACL, ALFTL and MCL; it causes a 3 + anteromedial rotatory instability, 2 + anterior drawer sign in NR, 1 + anterolateral rotatory instability, 2 + valgus instability, 1 + lateral pivot shift and a (1 +) recurvatum

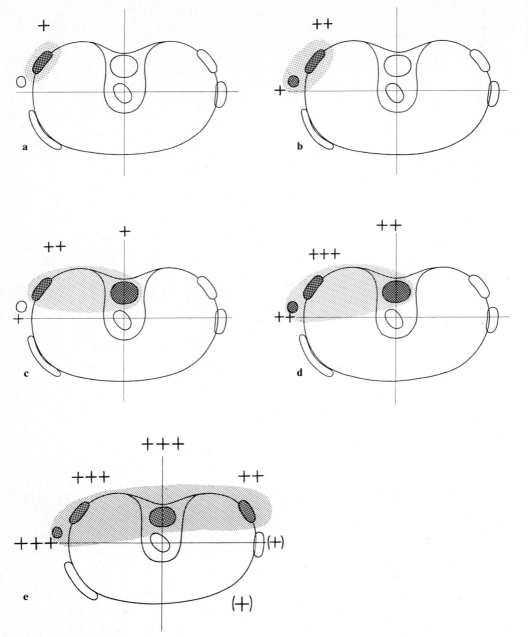

Fig. 181 a–e. Possible *posterolateral* instabilities, presented in order of complexity of the ligamentous injury. **a** The *monad* is an isolated lesion of the popliteus corner (popliteus, arcuate ligament complex, posterior horn of lateral meniscus); it causes a 1 + posterolateral rotatory instability. **b** *Duad A* is a combined injury of the popliteus corner and LCL; it causes a 2 + posterolateral rotatory instability and a 1 + varus instability. **c** *Duad B* is a combined injury of the popliteus corner and the PCL; it causes a 2 + posterolateral rotatory instability, 1 + posterior drawer sign in NR and a 1 + varus insta-

bility. **d** The *triad* is a combined injury of the popliteus corner, PCL and LCL; it causes a 3 + posterolateral rotatory instability, a 2 + posterior drawer sign in NR and a 2 + varus instability. **e** The *tetrad* is a combined injury of the popliteus corner, PCL, POL and LCL; it produces a 3 + posterolateral rotatory instability, 3 + posterior drawer sign in NR, 2 + posteromedial rotatory instability, 3 + varus instability, (1 +) valgus instability, (1 +) anteromedial rotatory instability and a 1 + recurvatum

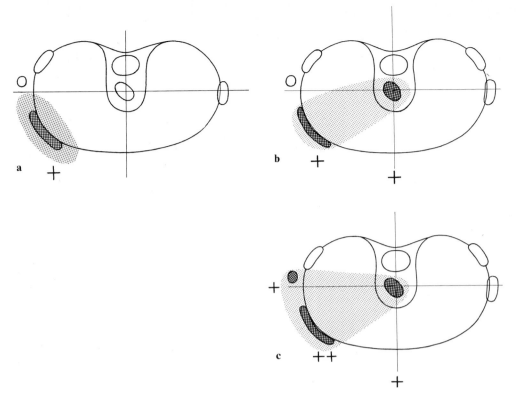

Fig. 182 a–c. Possible *anterolateral* instabilities, presented in order of complexity of the ligamentous injury. **a** The *monad* is a solitary lesion of the ALFTL; it causes a 1+ anterolateral rotatory instability. **b** The *duad* is a combined injury of the ALFTL and ACL; it causes a 1+ anterolateral rotatory instability, 1+ anterior draw-er sign in NR and 1+ lateral pivot shift. **c** The *triad* involves injury to the ALFTL, ACL and LCL and causes a 2+ anterolateral rotatory instability, 1+ anterior drawer sign in NR, 1+ lateral pivot shift and 1+ varus instability

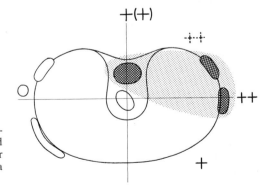

Fig. 183. The *posteromedial* instability. This involves a combined injury of the POL (semimembranosus corner), PCL and MCL. It causes a 2+ posteromedial instability in IR, a 1+ (or 2+) posterior drawer sign in NR, a 2+ valgus instability and a 1+ anteromedial instability

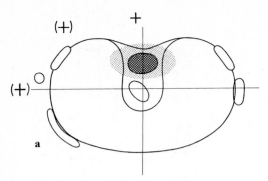

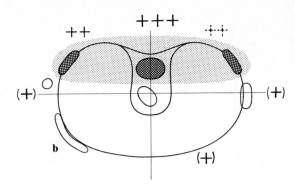

Fig. 184a, b. Other possible *posterior* instabilities. **a** A lesion of the PCL alone leads to a 1+ posterior drawer sign in NR, (1+) posterolateral rotatory instability and (1+) varus instability. **b** The "global posterior instability" involves a combined injury of the POL (semimembranosus corner), PCL and Po (popliteus corner). It creates a 2+ posteromedial instability, 3+ posterior drawer sign in NR, 2+ posterolateral instability, (1+) valgus instability, (1+) varus instability, (1+) anteromedial rotatory instability and a 1+ recurvatum

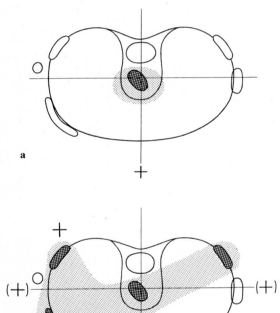

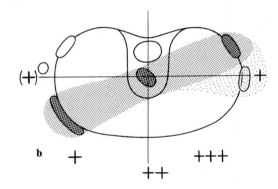

Fig. 185a–c. Other possible *anterior* instabilities. **a** An isolated lesion of the ACL causes a 1+ anterior drawer sign in NR. **b** The "global anterior instability" is usually a result of chronic anterior instability and involves injuries of the POL, ACL and ALFTL. It causes a 3+ anteromedial rotatory instability, 2+ anterior drawer sign in NR, 1+ anterolateral rotatory instability, (2+) valgus instability, (1+) varus instability, 1+ lateral pivot shift and 1+ recurvatum. **c** A combined injury of the POL, ACL, ALFTL and Po (popliteus corner) leads to a 3+ anteromedial rotatory instability, 2+ anterior drawer sign in NR, 2+ anterolateral rotatory instability, (1+) valgus instability, (1+) varus instability, 1+ posterolateral rotatory instability, 1+ lateral pivot shift and 1+ recurvatum

144

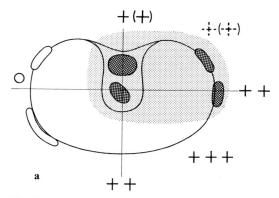
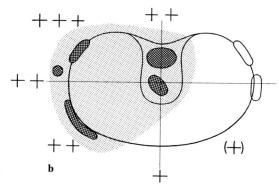

Fig. 186a,b. Possible *combined anteroposterior* instabilities. **a** The medial anteroposterior instability represents a combined injury of the ACL, PCL, POL and MCL. It causes a 2+ anterior drawer sign in NR, a 1+ (2+) posterior drawer sign in NR, 3+ anteromedial instability, 1+ (2+) posteromedial instability and 2+ valgus instability. **b** The lateral anteroposterior insta-

bility is a combined injury of the ACL, PCL, Po (popliteus corner), LCL and ALFTL. It causes a 1+ anterior drawer sign in NR, 2+ posterior drawer sign in NR, 2+ anterolateral instability, 3+ posterolateral instability, 2+ varus instability and (1+) anteromedial instability

produces a positive posterior drawer test in NR but also causes a mild posterolateral rotatory instability [359] and a marked varus instability.

When a tear of the PCL is combined with injury of the semimembranosus corner and the popliteus corner, a genu recurvatum is produced along with the objective instability signs (Fig. 184b). Because there is little varus or valgus opening in such cases, this injury may pose problems in terms of surgical access.

Anterior Instabilities

Besides the simple isolated anterior cruciate tear (Fig. 185a) with its mildly positive drawer test in NR, we have also shown the combined injury that is responsible for "global anterior instability." In the milder form (Fig. 185b) the popliteus corner is not yet involved, as it is, for example, in Fig. 185c. This latter combination is usually a late stage of chronic instability, in which the popliteus corner with its few purely passive ligamentous elements has also become stretched. This component of the instability must not be overlooked during reconstruction.

Clinically these combined injuries are marked by a lateral pivot shift sign and, especially in longstanding cases, by genu recurvatum.

Anteroposterior Instabilities

Both cruciate ligaments are ruptured, as are the medial ligaments (Fig. 186a) and the lateral ligaments (Fig. 186b). This is a very severe and debilitating injury. The next step is dislocation.

Dislocations

These complete lesions of all ligaments are not included in the illustrations. Remarkably, secondary instabilities after such dislocations are often rather mild. According to operatively verified cases, this is due to the fact that the entire capsuloligamentous apparatus often is preserved as a unit. Either the femoral condyle is torn out of the capsule by the injury, like a foot out of a stocking, or the joint capsule is torn off the tibial head like a cap.

145

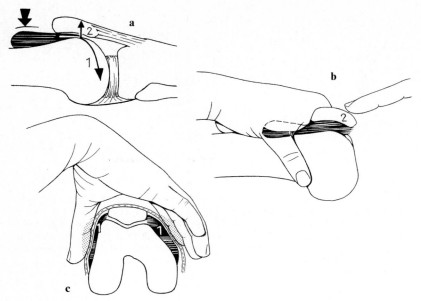

Fig. 187 a–c. Testing the knee joint for effusion. **a** Pressure on the suprapatellar pouch forces the effusion fluid around the femoral condyle (*1*) and beneath the patella (*2*). **b** Much effusion will raise the patella and is easily recognized by the sign of the "dancing patella." **c** Little effusion cannot raise the patella but fills the pouches next to the "cheeks" of the femoral condyles. There it can be verified by palpation as a fluctuating mass between the capsule and bone (after Smillie [328])

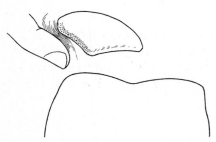

Fig. 188. Examination method for detecting patellar chondromalacia. The patella is pushed medially with the fingers, so that pressure can be applied to the lower facet with the thumb. Pressure is thus exerted on the soft tissues of the integrument, the inflamed synovium near the chondromalacia, and the alar fold. The resulting pain originates not only from the patella, but also from these soft tissues. Nevertheless, this method is of much diagnostic importance

Instability – Disability

An instability alone says nothing about the severity of the associated disability. The discrepancies can be great. Besides subjective complaints, objective signs such as effusion and patellar chondromalacia may accompany the instability. The connection between chondromalacia and instability has been particularly stressed by Ségal [314].

The effusion (Fig. 187) is seldom massive. A "floating" patella is present only on occasion, although the fluid mantle next to the femoral condyle is palpable.

Because patellar chondromalacia is such a troublesome factor in the disordered knee (for details see Rehabilitation, p. 267), the diagnostic maneuver to demonstrate patellofemoral pain (Fig. 188) should not be omitted from the examination.

Part II

Injuries of the Ligaments and Capsule

General

The layers of the capsule, ligaments, fasciae and tendinous expansions are not as easily recognized in situ as one might gather from our theoretical discussions of anatomy, physiology and kinematics. While the basic structural patterns remain essentially the same, individual differences can make recognition difficult. For example, as mentioned earlier, Laurin and Beauchamp [195] and Marshall's group [107] have found significant differences in the length ratio of one cruciate ligament to the other.

None of this alters the kinematic laws. Nevertheless, every knee, by virtue of the length of its cruciate ligaments and spatial distribution of their insertions, will exhibit a unique contour of the femoral condyle and tibial plateau. The Burmester curve, too, will have an individualized shape.

This means that every knee joint has its own ideal lines of ligamentous insertion.

The degree to which the different layers blend together also varies from one knee to the next. Thus, in some cases the medial longitudinal patellar retinaculum is well defined, and posteromedially the superficial fascial layer, which also envelops the pes anserinus tendons, can be separated easily from the deeper layer of the MCL back to the attachment of the semimembranosus. In other cases there is simply a broad fibrous capsulo-fascial layer running posteromedially, with no distinct retinaculum. Similarly, the connections from the MCL to the vastus medialis and adductor tendon may be prominent or ill-defined. Besides functioning as tension receptors and transmitters, relaying the signals that initiate defensive muscular contractions, these connections also provide an important means of exercising additional active control over the ligaments. Patients with intact connections between the ligaments and muscles are better able to stabilize their knee joints actively, even when

---

Individual cruciate ligament length and proportions determine the individual shape of the tibial plateau and femoral condyle.	Every knee joint has its own ideal lines of insertion for all its capsuloligamentous structures.

Hence, the collateral ligaments may course at various angles and may insert farther posteriorly at their proximal ends or farther anteriorly at their distal ends than in the basic model. The operator who performs reconstructive surgery for a recent injury or chronic instability must know the individual "laws" of the operated knee and look for the ideal lines of ligament attachment in order to ensure fiber isometry during knee movements.

there is a relative insufficiency of the purely passive ligaments. Therefore, special care should be taken to spare these important connecting structures during knee operations, for they provide the patient with his most efficient means of self-stabilization. Whenever possible, longitudinal structures should be incised parallel to their fiber course, avoiding transverse cuts that disrupt the continuity of the "functional chains."

Active, dynamic connecting structures should not be disrupted, so that the functional chains for active compensatory stabilization will remain intact.

The Layers of the Medial Capsuloligamentous System

Even the medial half of the quadriceps complex, with its pull across the patella and patellar ligament, serves to enhance medial stability by the active compression that is applied from the femur to the tibia. Just medial to the patella is the medial longitudinal patellar retinaculum (MLPR) (Figs. 1 and 2). It arises broadly between the patella, vastus medialis and the proximal insertion of the MCL, narrowing as it descends to insert on the upper tibia proximal and anterior to the distal MCL insertion. For kinematic reasons a femorotibial *ligament* could not exist in this location, which is why this *tendon* joins the vastus medialis with the tibia in the anteromedial quadrant.

The retinaculum is continued posteromedially in two layers (Fig. 189):

1. One is the superficial fascial layer, which joins farther posteromedially with the layer of the pes anserinus tendons and continues posteriorally as a common sheath, the popliteal fascia.

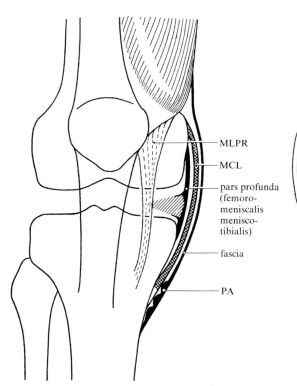

Fig. 189. Schematic representation of the medial ligamentous layers. The most anterior structure is the strip of the medial longitudinal patellar retinaculum controlled by the vastus medialis (*dashed lines*). Its dynamic attachment with the vastus medialis, which can move backward like the patella throughout flexion-extension, circumvents the law of insertion on the Burmester curve. Farther medially we see the medial meniscus with its femoromeniscal and meniscotibial fibers, and directly adjacent the deepest direct femorotibial fibers, which pass by the meniscus. There follows the true MCL, which is not adherent to the deep layer. Farther medially and superficially are the fascia and the pes anserinus tendons, which are included in the fascial layer

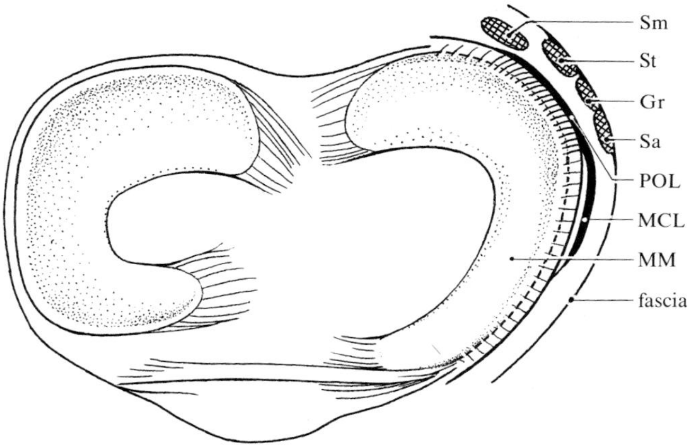

Fig. 190. This cross-sectional view completes our representation of the topographic relations of the ligamentous, tendinous and fascial layers. At this level, just proximal to the menisci, the tendons of the pes anserinus lie posteriorally in the semimembranosus corner

2. The other, which is separate from the MLPR and lies deep to the fascia, is the MCL. The posterior extensions of the MCL lie behind the Burmester curve and so would become lax during flexion if they were purely passive structures. However, being attached to the tendon of the semimembranosus muscle, they are actively tensed (dynamized) when the knee is flexed. The "superficial arm" of the posterior oblique ligament [136] belongs to this attachment between the semimembranosus tendon and posterior edge of the MCL (see also p. 72). The MCL itself, as mentioned earlier, requires an adhesion-free path of 1.5 cm on the upper tibia along which it can glide independently during flexion (Figs. 49 and 50). This is why there must be a *third, deep* layer, separate from the MCL, containing the femoromeniscal, meniscotibial, and femorotibial fibers. At the posterior edge of the MCL this deep layer unites with the posterior extensions of the MCL to form the POL. It is in this region that the medial meniscus has its firmest attachment with the ligamentous apparatus and the tibia (Fig. 190).

If this rigid femoral-meniscal-tibial ligamentous attachment remains intact, injury usually occurs within the substance of the meniscus itself.

The semimembranosus corner is under the most tension during automatic terminal rotation, when the medial femoral condyle glides backward and inward. A lesion of this corner invariably leads to pain and locking on extension.

In the extended knee all medial capsuloligamentous elements contribute to stability, and so tests for rotatory instability will be negative even if the POL is torn. In flexion, on the other hand, such a lesion will double the normal range of external rotation as reported by Brantigan and Voshell [34, 35].

In ER the collateral ligaments are stretched tight by virtue of their geometry. At the start of flexion, when there is an automatic IR of 15°, the entire collateral ligament system becomes slackened, and rotatory laxity is increased.

In intermediate flexion there is a further physiologic loosening of the medial ligament system (Fig. 45). If valgus stability is tested at this flexion angle in NR or IR, this physiologic loosening may be misinterpreted as a mild instability. But when the same test is done in ER, as is proper, normal medial closure is found.

According to Horwitz [quoted in 380], the longest fibers of the MCL are most tense in 90° flexion, which is consistent with Menschik's model of MCL tension (see p. 32). Brantigan and Voshell [34, 35] state that the MCL is "taut but not tight" in intermediate flexion, though it should be added that an intact ligament is never really lax in any position.

The problem of ligament tension is an important one from the standpoint of operative tactics. Every ligament suture should be tested functionally in both extension and flexion before it is definitively tied. If it tears or becomes lax, it has been incorrectly placed and must be moved to the correct location.

As Smillie [328] points out, all ligaments act in concert to stabilize the knee. Therefore all must be restored to their proper length during surgical repair, and all must be tight on full loading.

Medial Ligamentous Injuries with Disruptions of Bone and Ligament Continuity

In repairs of the medial ligament system, it is important that all lesions be attended to (Fig. 191). Thus, it is not enough to repair the MCL while neglecting tears of the deep femoromeniscotibial and femorotibial fibers of the POL.

Lesions with *bony avulsions* (Fig. 192a) are clearly delineated. Of course the form depicted is exceptional and could result only from a pure valgus trauma with the knee in 90° flexion, without a concomitant tear of the deep layer. In most cases there would be at least a moderate sprain of these deep fibers. Avulsions of this type are most common before epiphyseal closure is complete and can lead to growth disturbances due to the for-

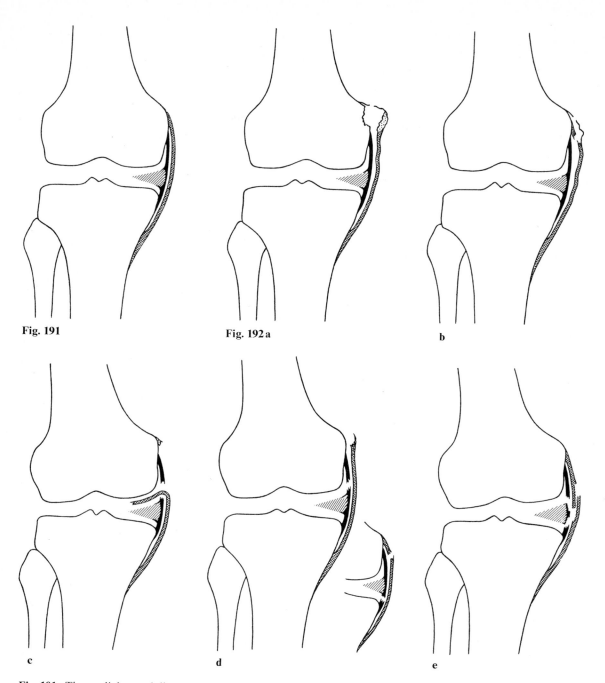

Fig. 191

Fig. 192 a

b

c

d

e

Fig. 191. The medial capsuloligamentous apparatus, reduced here to its purely passive stabilizing elements

Fig. 192a–e. Possible capsuloligamentous lesions with rupture or disinsertion of the MCL above the meniscus. **a** Bony avulsion of the MCL at the femur. **b** Ligamentous periosteal avulsion of the MCL at the femur. **c** Proximal ligamentous rupture of the MCL with displacement of the torn ligament into the joint. **d** The tear of the MCL and deep layer may be proximal to the meniscus, or the MCL may tear proximal to the meniscus and the deep layer distal to it. **e** This staggered tear through the MCL and deep layer with rupture of the femoromeniscal and meniscotibial fibers leads to the ligamentous detachment of the meniscus

151

mation of bony bridges across the epiphyseal plate. In adults a "Stieda-Pellegrini shadow" can develop during the healing period after injuries with a minimal avulsion of bone surface.

Bony ligament avulsions are favorable from an operative standpoint, for the fragment can be stably reattached, and the ligament restored to its ideal length and position, by means of screw fixation.

The next stage of severity, according to Palmer [279] and Ficat [85], is a *ligament rupture near the bone*. The extent of this lesion is more difficult to define, since the ligament is usually stretched and frayed at the rupture site. Repositioning and proper refixation are more difficult to achieve (Fig. 192 b).

The next stage is the *rupture of both the deep and superficial layers*. The fringed and frayed ligament elements are tangled and are often trapped in the joint space; moreover, they may have already become reattached to the wrong layer if some time has passed since the injury (Fig. 192 c). It be-comes more difficult to match up the torn ligament ends. An accurate knowledge of normal fiber anatomy and joint kinematics is a great aid to correct repositioning of the ligaments and their refixation with sutures or with a screw and toothed washer.

A *multilevel rupture* in which individual layers are torn at different levels (Fig. 192 d) is not uncommon and can be misleading, for a proximal tear of the long fibers will often mask a detachment of the coronary ligament from the tibia. If the deep lesion is neglected, a severe anteromedial rotatory instability can be anticipated, though straight valgus stability will be relatively unimpaired.

The closest thing to total destruction of the medial capsuloligamentous apparatus is the *detachment of the medial meniscus* from the femoromeniscal and meniscotibial fibers (Fig. 192 e). As the drawing indicates, this is not a true meniscal injury, but a ligamentous one. The cartilaginous substance of the meniscus (shaded) is undamaged; only its outermost ligamentous ring is torn. Note also the presence of a relatively large number

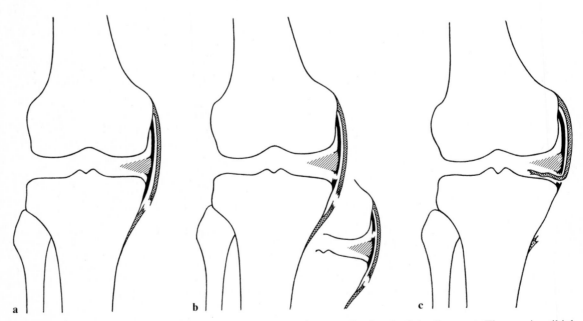

Fig. 193 a–c. Possible distal ruptures of the MCL. **a** Isolated distal rupture (rare). **b** Distal rupture of MCL with associated tear of the meniscotibial or femoromeniscal fibers. **c** Frequent form with incarceration of the torn distal end of the ligament. The meniscotibial layer has opened, allowing the avulsed portions of the MCL to become displaced far into the joint

of femorotibial ligament fibers in the deep layer, in addition to the femoromeniscal and meniscotibial attachments.

Figure 193 shows analogous situations associated with more distal ruptures of the MCL. Both the proximal (Fig. 192 a–c) and distal ruptures (Fig. 193) are common. Presumably their mechanisms of occurrence differ. It is our impression that skiing injuries are more apt to cause proximal tears, while soccer injuries tend to cause tears in the long fibers distal to the joint line.

We have found that the prognosis is better for distal tears than for proximal ones. Presumably this is because distal tears do not disrupt the delicate connections of the proximal MCL with the fascia of the vastus medialis and the adductor magnus tendon, which appear to be crucial for the control of medial stability.

This should teach us to be especially gentle when repairing these proximal tears, and not to underestimate the importance of the attachments with dynamic elements. The medial articular nerve also must be protected when operating in the area of the proximal MCL.

The Ligamentous Injury as a Function of the Force and Rate of Deformation

As mentioned, an intact collagenous ligament is reversibly distensible for up to 5% of its length [261]. If stretched beyond this limit, the ligament will irreversibly elongate or tear.

Kennedy et al. [175] have done several studies on the modalities of ligament rupture under various conditions with their test apparatus. By applying tension slowly and smoothly, a ligament can be stretched to twice its normal length before its continuity is destroyed by rupture. A sudden, quick pull, on the other hand, will snap the ligament even without elongating many of its collagenous fibers. The extreme case is the bony avulsion of the ligament at its site of attachment. The six classic examples of this type of injury are:

- proximal avulsion of the MCL from the medial femoral condyle;
- avulsion of both cruciate ligaments with the intercondylar eminence;
- avulsion of the anterior cruciate ligament with the anterior part of the intercondylar eminence;
- avulsion of the posterior cruciate ligament with the posterior part of the intercondylar eminence;
- avulsion of the posterolateral to lateral capsule with the fragment of Segond;
- avulsion of the lateral collateral ligament with the fibular apex.

The Three Degrees of Severity of Ligamentous Injuries (Fig. 194)

First-Degree Ligamentous Injury (Mild Sprain, "Stretch")

The continuity of the ligament is preserved. It is lax in situ and allows abnormal displacement of the joint ends. At operation these segments appear glossy and swollen with traces of ecchymosis.

Second-Degree Ligamentous Injury (Moderate Sprain, Partial Rupture, Interstitial Tear)

Gross continuity is maintained, but torn fiber bundles hang loosely from the ligament. Some areas are overstretched and there are varying degrees of ecchymosis, again associated with marked edematous swelling. The ligament is elongated and can no longer ensure stable joint closure.

Third-Degree Ligamentous Injury (Severe Sprain, Rupture)

Complete disruption of continuity by either a straight or multilevel tear. The torn ends can be reflected and lie loosely within the joint.

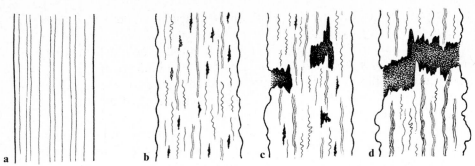

Fig. 194 a–d. The three degrees of severity of ligamentous injuries (schematic). a Normal ligament. b *First-degree injury:* Mild sprain in which the ligament has been "overstretched" beyond its 5% elastic reserve. Grossly the ligament appears intact, but microscopic examination reveals hemorrhages and minute tears; under the electron microscope the collagen fiber bundles have the appearance of overstretched springs. c *Second-degree injury:* Moderate sprain with overstretching accompanied by gross tears and hemorrhages at various levels. The continuity of the ligament is preserved, but its strength is greatly diminished. A ligament in this condition can easily be pulled apart along its longitudinal axis. d *Third-degree injury:* Severe sprain with complete disruption of continuity. Next to the rupture site there are additional small tears, hemorrhages and overstretched areas

Evaluation of the Three Degrees of Ligamentous Injury for Therapy

First-degree injuries with no disruption of continuity have the best prospect for spontaneous healing with full functional recovery. This presumes, of course, that the injured ligament is not constantly stretched to its "new length" with resultant healing in an elongated state. Mobilization may be allowed but should stop short of subjecting the healing ligament to true functional loads. Under cautious functional therapy the damaged collagen will be strengthened by the formation of new collagenous fibers, which will become organized into bundles as they mature. In this way the ligament will regain its former strength while retaining a normal length. Four to eight weeks are needed for complete healing.

In *second-degree injuries* some ligament continuity is preserved. Under proper conditions the granulation tissue and collagenous scar tissue will form a stress-resistant cicatrix which has the same orientation as the ligament. Mechanical rest is necessary for this to occur. If the ligament is continually overstretched while in its weakened state, adequate scar formation cannot take place. On the other hand, because we know that limited physiologic movements do not stress the ligaments beyond their elastic reserve [39], a moderate sprain must not necessarily be immobilized in plaster. Cautious functional therapy is not only possible but desirable.

A partial rupture can be critical in the case of an isolated ligament. A typical example is the anterior cruciate. This is a relatively delicate structure whose position in the joint makes it difficult to protect mechanically. An extensive partial rupture cannot scar properly if exposed to undue stress. A chronic, disabling instability is especially likely to develop if a second ligament also heals in a functionally incompetent state.

In *third-degree injuries,* or complete ruptures, the situation is definite. There is no chance that the torn ends will spontaneously reappose and form an adequate scar, and only surgical repair can ensure a complete functional recovery.

In reality it is not alway easy to classify a ligamentous injury as first-, second- or third-degree. Even in partial and complete ruptures, the ligament usually shows mild spraining elsewhere in its course. Thus, it is common for a ligament to be completely ruptured at one point while showing considerable elongation in other segments. The therapeutic implications of this must not be overlooked during operative repair.

General Operating Technique

Suturing Technique for the Various Degrees of Ligamentous Injury

Fig. 195 shows a schematic drawing of a ligament tear repaired with simple approximating sutures. Although continuity has been restored, sprained portions of the ligament remain elongated, rendering it insufficient for mechanical guidance of the joint. Therefore, approximating sutures should be reinforced with *tension sutures*. The pattern of the stitch is square or rectangular, in the manner of a mattress suture, its purpose being to restore normal length to the ligament while protecting the area of the tear (Fig. 196). These sutures may encompass a large or small area. The large dimensions of the knee ligaments sometimes make it necessary to place several such tension sutures, one within the other. However, their direction of pull must align precisely with the course of the ligament fibers if they are to perform their intended function – the more rapid restoration of an ordered collagenous fiber framework. These sutures may even be placed in overlapping fashion, as long as each is parallel to the local fiber axis. Like other sutures, they must be tested for correct functional placement and isometry during flexion-extension before they are definitively tied. If they become lax or cut into the tissue, their placement is incorrect. Tension sutures that do not follow the fiber axis will interfere with collagenous healing.

The Fixation of Avulsed Ligaments with a Screw and Toothed Washer (Fig. 197)

The screw and toothed washer are intended for use only at sites of broad ligamentous attachment to the bone (Fig. 197b). The ideal case is the superficial bony avulsion of an otherwise intact ligament (Fig. 197b, center). After refixation with the screw and washer, normal anatomic relations are restored. Even with a purely ligamentous rupture (Fig. 197b, left), the screw and toothed washer will provide good fixation. In these cases the bone appears denuded where normally it would be covered by the ligamentous expansion.

Design and Use of the Toothed Washer

We created the concept of the toothed washer about 10 years ago and since then have made several improvements leading to the design currently in use. The new washer has almost the same outside diameter as the old washer, but its teeth are located closer to the periphery and are more numerous, creating a larger area of contact (see schematic comparison of old and new washers in Fig. 197d). Each tooth consists of a cylindrical pedestal topped by a conical spike (Fig. 197c). The diameter of the cylinder is greater than that of the cone at its base. This creates a "shoulder" which minimizes the area of tissue compression with moderate tightening, allowing a normal microcirculation to be maintained below the washer and between the cylinders. Histologic studies of the tissue beneath experimentally-removed washers revealed no trace of pressure necrosis when the new washers were used. With flat metal washers or the early models made of plastic, fibrinoid necrosis and sclerosed connective tissue were found. The new washer, made of high-density polyethylene, has a metal ring embedded in its periphery. This provides contrast for roentgenographic visualization while remedying

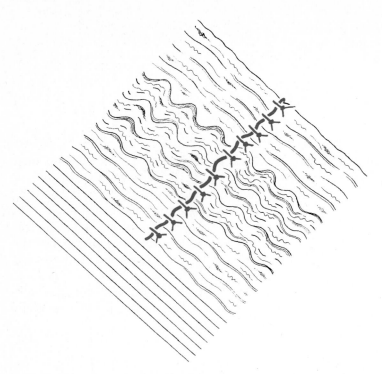

Fig. 195. Schematic representation of a suture through a torn ligament. In reality a ligament is rarely divided smoothly, as with a sharp knife. Even ligaments with third-degree sprains normally show additional first- or second-degree lesions above and below the rupture site. Thus, simple approximation of the tear cannot in itself restore the ligament to its original length

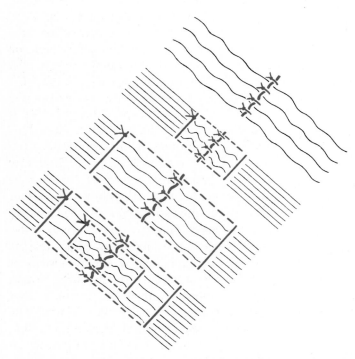

Fig. 196. We reinforce all approximating sutures with tension sutures placed parallel to the fiber axis of the ligament

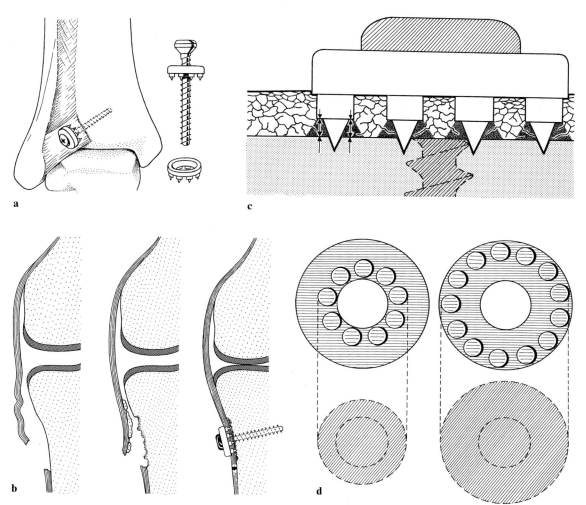

Fig. 197 a–d. The reattachment of avulsed ligaments with an AO screw and toothed washer. **a** Example showing reattachment of the anterior tibiofibular syndesmosis to the tubercle of Chaput. **b** Refixation of an avulsed ligament, with or without a bony fragment. **c** The washer is designed so that it grips the ligament and bone over a broad area with its peripherally arranged teeth, compressing and fixing them within the limits defined by the stop on each tooth. Little pressure is exerted on the tissue next to and between the teeth. The microcirculation in these areas of the ligament is normal; it is embarrassed only in the compressed areas represented by the *dark-colored trapezoids*. **d** An earlier model with a central tooth arrangement (and without stops), compared to the new model with peripheral teeth for more secure fixation

the problem of washer penetration by the screw head. The washers are available in two sizes, and the central perforations are shaped such that each washer is compatible with various-size screws from the AO/ASIF[3] inventory. Thus, the large washer can be fixed with the 35-mm small-fragment screw, malleolar screw, 45-mm cortical bone screw, or even with the 65-mm cancellous bone screw. If necessary the central perforation can be enlarged somewhat by drilling.

Similarly, the smaller washer is compatible with the 35-mm small-fragment cortical bone screw as well as with screws of smaller caliber and the corresponding screw heads.

---

3 AO = Association for the Study of Internal Fixation (*Arbeitsgruppe für Osteosynthesefragen*)

1. The ease with which ligaments can be anchored to the bone with screws might tempt the surgeon to use them in inappropriate sites, resulting in postoperative pain on movement and disability.

2. It is not difficult to overtighten screws, in which case the safety "shoulders" might not prevent the washer from crushing the tissue, especially in thick ligaments. The need for excessive tightening is remedied by using screws *and* sutures for accurate, atraumatic fixation.

3. Screws eventually have to be removed and so should be used sparingly and only where indicated.

Surgical Approaches

Abbott and Carpenter [1] reported extensively in 1945 on the various surgical approaches to the knee, summarizing the methods of Brackett and Hall, Coonse and Adams, Fisher and Timbrell, Henderson, Henry, Kocher, von Langenbeck, Ollier, Payr and von Volkmann. Other fundamental works on this subject were published by Bosworth [30], Campbell [45, 46], Honnart [131], Kaplan [166], Lange [190, 191], O'Donoghue [265], Trickey [345], Trillat and Rainaut [356] and Wilson [387].

The approaches have become fairly standardized and are based upon sound anatomic and physiologic criteria. Nevertheless, the surgeon must be able to tailor the approach somewhat in accordance with individual circumstances.

The topographic relations of the knee structures change greatly during joint movement. Some points are fixed, while others are mobile. To quote Kaplan: "The relative location of structures shifts when the position of a joint changes" [170].

Building on Kaplan's earlier work, we have systematically compared kinematic laws and functional anatomy with our own observations. In addition, we have studied the neurovascular anatomy of the knee, and have concluded our clinical and scientific research with a careful analysis of each operative procedure, including an evaluation of the postoperative course and outcome.

We reiterate Kaplan's [166] four prerequisites of an adequate surgical approach to the knee joint:

1. Precise knowledge of the anatomy of the region.
2. Selection of the most direct exposure of the structures requiring surgical treatment.
3. Rapid orientation, if extension of the original incision proves necessary.
4. Consideration of immediate and final postoperative function with minimal sacrifice of structures consistent with the requirements of the operation.

Vessels and Nerves

It is well known that structures deprived of their blood supply cannot carry out their normal function. Moreover, unless the structures are revascularized and given an opportunity for recovery, they will succumb to necrosis.

Similarly, structures that are deprived of their nerve supply fail to produce or transmit necessary reflexes, causing them to become excluded from the functional sequences to which they normally contribute.

The nerves also perform an important trophic function; together with the vessels, they are essential for a good result. This is why we place such emphasis on their atraumatic handling during operations.

Nerves and vessels tend to occur in areas that are subject to little relative movement, and with good reason: If they were to cross layers that move much relative to surrounding structures, they would be constantly folding and unfolding like an accordion. Instead, they course through muscles, bones, ligaments and tendons in areas where these structures are subject to the least movement relative to surrounding tissues, or where the surrounding soft tissues move the least relative to bones and joints. Therefore, natural discontinuities where tissue layers glide freely past each other provide ideal avenues of approach from the standpoint of avoiding neurovascular trauma.

The extent of a surgical operation is not necessarily a measure of its traumatization. A small "transverse" incision will sever many more important structures than will a longitudinal approach along natural discontinuities, which allows the surgeon to go in quite deep without having to divide a nerve or vessel.

Neurogenic Osteoarthropathy ("Charcot's Joint")

A joint that has lost its deep sensation and fine proprioceptive control is subject to a chronic degenerative process like that associated with various neurologic disorders. Diabetic neurogenic osteoarthropathy affects mainly the lower limbs, whereas syringomyelia with a loss of sensation in the upper limbs can precipitate an osteoarthrolytic process in the elbow joint. The knee, like the elbow, is a joint between long bony lever arms.

The knee joint is also subject to occasional severe postoperative deterioration of unclear etiology. In most cases this change bears no relation to prior trauma or residual instability. It is very similar in its osteolytic component to the changes associated with the neuroprival osteoarthropathies.

Fortunately we have not had to deal with such cases as yet, and so we are unable to correlate them with our operative procedures and evaluate them analytically. However, we share the opinion of other surgeons that these osteoarthropathies are referable to disturbances of nervous function, and this is why we take special care to spare the nerves at operation.

The Vascular Anastomosis Around the Knee Joint

The arterial anastomosis about the knee has a relatively simple structure. Proximal to the joint space the popliteal artery gives off the medial and lateral superior genicular arteries, and distal to the joint space it gives off the medial and lateral inferior genicular arteries. All four arteries pass forward, enveloping the knee and forming the rete articulare genus in front of the patella.

The anterior tibial recurrent artery rises laterally from the anterior compartment to join the anastomosis (Fig. 198).

Finally, the middle genicular artery arises directly from the popliteal artery in the popliteal fossa between the superior and inferior genicular branches and passes into the joint. It supplies the important "central pivot" of the cruciate ligaments and the posterior capsule. Two of its branches run medially and laterally forward about the periphery of the menisci to communicate again with the anterior anastomosis at the level of the anterior meniscal horns.

The anterior arterial anastomosis has *two layers:* one is situated *superficial to* the prepatellar bursa, if present, and the second is situated *deep to* this bursa, directly in and closely upon the galea aponeurotica of the patella with the adjacent patellar retinacula.

The first of these two layers, which lies in and upon the superficial fascia, is responsible for cutaneous circulation. If it is at all damaged when skin flaps are developed, the dreaded prepatellar skin necrosis will result.

The main arterial supply vessels do not run superficially near the cutis, but course directly on the basal layer of the subcutis, the superficial fascia. This circumstance must be taken into account during all skin incisions in orthopedic surgery, but particularly those which may jeopardize healing.

Consequently, *subcutaneous dissection must be avoided.* Only if the superficial fascia is left attached to the subcutis will the superficial arterial network remain intact, allowing wound healing to proceed undisturbed.

In many cases this layer is also the *subfascial prepatellar bursa,* which is of no significance for the postoperative course. In the great majority of cases there is no true subcutaneous or subfascial prepatellar bursa –

159

only a weblike, very loose and practically avascular connective tissue layer which, like the bursa, enables the necessary relative movement between structures.

If a prepatellar bursa is present, it may be *subcutaneous* or *subfascial*. The subcutaneous bursa should *not* be used as a surgical access layer, for the attendant risk of damage to the cutaneous vessels is too great. In doubtful cases access should be sought beneath the fascia.

Two fasciae may also be present: the *superficial* genicular fascia and, in a deep layer, the *anterior* genicular fascia. The deep layer should always serve as the avenue of approach.

layers (the obturator nerve with its terminal branches, the tibial nerve, peroneal nerve, saphenous nerve and branches from the vastus lateralis, vastus intermedius and vastus medialis muscles).

The most important branch to be identified on the medial side is the 1-mm-thick medial articular nerve (n. articularis proprius genus medialis), which descends across the adductor tubercle, closely overlies the proximal attachment of the MCL along with two accompanying vessels, and continues downward and anteriorly into the joint. It has an important branch that passes deep into the joint capsule to the fat pad and below the patellar ligament to the lateral side. We

---

Hence, lateral undermining should always proceed *beneath* the superficial fascia. Flaps should be developed just superficial

to the galea aponeurotica of the patella to avoid the danger of necrosis.

Nerve Supply of the Knee Joint (Fig. 199)

1. *Femoral nerve.* On the medial side the anterior cutaneous branches of the femoral nerve descend with the vastus medialis muscle to the proximal medial quadrant of the knee joint. Above the joint space they pass across the midline to the lateral side.

2. *Saphenous nerve.* The branches of the saphenous nerve pass down the medial side of the leg, the best known being the infrapatellar branch and the medial crural cutaneous branch. They also cross the midline to supply the skin, subcutis, capsule of the knee, infrapatellar fat pad and iliotibial tract.

3. *Lateral branches:* In the proximolateral quadrant these may be branches of the lateral femoral cutaneous nerve, followed more distally by the lateral crural and lateral sural cutaneous branches. These lateral branches are far less important surgically than those on the medial side.

4. *Nerve supply of the actual joint.* All the main nerve trunks that pass the knee give off branches to the joint capsule and deeper

always expose this nerve when dissecting in the area of the proximal MCL and protect it by carefull snaring it with a rubber drain.

Medial Incisions

The Medial Parapatellar Incision

This is the basic incision for exposures on the medial side. This simple incision between the patella and medial longitudinal retinaculum, which normally ends 1 cm below the joint space so that the infrapatellar branch of the saphenous nerve is not endangered, is the most suitable approach for an arthrotomy in medial meniscus injuries or other simple indications for arthrotomy. The incision can be extended distally past the tibial tuberosity as needed, though this entails division of the twigs of the infrapatellar branch, which will result later in an area of anesthesia with dysesthetic sensations when kneeling on the tibial tuberosity.

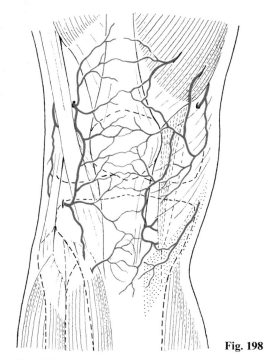

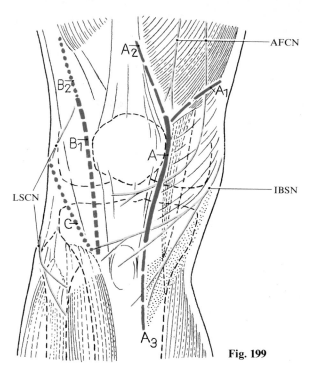

Fig. 198. Semischematic drawing of the rete articulare genus on the anterior side of the knee joint. The network is formed by arterial branches which arise both

Fig. 199. The medial or lateral (Fig. 203) parapatellar incision is favorable in terms of associated nerve disruption, for it divides the nerves near their terminations. *A* The basic medial parapatellar incision, *A1* posteromedial extension, *A2* proximal extension, *A3* distal extension; *B1* and *B2* lateral auxiliary incisions, which al-

proximal and distal to the joint line and pass forward on both the medial and lateral sides. Hence, a median incision which spares these supply vessels is preferred

low *B1→B2* or *B2→B1* modes of extension; *C* posterolateral auxiliary incision. AFCN anterior femoral cutaneous nerve branches; LBSN infrapatellar branch of sapheneous nerve; LSCN lateral sural cutaneous nerve branches

The incision may be extended proximally in two directions:
- in the direction of the quadriceps tendon and as far up the thigh as needed,
- posteromedially along the border of the vastus medialis muscle.

These extensions (see Fig. 199) can provide access to any point on the medial side of the knee back to the semimembranosus corner and even to the tibial attachment of the posterior cruciate ligament. Following direct entry into the knee joint (Fig. 200, straight arrow), the surgeon dissects back below the superficial fascia. Often it is difficult to separate the layers in the area of the longitudinal and transverse patellar retinacula, but by moving farther medially it should be possible to get below the fascia

and reach the collateral ligament structures without difficulty. If the approach proves difficult and it is anticipated that further exposure will be needed in the area of the semimembranosus corner, the bony insertion of the pes anserinus should be detached for a length of about 3–4 cm and width of 0.75 to at most 1 cm (Fig. 201). This is necessary because the superficial fascia blends directly with the pes anserinus layer. If the dissection is carried medially beneath this layer, it will pass safely below the entire neurovascular supply of the flap with the subcutaneous tissue (Fig. 201).

Caution is advised when chiseling off the pes anserinus attachment in situ, for its area of insertion is small and very close to the distal attachment of the medial collateral liga-

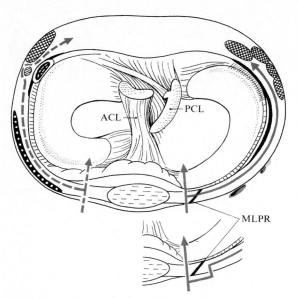

Fig. 200. Transverse section through the knee joint just proximal to the menisci. The lateral parapatellar approach, combined with distal detachment of the iliotibial tract at the tubercle of Gerdy, provides good access to the LCL, biceps tendon, popliteus tendon and arcuate ligament. The medial parapatellar approach below the superficial fascia provides access to the semimembranosus tendon, POL and medial gastrocnemius border along a plane containing few nerves and blood vessels. The major veins, arteries and nerves course external to the fascia, which therefore should be left attached to the subcutaneous tissue. If there is much fusion between the medial longitudinal patellar retinaculum and fascia, the latter is divided parallel to its fibers and retracted; it is repaired at the end of the operation

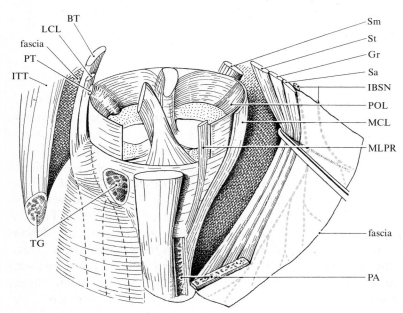

Fig. 201. The major ligaments are located on the medial, posteromedial and posterolateral sides of the knee. Considerable dissection is needed for adequate exposure. On the lateral side this is obtained by detachment of the tubercle of Gerdy (Fig. 200). On the medial side, access to the MCL and semimembranosus corner is gained by detaching the pes anserinus insertion and reflecting the pes tendons and fascial flap. The twigs of the infrapatellar branch of the saphenous nerve as well as the arterial and venous vascular system lie outside the reflected fascial flap

ment. We first isolate the pes anserinus tendons by inserting an elevator between them and the MCL at the attachment of the MLPR and passing it down to the *insertion of the tendons,* so that *it alone* can be chiseled free. When the tendons are retracted and the MCL is seen, there should be no difficulty in advancing bluntly to the semimembranosus and border of the gastrocnemius. The MCL/POL system can now be easily inspected. Exposure can be maintained with Hohmann retractors on the semimembranosus muscle and tendon on the posterior tibial plateau and in the region of the adductor tubercle on the femur (taking care not to injure the medial articular nerve; Fig. 202). The more the knee is flexed in this position, the more the medial retracted structures are relaxed, allowing the surgeon to get as far back as the posterior cruciate attachment to the tibia without tension (this may prove necessary in the case of large tears). As long as one keeps close to the bone and joint capsule in such a situation, there is no danger of injury to popliteal structures. In any case these structures are lax when the knee is flexed and so are not especially prone to injury.

Figure 202 shows the course of the medial articular nerve in the operative field as well as the line of incision at the posterior edge of the POL that must be used if further posterior access is required. This may be the case in unclear meniscus lesions with detachment of the posterior horn or during the repair of old injuries where there is no existing traumatic aperture in the semimembranosus corner. At the end of the operation the pes anserinus insertion can be reattached with two small-fragment cortical bone screws and washers securely enough that no postoperative immobilization is required.

Secondary Posterior Incision to Supplement a Minimal Medial Parapatellar Approach

If a detached posterior horn makes it necessary to employ a secondary incision, the skin is incised proximal from the tibial attachment of the semimembranosus, parallel to the pes anserinus tendons, taking care to locate and spare the saphenous nerve and its branches. Then the fascia is divided parallel to its fibers, and the underlying posterior edge of the POL is bluntly dissected free, the incision now proceeding in the same manner as after detachment of the pes anserinus (Fig. 202).

Lateral Incisions

The Lateral Parapatellar Incision

Running parallel to the patellar ligament and anterior to the course of the iliotibial tract, this incision is far less traumatizing to the nerves than the medial approach (Figs. 199 and 203). Operations on the lateral side also have a much smaller incidence of troublesome and painful neuromas than on the medial side, where such lesions can often be a real problem.

The lateral incision may be extended as needed proximally in the direction of the iliotibial tract or the quadriceps muscle. As Fig. 203 shows, it may also be extended as far distally as needed in front of the anterior compartment lateral to the anterior border of the tibia.

The Lateral Incision as a Supplement to a Medial Approach

This secondary incision is placed at the posterior border of the iliotibial tract (Fig. 199) and allows access to the posterior femoral condyle and metaphyseal shaft of the femur for proximal reinsertion of the anterior cruciate ligament. The lateral portion of the joint anterior to the popliteus tendon can also be readily inspected through this incision.

If it is necessary to expose the deep structures of the lateral side, as for example in a complex posterolateral injury, the tubercle of Gerdy (Fig. 201) with the attachment of the iliotibial tract is chiseled from the tibia. To avoid weakening of the femorotibial por-

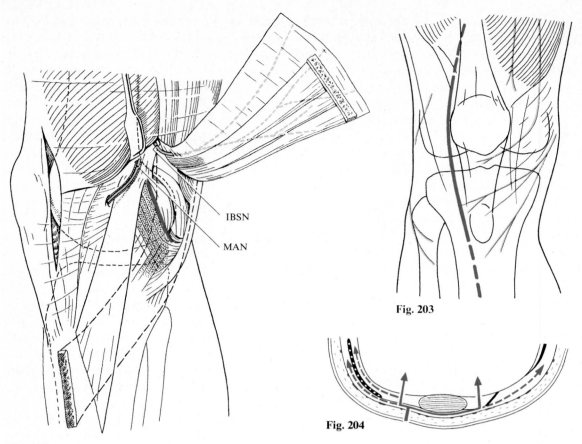

Fig. 202

IBSN

MAN

Fig. 203

Fig. 204

Fig. 202. The medial capsuloligamentous structures, as demonstrated by detachment of the pes anserinus and reflection of the associated fascial flap. The medial longitudinal patellar retinaculum has been left intact. From the adductor tendon the medial articular nerve (MAN) with its two accompanying vessels courses over the femoral attachment of the MCL, disappears anterior to the MCL into the deep capsular layers, and continues into the soft tissues of the anterior half of the joint. If an additional arthrotomy is necessary behind the MCL, it must be done at the posterior edge of the POL

Fig. 203. The lateral parapatellar incision, which may be extended proximally or distally as needed, avoids troublesome sensory losses in front of the patella and tibial tuberosity

Fig. 204. From the lateral parapatellar incision, the fascia is divided in the same direction as the skin. The approach can be carried medially or laterally beneath the fascia, and access can be gained for a medial or lateral arthrotomy or for operations on the semimembranosus or popliteus corner. Lateral structures may be approached either *over* the iliotibial tract or *beneath* it (e.g., after detachment of the tubercle of Gerdy)

Fig. 205. Trickey's posterior approach to the knee. The skin incision crosses the popliteal flexion crease in a curving, oblique fashion. Following blunt separation of the medial and lateral muscles, the blood vessels are retracted to the side with the lateral muscle group. The medial head of the gastrocnemius is transversely sectioned in its tendinous origin on the medial femoral condyle in such a way that the neurovascular bundle supplying the medial gastrocnemius is preserved and the muscle can later be easily resutured to the proximal tendon stump. The capsule is incised vertically next to the medial femoral condyle, at the same time dividing the oblique popliteal ligament. This affords direct access to the posterior cruciate ligament, which is sometimes difficult to reach by any other route

Fig. 206. Transverse section through the knee joint at the level of the femoral condyles. The *solid red arrow* represents the approach of Trickey [345]. The *dashed arrows* indicate how the semimembranosus and popliteus corner can also be reached in this situation

164

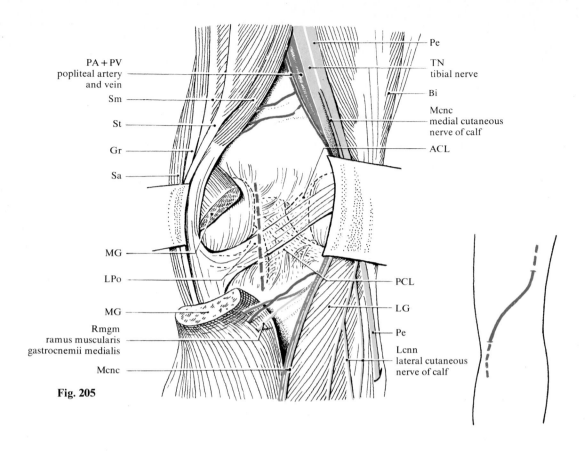

PA + PV
popliteal artery
and vein

Sm

St

Gr

Sa

MG

LPo

MG

Rmgm
ramus muscularis
gastrocnemii medialis

Mcnc

Fig. 205

Pe

TN
tibial nerve

Bi

Mcnc
medial cutaneous
nerve of calf

ACL

PCL

LG

Pe

Lcnn
lateral cutaneous
nerve of calf

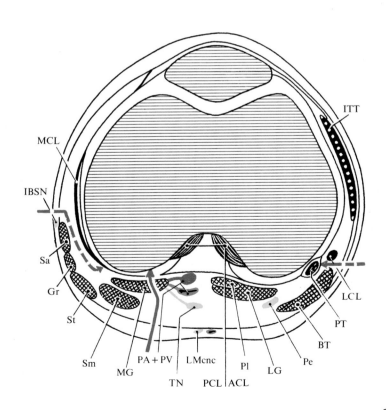

ITT

MCL

IBSN

Sa

Gr

St

LCL

PT

BT

Sm

MG

PA + PV

LMcnc

TN

PCL

ACL

Pl

LG

Pe

Fig. 206

165

tion of the iliotibial tract after refixation, the osteotomy must be carried out *directly below the coronary ligament of the meniscus.* In this way the detached bone fragment will include all the femorotibial fibers, and it will be unnecessary later to cut these all-important tract fibers from the upper tibia with a knife.

Below the flap thus raised, the extremely thin joint capsule can be incised anterior to the popliteus tendon. The entire fibular collateral ligament is now freely accessible and can be sutured at any level. The arcuate ligament complex can also be well visualized.

Replacement of the detached tubercle of Gerdy should present no difficulties at the conclusion of the operation. If the iliotibial tract is under much tension, it can be fixed temporarily with one or two 1.4-mm Kirschner wires before the fragment is definitively reattached with one or two small-fragment cortical bone screws and washers.

In some cases it is possible to leave the entire iliotibial tract in place, gaining access to deeper structures by incising along its anterior and posterior borders.

Lateral Long Parapatellar Incision

Figs. 203 and 204 show the topographic reference points for this type of incision. The more experience we have gained in knee operations, the more we have come to rely on this single long incision, even in cases where medial *and* lateral structures have to be repaired in the same operation. We have found that despite the length of the approach, a generally better result is obtained than with a primary medial incision combined with a secondary lateral incision – the major advantages being unaltered sensation in the anterior region of the knee and better trophism. However, one prerequisite in this approach is absolute respect for the superficial arterial network (see section on Vascular and Nerve Supply, p. 158, and Fig. 204).

If surgical scars exist from prior operations, we use this incision if possible in order to avoid zones of poor trophism between old

and new incisions and the attendant risk of necrosis. Short scars from earlier operations, as after a meniscectomy, do not represent an absolute obstacle to the broad lateral parapatellar approach.

Closure of the lateral incision requires careful drainage with Redon drains in all four quadrants of the operative field in order to avoid hematoma formation in the large cavities that have been created. The superficial fascia, which has been divided parallel to the line of the main incision, is closed with a continuous or interrupted Dexon suture of size 0–00. Without this tension-relieving fascial suture, the skin suture would come under too much tension, and subcutaneous hematomas could develop with tension necrosis of the wound edges and subsequent gaping.

Posterior Approach to the Knee Joint

The direct posterior approaches through the popliteal fossa have a higher incidence of postoperative complications such as hematomas, thromboses and disturbances of wound healing, and are more prone to the development of contractures, than are the anterior approaches.

In contrast to straight incisions on the extensor surface, incisions on the flexor surface must be S-shaped and must run either parallel or oblique to the popliteal fold, inasmuch as perpendicular incisions can cause flexion contractures.

The posterior incision for the knee was described by Abbott and Carpenter [1] and refined by Trickey [345], which is why the incision is often called the Trickey approach (Figs. 205 and 206).

The extended incision crosses the popliteal area diagonally in an S-shaped fashion, running either from proximomedial to distolateral [1] or from proximolateral to distomedial [345]. One must proceed carefully in the subcutaneous tissue to avoid nerve and vascular injury. Generally the medial sural cutaneous nerve is encountered first, running outside the fascia. Usually the fascia is divided, and the medial head of the gastrocnemius and its lateral border are reached by

166

blunt dissection. Special care must be taken with the neurovascular supply of the medial head of the gastrocnemius. The site of nerve entry is located only a few centimeters distal to the origin of the medial muscle belly on the femur or even at the level of the joint space in many cases.

As soon as the neurovascular status of the gastrocnemius head has been clarified, the medial head is cut in its tendinous portion behind the femoral condyle about 1 cm from the bone to permit an easy resuture. Now it will be easy to retract the important structures medially and laterally and incise the posterior capsule vertically just lateral to the medial femoral condyle and medial to the posterior cruciate ligament. It will be recalled that the cruciate ligaments are located not intraarticularly, but in a keel-shaped projection of the popliteal space. Therefore an incision placed too far laterally will enter not the joint but the cruciate ligament complex. Corresponding caution is advised during the dissection, for just lateral to the site of incision the middle genicular artery also enters the central pivot as its only major supplying vessel.

Because this approach has its pitfalls and does not allow access to the joint periphery, we rarely use it. In the great majority of cases the main approaches described earlier provide sufficient access to the popliteal space that we are able to reach the tibial attachment of the posterior cruciate ligament with little difficulty from both the lateral and medial sides. From the medial approach one can advance bluntly from the semimembranosus tendon and its insertions in the direction of the posterior tibial surface, easily reaching the belly of the soleus and popliteus muscles. The tibia and the indentation with the attachment of the posterior cruciate ligament can be easily felt with the palpating finger. If necessary the medial head of the gastrocnemius can be incised in its tendinous portion above the femoral condyle until adequate access is obtained for suturing or screw fixation (Trillat, personal communication).

Carefully placed Redon suction drainage is also necessary with the posterior Trickey approach, so that a hematoma will not delay healing, and contractures will not form as a result of scar contraction.

167

The Primary Repair of Special Injuries

Injuries of the Medial Side and Their Repair

General

Both Hughston [in 140] and Trillat et al. [359] have sought sites of predilection for ligament tears in the medial capsuloligamentous triangle.

Chambart [in 359] found the following prevalences in 44 consecutive cases:

50% – proximal rupture at the femur
33% – distal rupture at the tibia and
17% – rupture in the intermediate to posterior region.

Hughston [in 140] found these prevalences in his evaluation of 50 consecutive cases:

20% – isolated rupture of the MCL at the femur
56% – isolated rupture of the MCL at the tibia
24% – probable combined proximal and distal or mid-third rupture
40% – rupture of deep meniscofemoral fibers
42% – rupture of deep meniscotibial fibers
10% – rupture of deep meniscofemoral and meniscotibial fibers
 6% – rupture of deep intermediate fibers
 2% – overstretching of deep meniscofemoral fibers
12% – rupture of the POL at the femur
34% – rupture of the POL at the tibia
14% – rupture of the POL in the intermediate region
18% – rupture of the POL with the posterior capsule
 8% – overstretching of the POL (interstitial tear)
14% – intact POL.

The 8% of cases with overstretching of the POL and 14% with an intact POL appear to correspond to the 20% of cases reported by Chambat [in 359] in which the ligament was not ruptured, but was found to be overstretched with bloody imbition and edema. Presumably these cases involved slow distensions with first- to second-degree lesions. Objectification is difficult in such cases and relies in part on personal judgment.

The relatively high percentage of MCL tears from the tibia reported by Hughston [in 140] may be due to the large proportion of football injuries in his material, whereas the injuries evaluated by Trillat [359] had more diverse causes (see also p. 190).

The Normal Medial Aspect

Figures 207 and 208 show the normal medial structures of the knee. Depending on the angle of flexion, some 40% of the MCL and almost the entire POL are covered by the pes anserinus! Over 80% of the most important ligamentous structures are located in the posterior half of the medial side of the joint. Kaplan [167] writes that repair of the collateral ligament cannot restore full stability unless the semimembranosus expansion is also repaired. If one does not wish to detach the bony insertion of the pes anserinus, it may be sufficient, depending on the extent and complexity of the injury, to open the fascial space (parallel to the fiber course) between the longitudinal retinaculum and the proximal anterior border of the pes anserinus, taking care to spare the saphenous nerve branches (Fig. 207).

When the pes anserinus is raised, we also divide a portion of the fascia in the same layer at the posterior edge of the medial longitudinal retinaculum and reflect the flap upward. In Fig. 209 the reflection of the pes anserinus and fascia is exaggerated to show the complex of the semimembranosus corner in its entirety. In reality we maintain continuity between the pes anserinus fascia and the more distal crural fascia in order to preserve the advantage of the subfascial approach with regard to the avoidance of nerve trauma.

At the upper edge of the operative field the medial articular nerve descends over the proximal attachment of the MCL. The pas-

sage of this nerve over the ligament insertion explains why the MCL lesion is most painful over the adductor tubercle of the medial femoral condyle. This fact often masks the presence of coexisting distal lesions of the ligament. The degree of local tenderness is not a reliable indicator of the extent of a ligamentous lesion in this area.

The following figures show only the deep capsuloligamentous structures and semi-membranosus expansion, with the pes an-

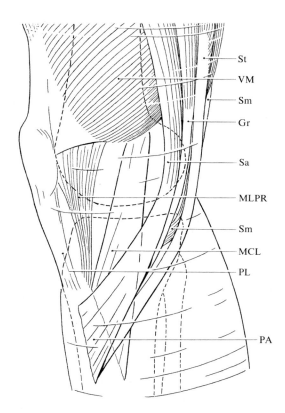

Fig. 207. Cross-section just proximal to the menisci showing the principal medial layers

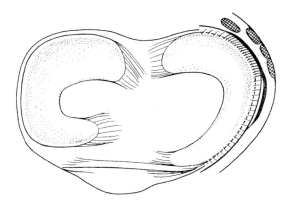

Fig. 208. The medial aspect of the knee joint with its anatomic structures

169

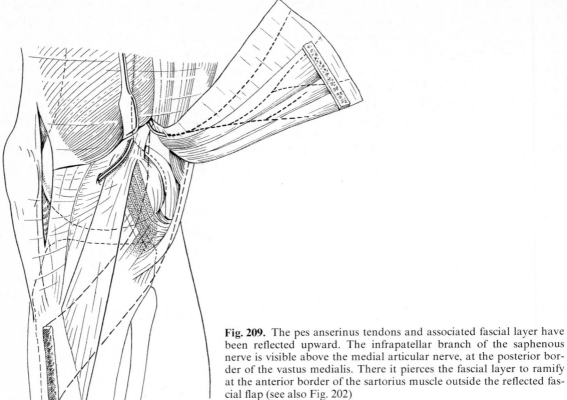

Fig. 209. The pes anserinus tendons and associated fascial layer have been reflected upward. The infrapatellar branch of the saphenous nerve is visible above the medial articular nerve, at the posterior border of the vastus medialis. There it pierces the fascial layer to ramify at the anterior border of the sartorius muscle outside the reflected fascial flap (see also Fig. 202)

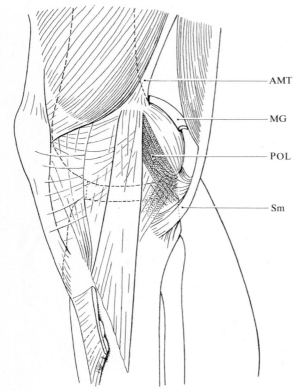

AMT

MG

POL

Sm

Fig. 210. The medial aspect of the knee joint, showing only the passive stabilizing elements

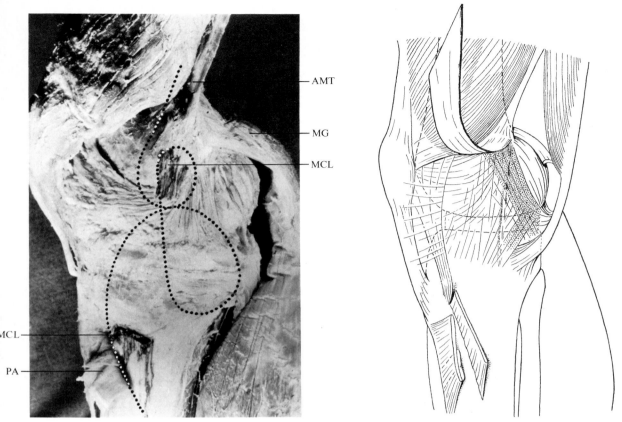

Labels on figure: AMT, MG, MCL (right side); MCL, PA (left side)

Fig. 211. Anatomic preparation of the deep femorotibial capsule with its ligamentous and fibrous structure. The MCL was removed to demonstrate the underlying structures. The Burmester curve is shown in its approximate location. Note the absence of femorotibial fibers anterior to this curve. All fibers which lie anterior to the crossing point of the curve have attachment with the patella and the quadriceps extensor apparatus. This enables them to maintain isometry during flexion, for the patella and quadriceps apparatus follow the posterior shift of the femur during each flexion movement. A knowledge of this fiber architecture is essential for the suturing techniques described below (v. Hochstetter)

Fig. 212. Semischematic representation of the deep layer (Fig. 211) in its topographic relationship to more superficial neighboring structures. The MCL is schematically divided near its distal attachment and reflected upward. The POL is *stippled* to set it off from the deep fibers. The line of fusion between these two ligaments is indicated by a *double dashed line*

serinus and fascia removed. Figure 210 shows the typical fiber architecture of the deep femorotibial layer, corresponding to the anatomic specimen in Fig. 211, on which the Burmester curve is superimposed. The photo clearly shows that no femoromeniscal ligamentous fibers can exist anterior to the Burmester curve; all capsuloligamentous elements located anterior to this curve have attachment with the transverse retinaculum.

In Fig. 212 the MCL is reflected upward to demonstrate the deepest femorotibial ligamentous structures. The various types of tear

described below are, except for the isolated tear, always combined with a rupture of the MCL. Tears of the MCL itself are discussed at the end of the section (Figs. 221 and 222).

Tears of the Deep Layer and the POL

Diagonal Tear, Posterosuperior to Anteroinferior

This tear is perhaps the easiest to recognize, causing medial opening of the joint space in

171

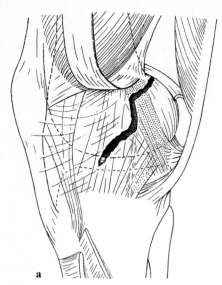

a

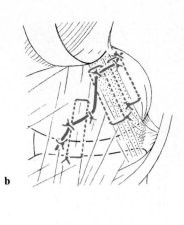

b

Fig. 213a, b. The posterosuperior-to-anteroinferior diagonal tear. **a** This tear of the deep layer and POL is frequently observed in complex medial ligamentous injuries. **b** Technique of suture repair

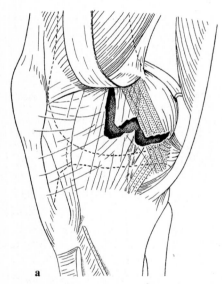

a

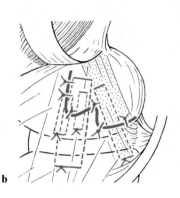

b

Fig. 214a, b. The anterosuperior-to-posteroinferior diagonal tear. **a** A common form limited to the femoromeniscal fibers. **b** Repair with overlapping tension sutures in the most severely stretched portions of the ligament

both flexion and extension. It represents the detachment of the entire posterior capsular plate (Fig. 213a). It begins with a tear below the gastrocnemius muscle, or through the muscle in extreme cases, and extends along the femur beneath the MCL and diagonally down through the capsule to the level of the joint space. It extends no farther anteriorally, because there are no more true femorotibial ligamentous connections beyond that point. Figure 213 shows the tear repaired with approximating sutures and tension sutures aligned with the local fiber axis and stress lines.

172

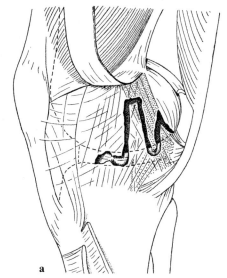

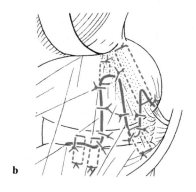

Fig. 215a, b. The zigzag tab tear. **a** This tear is often difficult to identify and repair, because the tabs are often tangled and separated from one another. The tears may extend across the meniscus to involve the meniscotibial fibers. **b** Technique of suture repair

Diagonal Tear, Anterosuperior to Posteroinferior

Figure 214a shows a diagonal tear of the femoromeniscal ligament fibers. The instability is similar to that caused by the tear described above, except that the present tear runs almost perpendicular to the first. The suturing technique is essentially the same. The tension sutures overlap and restore a normal length to the ligamentous structures (Fig. 214b).

The Zigzag Tab Tear

Tears running in zigzag fashion through the entire capsuloligamentous apparatus are more difficult to assess (Fig. 215a). Especially if the injury is not recent, it is often difficult to identify the ligamentous tab and reapproximate it correctly. In most cases, however, the tabs are more or less parallel to the main axis of the POL. This has an important bearing on the approximating sutures in Fig. 215b and on the placement of the tension sutures.

The Zigzag Tab Tear as Part of an Anteromedial Combined Injury

Figures 216a, d, e, show stages in an operation for a triad injury of the ACL, MCL and POL. The ACL is ruptured. An "over the top" repositioning suture for this tear is seen running through the intercondylar notch. Figures 216b, d, f, h show corresponding schematic drawings of the structures seen in the photos. Essentially the injury involves a tab tear like that shown in Fig. 217. Viewing these figures, it is easy to see why a meniscus injury was regarded as the third component of the "unhappy triad" of O'Donoghue. In reality a meniscectomy in such cases is unnecessary and even contraindicated, for the meniscus can be restored to its normal position and securely anchored without damage. The views in Fig. 216e, f confirm that the injury is purely ligamentous. In Figs. 216g and h the reflected flap of the POL is seen through a longitudinally-split MCL whose posterior portion is torn from the femur. The secondary closing sutures for the MCL are schematically shown.

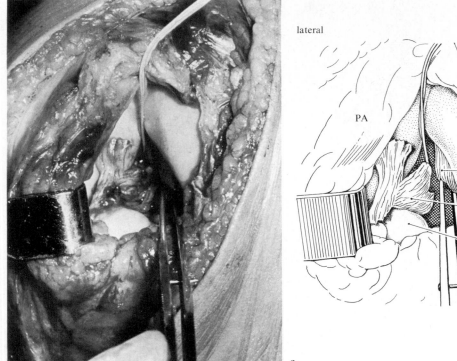

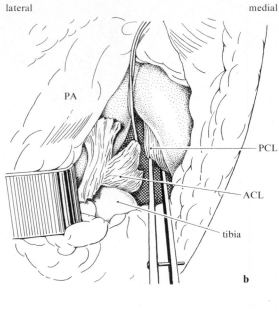

lateral   medial

PA

PCL

ACL

tibia

b

a

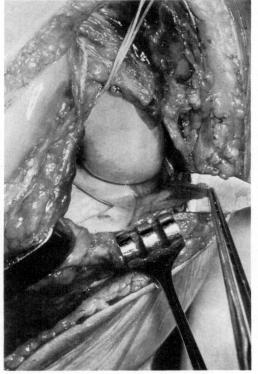

lateral

medial
MFC
medial femoral condyle

MM

POL

d

c

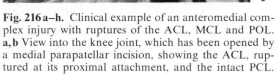

Fig. 216a–h. Clinical example of an anteromedial complex injury with ruptures of the ACL, MCL and POL. **a,b** View into the knee joint, which has been opened by a medial parapatellar incision, showing the ACL, ruptured at its proximal attachment, and the intact PCL.

c,d Another view through the same incision clearly showing the incarcerated meniscus on the tibial plateau in front of the femoral condyle. It is obvious that there is no true tear in the cartilaginous substance of the meniscus, but that the *ligamentous attachment* of the meniscus

174

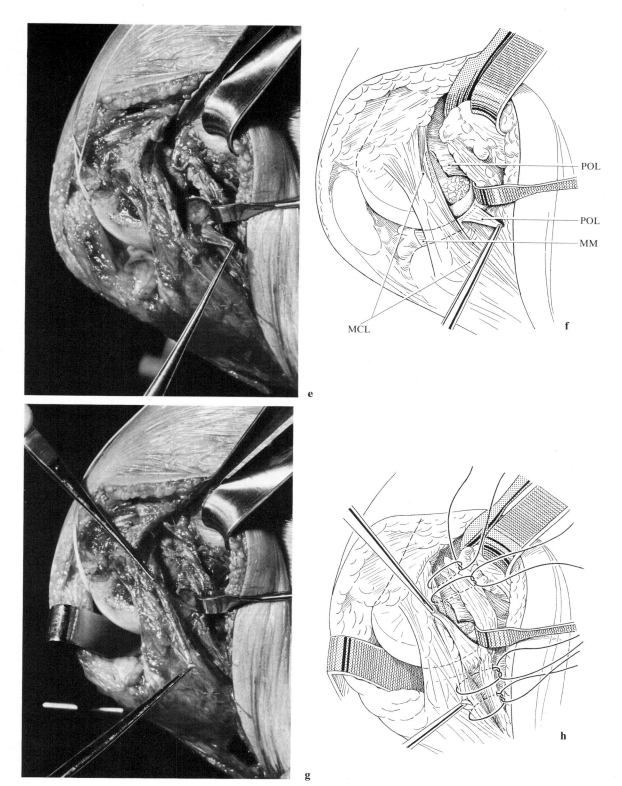

e

f

POL

POL

MM

MCL

h

g

has been avulsed, allowing luxation of the meniscus into the joint. **e, f** The same knee joint viewed from the side, showing the replaced meniscus and attached portion of the POL. After reduction of the meniscus the articular surfaces are again in proper relation, and the un-

damaged meniscus can be fully reintegrated by the peripheral repair. **g, h** The POL flap reflected with the *forceps* is sutured back into the associated deep layer before the preplaced approximating sutures in the superficial layer are tied

175

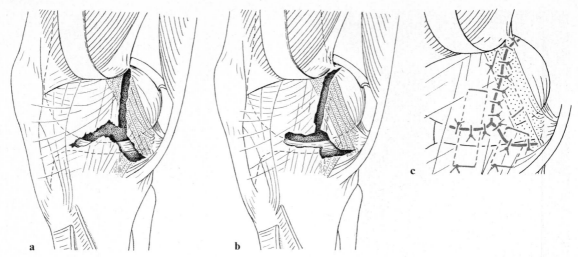

Fig. 217 a–c. The Y tear. **a,b** One limb of this tear may run horizontally and thus involve the peripheral menis-cal attachment with no damage to the meniscus itself. **c** Technique of suture repair for this type of Y tear

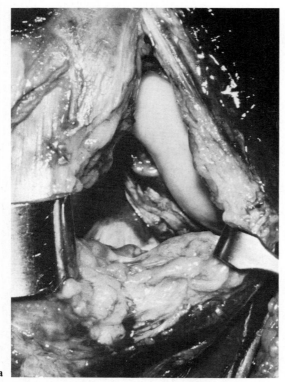

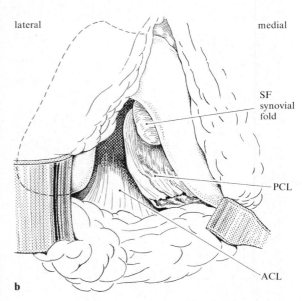

Fig. 218 a–f. Clinical example of a posterosuperior-to-anteroinferior diagonal tear in a posteromedial complex injury with ruptures of the MCL, POL and PCL. **a,b** View into the injured joint through a medial para-patellar incision. The ACL is intact, while the PCL is torn at its distal attachment and displaced forward be-tween the tibia and femur. A synovial fold (sf) belonging to the central pivot is swollen and prominent. **c,d** View of the lacerated ligaments of the medial side after de-tachment of the pes anserinus insertion. The medial ar-ticular nerve with its vascular bundle has been snared with a rubber strip and raised. * The denuded femoral condyle is visible through the tear below the articular nerve. **e,f** General view of the same aspect. The *clamp on the right* retracts the torn MCL while the stump of the POL, which has been torn from the femur, is pulled forward with the *two forceps*

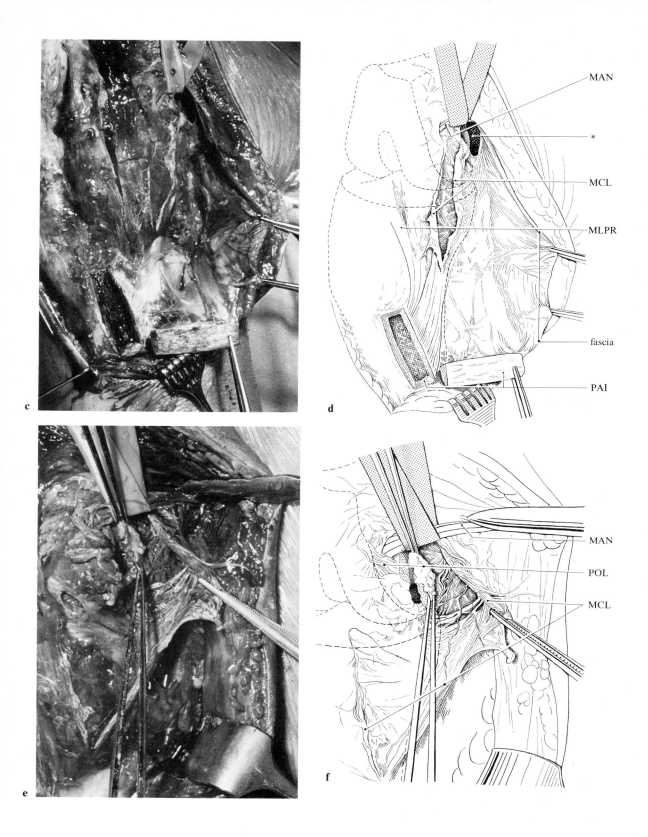

c

d

MAN

*

MCL

MLPR

fascia

PAI

e

f

MAN

POL

MCL

177

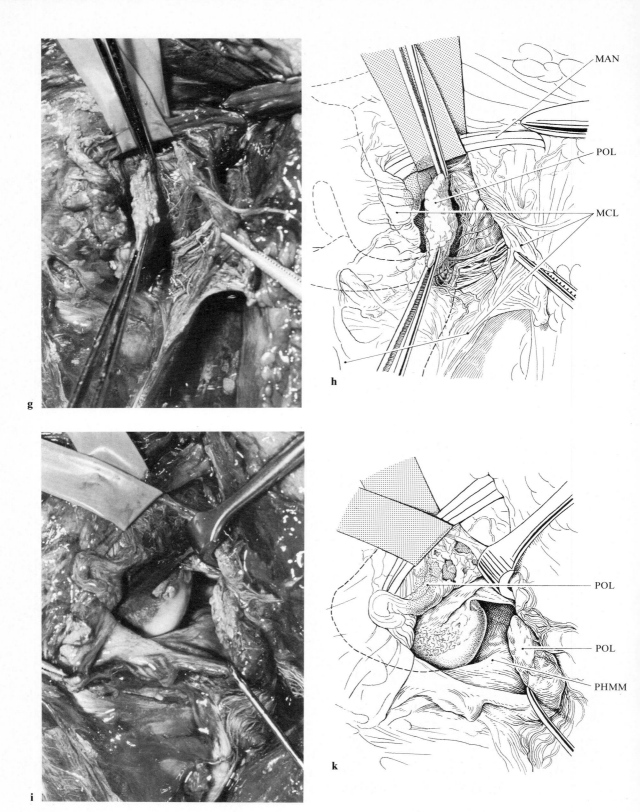

Fig. 218 g–k. On closer inspection the POL is seen even more clearly. It appears as a firm, well-defined ligament next to the tangle of torn and overstretched collagenous fiber bundles. The *stippled area* represents its approxi-

mate site of reinsertion on the femur. **i, k** Posteromedial view into the joint. The *hook at lower right* retracts the POL to demonstrate the posterior femoral condyle and posterior horn of the meniscus

178

The Y Tear

Tears that are Y-shaped or take an irregular forked course are not unusual. Such situations are deceptive, for the suturing of only two of the three limbs of the tear cannot restore stability. Usually the surgeon must examine the tear carefully in order to locate the third limb.

It is no coincidence that one of the limbs points toward the fixed point at the attachment of the semimembranosus, while another extends anteriorly. The distinctive feature of these lesions is the possibility of peripheral denudation of the meniscus. In the present case (Fig. 217a) the posterior part of the tear must be well repaired to prevent anteromedial instability.

The Y Tear with Meniscal Detachment

It is a small step from the situation in Fig. 217a to that in 217b. With more extensive denudation of the meniscus, even a purely ligamentous injury can produce a bucket-handle tear located not in the cartilage, as in the classic form, but in the fibroligamentous periphery of the meniscus. In contrast to a classic meniscus tear in the region of the cartilaginous degenerative zone, a meniscus torn from its ligamentous periphery should be carefully reattached. It is particularly important that the annular meniscotibial fibers of the coronary ligament be well repaired; absorbable suture material is especially good for this purpose. Only parts of the meniscus that are torn in the cartilaginous substance need be resected, taking care that the circumferential ring of ligamentous fibers is preserved for further ligament reconstruction and can be reintegrated into the ligament system. The suturing technique is illustrated in Fig. 217c. Note that the meniscotibial tension suture on the right is angled back anteriorly to conform to the course of the meniscotibial fibers of the POL (see also Figs. 210 and 212).

The Posterosuperior-to-Anteroinferior Diagonal Tear as Part of a Posteromedial Combined Injury

Figures 218a–k show a posteromedial combined injury of the triad type with tears of the PCL, MCL and POL. This injury is much rarer than the triad with avulsion of the anterior cruciate, but improved methods of examination are leading more frequently to its diagnosis and surgical repair. Figure 218b shows the intact anterior cruciate ligament rising into the intercondylar notch, and the posterior cruciate ligament, which is torn from its tibial attachment and reflected forward. A swollen, edematous synovial fold is visible on the roof of the intercondylar notch. Figures 218c, d show the approach with the pes anserinus detached and provide an overview of the entire medial and posteromedial ligament system. Figures 218e, f present a detail view showing how powerful the POL can be. In the present case the MCL is rather badly disrupted and is torn mainly in its proximal portion. Some of its anterior fibers are also torn from the tibia and lie crumpled in front of the rubber band. Figures 218g, h show how the POL is drawn forward and upward for repositioning.

The ligamentous injury shown here is so extensive that the retractor can be inserted far into the pocket of the posterior condylar plate, exposing it down to the bed of the meniscus (Figs. 218i, k). The femur itself exhibits a large denuded area from which all the femoromeniscal and many of the femorotibial fibers have been avulsed.

The two clinical cases of complex injuries depicted are interesting in several respects. On the one hand, they document the synergism of the semimembranosus corner with both the anterior and posterior cruciate ligaments. In both cases there is a concomitant tear of the MCL which completes the triad, and in both cases the MCL is longitudinally split and frayed.

Both series of figures also show that different mechanisms of injury result in correspondingly different combinations of in-

179

juries: A pure valgus trauma without rotation causes a medial collateral ligament lesion with or without a lesion of the semimembranosus corner. An ER injury, on the other hand, tears mainly the semimembranosus corner and anterior cruciate ligament – this before the MCL is injured.

The anteromedial triad of the first series was caused by a fall with the knee flexed and externally rotated, whereas the posteromedial triad of the second series occurred in an overweight young man who slipped and fell with the knee internally rotated.

A knowledge of functional relationships and synergisms provides valuable clues for localizing a presumed lesion in fresh as well as old injuries, and it is indispensable in planning the operation and locating the lesions during surgery.

Horizontal Tear through the Coronary Ligament

Figure 219a shows a rare type of injury in which the tear in the deep layer is limited to the coronary ligament of the meniscus and runs transversely through the entire meniscotibial attachment. The main part of

this ligamentous attachment is the angled posterior arm of the POL system that joins the meniscus with the medial surface of the upper tibia by the insertion of the semimembranosus. The tear in the coronary ligament must be systematically sutured, starting posteriorly and working toward the front; if necessary the repair is reinforced with tension sutures (Fig. 219b).

The extent of this injury may be difficult to discern, because even at operation the tear is not always obvious and often causes the patient little pain. Its surgical repair is indicated, however, because proper reconstruction offers an excellent prospect of full functional recovery, whereas a neglected tear of this type often leads to severely disabling anteromedial instability.

The Vertical Tear

Figure 220 shows a vertical tear extending through the entire posteromedial corner, accompanied by a 2nd-degree sprain of the MCL. This tear of the posterior capsule is caused mainly by excessive ER. The MCL fibers are best able to yield owing to their length and do not suffer a complete rupture.

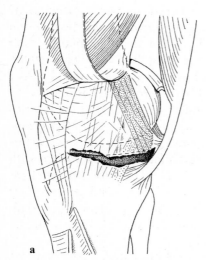

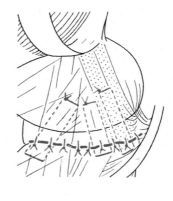

Fig. 219a,b. Horizontal tear through the coronary ligament. **a** In rare cases the tear is confined to the deep meniscotibial fibers, with complete division of the tibial fibers of the POL. **b** Repair with approximating and tension sutures; the latter extend above the rupture site to restore tension to overstretched areas

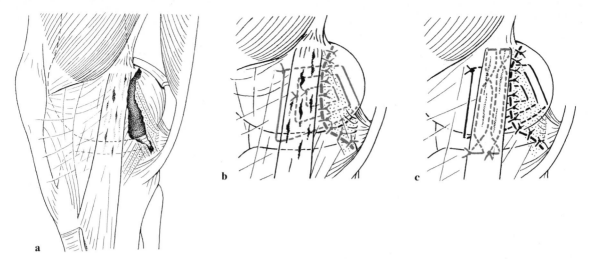

Fig. 220a–c. The vertical tear. **a** This tear through the semimembranousus corner, shown here with a typical associated injury of the MCL, reminds us that the tears discussed so far are almost always accompanied by lesions of the MCL. It is not unusual for 3rd-degree injuries of the deep layer to be accompanied by 1st- or 2nd-degree lesions of the MCL. **b** The tension suture pulls the semimembranosus corner anteriorally beneath the MCL. Often an additional tension suture must be placed to exert tension in a more anteroinferior direction. **c** Following repair of the deep layer, the MCL is repaired, here with the Bunnell suture technique

Surgical repair of this injury is essential, for it is practically always accompanied by an anterior cruciate rupture and causes severe anteromedial rotatory instability if not adequately treated. In these cases the tension sutures must be placed such that the posterior capsular plate and POL can again pass normally beneath the MCL. This suturing technique is similar to that used by Hughston and Eilers [136] in their repair of the chronically insufficient posteromedial corner (see Figs. 265–268). The next step in the surgical repair is shown in Fig. 220c, in which the MCL has also been reinforced

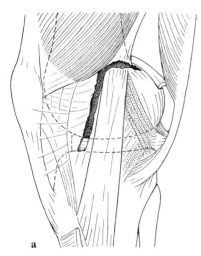

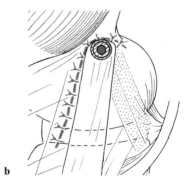

Fig. 221 a, b. The proximal global avulsion of both the MCL and POL. **a** This is the most easily repaired and most prognostically favorable of the combined medial ligamentous injuries. **b** Both ligaments can be reattached in mechanically ideal fashion with a screw and toothed washer. The remainder of the tear is repaired with approximating sutures

with tension sutures. Of course these are more superficial than the first tension sutures placed in the deep layer. According to Bunnell these sutures in the MCL often must be criss-crossed to keep them from cutting in between the longitudinal fibers and losing their effect.

Proximal Avulsion of Both Medial Ligaments

This tear usually follows an L-shaped course from the medial gastrocnemius tendon over the adductor tubercle downward and forward to the level of the joint space (Fig. 221 a). The femur is completely denuded in the area of the tear and presents a bare surface. This type of injury is most commonly associated with skiing accidents with a valgus-flexion-ER trauma. A concurrent tear of the anterior cruciate ligament is the rule.

This situation is ideal for fixation with a screw and toothed washer. After the bone is freshened, the screw and washer are placed precisely at the main insertion point of the entire medial capsuloligamentous apparatus at the adductor tubercle (Fig. 221 b). When this is combined with simple approximating sutures, postoperative ligament strength is practically normal. Functional aftercare may be instituted, provided there are no additional injuries requiring temporary immobilization of the limb.

Principal Tears of the Classic Medial Collateral Ligament

The medial collateral ligament is subject to varying degrees of sprain whenever the deep layer is injured. Because it overlies the deep layer, the tears discussed above are not as easily recognized as our schematic drawings would indicate. To gain access to the deep fibers for surgical repair, one should exploit existing tears in the MCL and avoid any additional division or traumatization of capsuloligamentous structures that are still in-

tact. This would only worsen circulatory and neurotrophic conditions and jeopardize a good end result.

After the sutures for repair of the deep layers have been definitively placed and tied, repair of the overlying MCL is begun. This is done by various techniques, according to the type of tear that is present.

The Simple or Double Z-Shaped Tear

In this injury proximal tears of some fiber bundles are combined with distal tears of others. The case shown in Fig. 222 a is a double Z tear of the MCL. The anterior and posterior fibers are torn in their proximal femoral portion, while the middle fibers are torn in their distal tibial portion. The posterior avulsed part is reattached to the bone with a screw and toothed washer at the ideal center of rotation, while the remaining, more intermediate tears are repaired with approximating and tension sutures (see also Fig. 222 b).

The Diagonal Oblique Tear

This tear typically runs from the posterosuperior edge of the ligament to the anteroinferior edge (Fig. 222 b). In the case shown the part torn near its distal attachment can be repositioned and fixed with a screw and toothed washer. The remaining parts of the tear are located in the intermediate area where the ligament must glide past the femur and tibia, and so must be repaired only with approximating and tension sutures as in Fig. 222 a.

The Intermediate Transverse Tear

In about two-thirds of cases this tear occurs at the level where the upper tibial diameter is greatest (Fig. 222 c), presumably due to a fulcrum effect at that location. Screw fixation is contraindicated at this level, for the ligament must have a free gliding path of 1–1.5 cm there during flexion-extension. Again, only approximating and tension su-

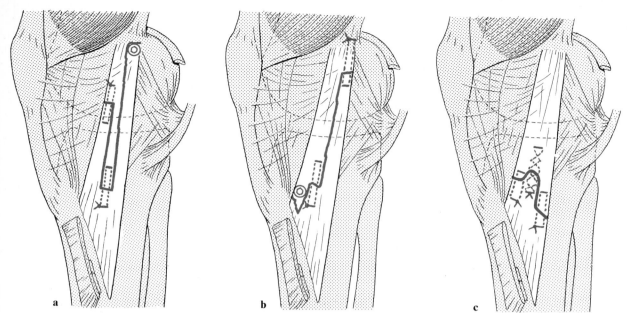

Fig. 222a–c. Tears of the medial collateral ligament. **a** The simple or double Z-shaped tear. Fibers torn at their proximal insertion can be fixed with a screw and toothed washer, as shown. Tears more distant from the insertion are repaired by suture. The approximating sutures may be reinforced with long tension sutures if necessary or desired. **b** The diagonal oblique tear. In this case the portion of the tear near the distal insertion of the ligament may still be fixed with a screw and toothed washer, but the rest of the tear must be repaired by suture to maintain physiologic movement of the MCL between the femur and tibia (see also Figs. 49 and 50). **c** The intermediate transverse tear. This tear, located between the upper border of the pes anserinus and the joint line, requires suturation (usually by the Bunnell technique) for a kinematically correct repair

tures are permitted in this region, the latter being placed by the Bunnell method. By using absorbable material, several sutures may be placed until the desired mechanical strength is achieved, without causing an accumulation of suture granulomas or late complications. It should be noted that these sutures alone are inadequate for unprotected early mobilization and functional aftercare and require additional protection from a temporary external fixation. Mobilization will depend, of course, on whether the MCL lesion is isolated or is one component of a complex injury.

Temporary Internal Splinting

Approximating sutures, which often tear easily, can be protected by temporary internal splinting with strong, nonabsorbable threads (e.g., Polydec size 3).

This is done by driving one screw each into two opposite corners of the ligament (roughly as in Fig. 222a and b). The thread is then looped around both of these "mooring posts" for 3 or 4 turns, so that a total of 6 or 8 thread lengths extend from one screw to the next. These turns encircle the necks of the screws (unthreaded!) in U-shape fashion and permit normal joint mobility on the ideal kinematic line.

If the knee joint is manipulated after the loops have been placed, it will be seen that the threads behave like the MCL, relaxing during IR and tightening during ER.

With joint motion thus guided, if possible without continuous immobilization, the microstructure of the healing ligament will gradually be restored without elongation. The screws and loops must be removed after about three months to avoid later mechanical disturbances.

A sutured ligament that has been badly lacerated can be protected by inserting screws into all four corners and then looping two threads about diagonally opposite screws to form a crossed linkage. The placement of the loops is kinematically correct if the threads passing from the anterior screw on the femur to the posterior screw on the tibia cross *under* those from the posterior femoral screw to the anterior tibial screw (see section on Kinematics, Figs. 40, 43, 63–65).

Typical Lesions Accompanying Injuries of the Medial Side

Rupture of the ALFTL

The anteromedial tetrad. Figure 223 shows an extensive anteromedial complex injury as seen at operation. Complicating the tears of the POL, ACL and MCL is the detachment of the ALFTL from the femoral condyle. The location and function of this ligament were described in detail in the introduction (p. 43, Fig. 57). Here we shall repeat only that it acts in concert with the anterior cruciate ligament and POL to control anterior drawer displacement of the tibia.

We were aware of these relationships in cases of extensive, chronic anterior instability in which we could demonstrate an anteromedial instability as well as an anterolateral instability and anterior drawer sign. During routine exposures of fresh "unhappy triad" injuries, we frequently found that they were actually tetrad injuries, the fourth component being a fresh lesion of the ALFTL. Because there was usually a proximal tear of the anterior cruciate ligament, and we employed the "over the top" suturing technique requiring that the iliotibial tract be split for making the drill holes, it was initially by accident that we found these fresh lesions. The injury is logical, however, and confirms the function of the ALFTL. Its reconstruction is discussed in the chapter on chronic anterior instability.

Because the ALFTL is protected by the powerful, more superficial layer of the iliotibial tract, it practically never tears. It may, however, be avulsed from the lateral epicondyle of the femur (Fig. 223 c, d) or suffer hemorrhagic edema in the area where the iliotibial tract joins with the intermuscular septum on the femur (metaphysealward from the lateral lip of the linea aspera).

No true rupture of the ALFTL need occur for an anterolateral rotational drawer sign to develop. It is enough if these fibers become elongated by 5–10 mm by distension or a continuity disruption. This femorotibial ligament, whose importance has been underestimated, must not be neglected at operation and must be reconstructed in its proper length. Based on cases referred to us for disability assessment, as well as on personal communications from experienced surgeons, we know of many instances in which "lateral repairs" performed by a variety of techniques have left considerable varus laxity on the lateral side with anterolateral and posterolateral rotatory instability.

Repair is relatively simple if the injury is recent. We first freshen the denuded bone somewhat with a drill and chisel. If the surrounding periosteum and adjacent intermuscular septum are firm, the ALFTL can be refixed with sutures in the usual fashion. Like other ligament sutures, they must be tested to ensure 1) that they follow flexion-extension movements well and 2) that an anterolateral rotational drawer sign can no longer be elicited in any position. Similarly, the tract tensed by these sutures must not become visibly lax at any flexion angle. If the ideal fixation point is not apparent, we recommend temporary transfixation of the tract segment in question with a 2.0-mm Kirschner wire, as in the ALFTL transfer. If the ideal point is located in this way, the tract can be fixed at the transfixation site by means of an AO small-fragment cortical bone screw and toothed washer, if appropriate.

Our experience with repairs of the ALFTL has taught us that individual differences are a particularly important con-

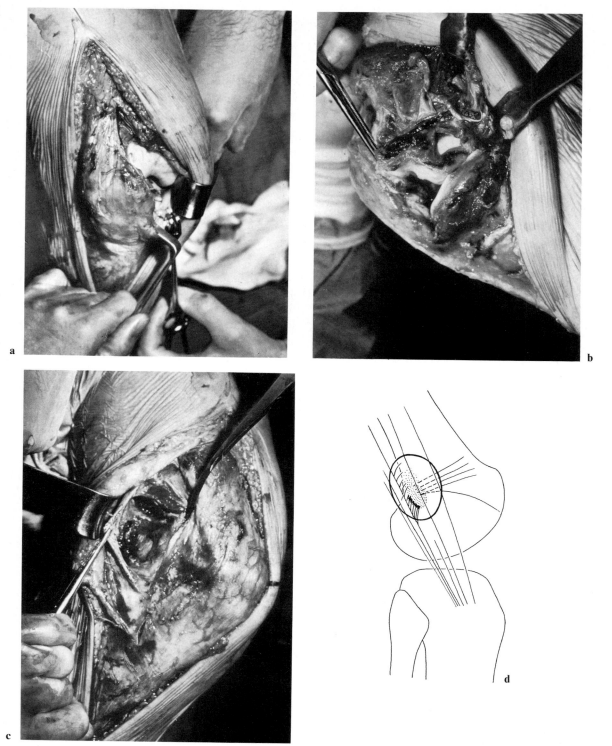

Fig. 223 a–d. Lesion of the anterolateral femorotibial ligament (ALFTL) in a complex injury of the "anteromedial tetrad" type. **a** Tears of the ACL, MCL, semimembranosus corner and ALFTL are found at operation. **b** View into the medial joint half with the MCL and semimembranosus-corner lesion. **c** View of the site of avulsion of the ALFTL. **d** Positional drawing for c; the *stippled area* represents the site of avulsion from the femur (see also Fig. 57)

sideration in such operations. In doubtful cases it is better to attach the inner, deep portion of the tract to the periosteum and septum over a large area, for a small fixation area that is not located at the ideal site cannot maintain stability for long.

tation. It follows, then, that the shortest fibers are among the most important passive rotatory stabilizers.

The drawing in Fig. 224 is based upon our own observations as well as an illustration in [172]. It demonstrates clearly how lesions of

---

The earlier concept of the "unhappy triad" denoted a complex injury of the ACL, MCL and "meniscus" (POL). We have found, however, that in many cases a lesion of the ALFTL constitutes a fourth component to the injury, thus making it a tetrad, rather than a triad.

Special Injuries of the Semimembranosus Corner

Pure Rotational Trauma with Peripheral Detachment of the Meniscus from the POL

In their experimental studies, Kennedy and Fowler [172] described examples of pure rotational injuries. The shortest fibers are the first to tighten during excessive rotation and are also the first to tear. The result is an immediate increase in the range of passive ro-

the capsular ligaments can occur in the absence of appreciable damage to the MCL. Though not always easily recognized, these injuries nevertheless demand attention during treatment. Arthroscopy is particularly useful in these situations if there is doubt concerning the nature and extent of the injury. Not infrequently, such lesions are combined with a rupture of the anterior cruciate ligament. The diagnosis of such a duad in a young, athletic patient constitutes an indication for surgical repair, whereas an isolated lesion of the deep layer and POL may be

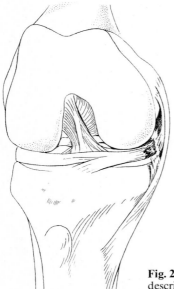

Fig. 224. External-rotation injury of the semimembranosus corner. Form of injury described by Kennedy and Fowler [172], in which the attachment between the meniscus and POL is torn purely by excessive lateral rotation

186

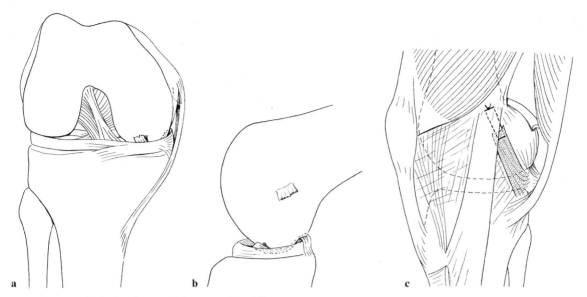

<table>
<tr><td>a</td><td>b</td><td>c</td></tr>
</table>

Fig. 225 a–c. The isolated tear of the posterior oblique ligament (POL). **a,b** These drawings illustrate a rare form in which the POL fibers (Fig. 224) have been torn at their proximal attachment, without concomitant in-jury to the MCL. Displacement of the torn ligament into the joint space mimics the clinical findings of a tab tear of the posterior meniscal horn. **c** Situation following suture repair

managed conservatively, provided it in-volves nothing more than a 1st- or 2nd-degree sprain or meniscus detachment.

If it is necessary to operate, repair is car-ried out on the femoromeniscal, menisco-tibial and femorotibial ligamentous struc-tures (fiber bundles) essentially as shown in Figs. 217b, c and 219. Because the MCL is normally intact, the placement of these su-tures may be difficult. However, in most cases the problem can be solved by combin-ing a standard medial parapatellar incision with an auxiliary posterior exposure at the semimembranosus corner (see p. 163).

Isolated Tear of the POL

Figure 225 illustrates a special situation that we have so far encountered on three oc-casions. The first case, involving a fresh ro-tational trauma during a soccer game, had all the features of a classic meniscus injury. A stress-independent effusion was present, and the grinding test of Appley and the Mc-Murray test elicited a clicking sign like that ordinarily associated with tab tears of the posterior meniscus horn. To our amazement we found at operation an intact meniscus with normal tibial attachment, over which lay a loose, noncartilaginous tag of tissue that could be interposed between the femur and tibia. Additional exposure through a posterior incision at once revealed a defect in the deep capsule with a tear of the POL near its femoral attachment below the long fibers of the MCL. The case was managed by suture repair followed by functional af-tercare with progressive weight-bearing, and within two months the patient was able to resume soccer playing without functional difficulty. Several months later the knee exhibited no signs of anteromedial rotatory instability.

First- to Second-Degree Sprain of the Semimembranosus Corner with Contraction and Gradual Loss of Extension

Each year, usually after the skiing season, we are confronted with several ligamentous lesions of a special type. The patients are generally women. If seen days or weeks after the injury, they exhibit a loss of extension of 30–40°. Any attempt at active or passive extension is met with firm resistance and considerable pain. The resistance is much harder and less elastic than in the case of an incarcerated meniscus. The area of the semimembranosus corner over the POL is swollen and tender. The joint itself shows a slight increase in its fluid content, but no significant effusion is present. The mobility in flexion is usually better, but it, too, is limited and is inhibited at about 110–120°. There are no marked signs of instability, though there may be mild valgus laxity and an anteromedial drawer of 1–3 mm compared to the healthy side. Operative inspection or arthroscopy reveals an undamaged joint interior with no signs of meniscus pathology. Tissue structures in the area of the POL and semimembranosus expansion are thickened by hemorrhagic swelling with no manifest tear.

Based on these operative findings, we now take an essentially conservative approach in the management of these cases. But whether treatment is operative or conservative, we have found that the loss of extension often stubbornly persists for months, despite a sound program of physical therapy. Therefore we have adopted the practice of restoring extension relatively early by the use of corrective casts that are changed weekly if the patient does not progress well during active physiotherapy.

Both Trillat (personal communication) and we have observed ectopic ossifications of the posteromedial ligament as a late sequela of these injuries (Fig. 226). These are especially likely to occur if there have been attempts to extend the limb forcibly under general anesthesia.

We assume that the clinical symptoms are the result of scar contractures secondary to a 1st- or 2nd-degree sprain of the postero-

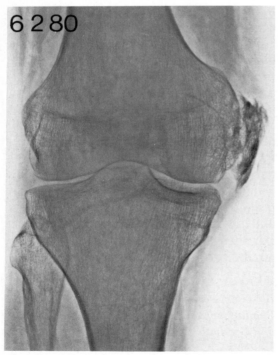

a

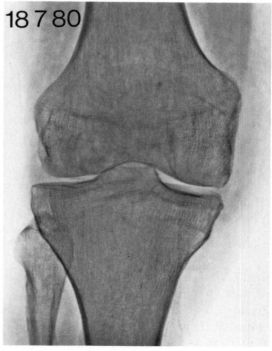

b

Fig. 226a, b. Ectopic ossification in the region of the POL and capsular ligaments following mobilization under general anesthesia (St. Elsewhere case), due apparently to spraining and scar contraction in the semimembranosus corner. **a** Status prior to secondary surgical ar-

throlysis with a mobility of 60—20–0°. **b** Status 6 months after arthrolysis with a motion range of 100–5–0°. One month later the final motion range was 120–0–0°, which represents a 60° gain of flexion and 20° gain of extension over the prearthrolytic state

188

medial corner. As mentioned earlier, the capsular portions of the semimembranosus corner are especially tense during the final degrees of extension, when the medial femoral condyle is "screwed home." Presumably the highly specific loss of extension is referable to this physiologic circumstance. The relation of the adjacent medial articular nerve to symptoms remains unclear.

All cases treated to date have healed with normal stability, even the two that were treated by exploratory repair. A mild extension loss of about 5° persisted in some cases.

We cannot dismiss the possibility of an algodystrophy along the lines of Sudeck's disease, and so we routinely administer the triple drug combination (see p. 284) in such cases as well as in difficult postoperative situations.

Concluding Remarks on Medial Injuries

Because most types of injury discussed thus far do not represent isolated lesions but are accompanied by lesions of the cruciate ligaments, it is always necessary to make a careful plan of operation, taking into account all the lesions present and designating the sequence in which the repairs and reconstructions are to be carried out. Remember that pathologic laxities can be exploited to gain access to difficult areas.

As a rule, the first sutures are passed through the cruciate ligaments, assuming they are accessible. These sutures are then brought through the definitive transosseous drill holes and positioned at the correct pull-through sites in the capsule before any sutures are placed in the periphery. The cruciate ligament sutures and other hard-to-place sutures are not tied until the very end, so that additional manipulations of the injured joint will not tear out or loosen the sutures that have already been placed. When all peripheral sutures are securely in place and stability has been verified in all four quadrants as well as under varus, valgus and anteroposterior stress, the cruciate ligament

sutures may be carefully tightened and tied; from that point on they will be protected by the synergistic peripheral ligaments, even if these structures themselves have been sutured (see Figs. 238 b–250 d).

Injuries of the Lateral Side and Their Repair

General

The conditions of movement and stabilization are fundamentally different on the lateral side than on the medial. Kaplan [166] relates this to the fact that the medial structures are more responsible for stabilization in extension, and the lateral for stabilization in flexion.

The lateral structures stabilize the knee in extension too, but the difference lies in the fact that *stability in extension* is for the most part *passive*, whereas *in flexion* it is chiefly *active*. Thus, on the more mobile lateral side, the principle of dynamic stabilization prevails. Even a century ago Duchenne [166, 167] recognized the importance of agonists and antagonists (e.g., biceps' – semimembranosus/semitendinosus) in stabilization and rotational control.

It is known that voluntary rotation becomes possible when the knee is flexed, and that the center of this rotation lies on the medial side of the central pivot. Consequently the lateral plateau makes much greater forward and backward excursions during knee movements than does the medial plateau. As a result, the purely passive ligamentous structures on the lateral side cannot be as rigid as on the medial side. As will be seen, almost all the lateral ligaments have a powerful active component or partner. Presumably it is this greater overall mobility of the lateral side that explains why both ligamentous and meniscal injuries are far less common on this side than in the medial half of the joint.

The lateral collateral ligament relaxes considerably during flexion, when the femoral condyle rolls down posteriorly over the convex tibial plateau. As a result, considerable internal or external rotation of the knee is required for this ligament to tighten or become torn. Among our patients, for example, lateral lesions account for only 5% of all ligamentous injuries. The literature, too, contains few reports on this type of lesion. Presumably this is due not just to its rare occurrence, but also to the fact that the results of treatment in this half of the joint are poorer than on the medial side.

Because the system of active-passive stabilization on the lateral side is extremely delicate, the restoration of normal anatomic conditions is a prime concern during surgical repairs. When we compare our results today with those of a decade ago, we find that as our knowledge of anatomic relationships improved, so did our surgical results. We shall cite two cases to illustrate this.

The first case involved a soccer player who had sustained an injury of the varus-flexion-IR type: The posterior cruciate ligament was completely torn from the tibia, while the anterior cruciate still had some continuity in one third, though even this segment was badly damaged. Damage on the lateral side was total. The iliotibial tract and popliteus muscle and tendon were ruptured, the lateral collateral ligament was extensively torn, and the biceps tendon and arcuate ligament complex were avulsed together with the capsule below the attachments of the gastrocnemius. One by one, each structure was carefully repaired and reattached, and today the patient has been playing competitive soccer for three years with practically normal lateral knee stability.

The second case involved a schoolboy who was injured when jumping from a mini-trampoline. In this case the combined injury was even more severe, though fortunately the peroneal nerve was undamaged. Both cruciate ligaments were ruptured, and there were 2nd- and 3rd-degree injuries of the iliotibial tract, popliteus tendon, lateral collateral ligament and biceps tendon. In addition, the entire joint capsule was avulsed from the femur, forming hanging tissue

shreds that obscured the field and necessitated careful study before repairs could be performed. But the damage did not end with these structures. The tears in the capsular region extended farther posteriorly. Even the lateral head of the gastrocnemius and insertion of the plantaris longus lay avulsed in the popliteal fossa. Again, working from the back toward the front, each structure was systematically taken, anchored transosseously, and restored to its original length and position by a variety of suturing techniques. At nine months postoperatively the result is not perfect, but the knee is compensated with no serious instability or functional disability.

The lateral injuries which we observed were practically always complex and involved concomitant damage to the cruciate ligaments. Solitary lesions are somewhat rare and will heal without treatment.

From the clinic of Trillat, Lerat et al. [199] report on 31 ligamentous tears of the lateral side treated by surgical repair. Twelve of these injuries were accompanied by tears of both cruciate ligaments, 10 by tears of the anterior cruciate ligament only, and 7, surprisingly enough, by tears of the posterior cruciate only.

According to Lerat, the lateral ligaments can sustain only partial ruptures without associated tears of the cruciate ligaments. Interestingly, bony ligament avulsions were found in 19 cases. The frequent involvement of the peroneal nerve is unfortunate. Lerat's statistics show 7 such cases; in 4 of these the nerve failed to recover spontaneously. Among our patients we have often seen the nerve altered by hemorrhagic swelling, but we know only 2 cases in which permanent paralysis ensued. One case involved a runner who inadvertently stepped in a hole and sustained a total complex injury of the lateral ligaments with ruptures of both cruciates. The peroneal nerve was torn and lacerated for a length of 15 cm (!). A secondary nerve graft was performed, which has at least resulted in improved sensibility and trophism. Pure passive stability is good, but the motor loss in the peroneal region has left the patient with a severe impairment of active stabilization.

According to Lerat [199], little is known about the mechanisms of injury. His series includes 23 multiple injury patients, but hardly any represent athletic injuries. Our material, on the other hand, includes several typical sports injuries.

While on the whole there is little hope of a very good end result, Lerat nevertheless states, based on his experience, that the complex lateral ligamentous lesion with a tear of the *anterior* cruciate ligament offers a better chance of recovery than an injury involving the *posterior* cruciate.

The Major Passive and Active Stabilizing Structures of the Lateral Side
(Figs. 227 and 228)

Besides the posterior cruciate ligament, which belongs mainly to the lateral, "ro-tational" group, the main structures responsible for passive stability are, from behind forward, the arcuate ligament complex, the lateral collateral ligament, and the iliotibial tract with its ALFTL.

In addition to these ligamentous structures, there is a ligament-like thickening of the capsule which runs roughly parallel to the popliteus tendon, extending to the posterior meniscus horn and from there to the tibia (the "posterior lateral collateral ligament" [226]). Because the posterior cruciate ligament is important as a pivot point for rotation, its injury, together with that of the lateral rotational stabilizers, has severe functional consequences. From the middle of the joint forward the lateral capsule is quite thin above the meniscus and consists essentially of a synovial duplication.

The principal active stabilizers supplementing the passive system are, from behind forward, the lateral gastrocnemius, the popliteus muscle and tendon, the biceps with

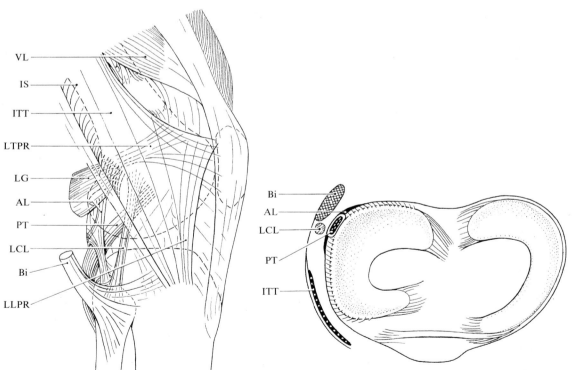

Fig. 227. Lateral aspect of the knee joint showing the anatomic structures important for ligamentous repairs

Fig. 228. Transverse section through the knee joint above the menisci, showing the structures important for lateral stability

191

its tendinous expansions to the fibular head and tibia (the main stabilizer against varus in extension and against IR in flexion), and finally the iliotibial tract, which is tensed by the tensor fasciae latae and gluteus maximus and serves as a powerful active stabilizer against lateral opening in extension and against excessive IR in flexion. For completeness we should also mention the transverse and longitudinal patellar retinacula as well as the meniscopatellar ligament of Pauzat [in 164, 166].

Anatomic Variants and Individual Differences

Earlier we pointed out the wide range of anatomic variation on the lateral side of the knee. The structural principles remain unchanged, but their individual "embodiment" varies. For example, we have seen patients with a poorly developed LCL and a correspondingly more powerful popliteus tendon, while in other cases the opposite was true. We have also seen cases in which the connection between the fibula and fabella was very strong while the remaining capsular structures and arcuate ligament were proportionately weaker.

The Fabella as a Stress Nodal Point

The fabella is "only" a small sesamoid bone that is present in about 20% of the population. Nevertheless, its special location in the lateral gastrocnemius tendon is no accident. Proximal to it the deep layer of the gastrocnemius tendon simultaneously forms the posterior joint capsule (condylar plate); distal to it the posterior capsule and gastrocnemius tendon can again be resolved into two separate layers. The fibers of the posterior capsule converge upon the fabella from all directions. As stated earlier (see p. 96), the fabella is analogous to the patella in that it lies at the intersection of lines of tensile stress. The following structures terminate at or on the fabella: the oblique popliteal ligament arising from the semimembranosus

muscle, the arcuate ligament from the popliteus muscle, the main tendon slips of the gastrocnemius muscle from above, and the fabellofibular ligament (termed the "short lateral collateral ligament" by Kaplan [169]) from below.

Because bone can form only in areas of sufficient mechanical rest [285], the site of the fabella must represent a kind of neutral point in the capsuloligamentous apparatus. This has important surgical implications, for such a site would also make an excellent anchoring point for reconstructive procedures and repairs.

Injuries of the Lateral Collateral Ligament (LCL)

This thin fibular collateral ligament is often overrated in comparison to its medial counterpart. Because the fibula is attached elastically, rather than rigidly, to the tibia, every varus stress does not act immediately on the LCL alone, but also on the fibula and tibiofibular attachment.

Tears of the Lateral Collateral Ligament

Thus, it is no coincidence that in avulsions of the fibular apex, often both the insertion of the biceps tendon and that of the LCL come away with the avulsion fragment (Fig. 229 a). The tension of this muscle supposedly stabilizes the lateral side against varus-producing forces while preventing ligamentous injury. But the more extended the knee is when the varus stress is applied, the greater is the likelihood that the biceps will avulse the fragment at the fibular apex. As the degree of flexion is increased, the injury will tend to occur in the ligament itself (Fig. 229 c, d). In bony avulsions, refixation can be accomplished with a lag screw, a wire suture or a tension band, depending on the location of the fragment and hardness of the bone. Screw fixation is simpler, because it requires no additional exposure of the peroneal nerve. But because the screw alone cannot safely with-

192

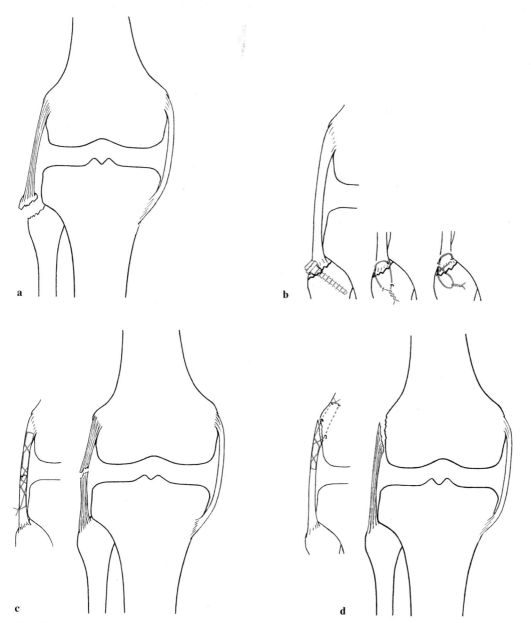

Fig. 229 a–d. The various injuries of the lateral collateral ligament and the standard techniques for their repair. The techniques are analogous for tears of the popliteus tendon and arcuate ligament

stand the pull of the biceps and may become dislodged from the bone, this pull should be neutralized by means of an additional wire-loop tension band. When making the drill holes for the tension-band loops, the peroneal nerve must first be identified, carefully exposed and protected during the drilling. Despite the increased time and effort, reinforcement with a tension band is recom-

mended in cases where the biceps tendon is attached to the bony avulsion fragment (Fig. 229 b).

Less frequently the LCL is torn in its mid-portion (Fig. 229 c) or proximal half. The smooth transverse tear shown in the drawing is rare; usually the tear has an elongated Z shape. The distal half of the ligament is identified as a round cord enveloped by a "pseudo-sheath." The proximal half is blended with the capsular tissue. Usually the distal cord remains intact, while fraying takes place in the part blended with the capsule. It may be quite difficult to identify the proximally avulsed tags and corresponding tear sites in the capsular tissue and re-approximate them.

A proximal tear near the bone is shown schematically in Fig. 229 d. At operation the bone looks as if it has been exposed with a periosteal elevator. We have yet to find a true bony avulsion at this site. Normally the ligament broadens where it inserts on the bone. It can therefore be securely engaged with a criss-cross Bunnell suture and fixed to the freshened bone through drill holes. The refixation sutures must be placed such that the knots are extraarticular, outside the gliding surface on the femoral condyle. Because of the extreme importance of these sutures, we generally use nonabsorbable material or even a pliable braided wire.

Particular care must be taken in lateral repairs that gliding surfaces are not damaged by knots, drill holes, etc., lest postoperative adhesions develop that could hinder functional recovery.

Combined Injuries

Simple injuries of the LCL are almost always associated with a capsuloligamentous lesion of the posterolateral corner. The popliteus tendon itself is sufficiently mobile to remain intact in many combined lateral injuries. However, one must always be alert for possible distension of this tendon in the 2 cm segment just before its femoral insertion.

In view of the limited case data and the numerous variants that occur, we cannot present the sequence of injuries as systematically as on the medial side.

The joint capsule is thickened in the popliteal tendon area to form a ligament-like structure which Meyer [226] calls the "posterior lateral collateral ligament." We have not adopted this term, because the junctures in the arcuate ligament complex are difficult to discern. For its part the arcuate ligament extends from the posterolateral tibia and fibula to the middle of the joint capsule and upward to the fabella and has an attachment with the meniscus. The broad, flat part of the bipartite popliteus tendon is joined to this ligament and can exert tension on it in any position. The thin anterior half of the lateral joint capsule is devoid of further ligamentous attachments. Lateral to the popliteus tendon and especially between the meniscus and tibia, the capsule is firm and may be torn in lateral complex injuries.

Figures 230 a–d show the less common variant with a proximal tear of the deep capsule and LCL at the femur, as may occur during severe dislocation-type injuries. The severed posterior cruciate ligament reminds us of the central-pivot lesions that usually accompany such injuries.

The more frequent combination (Figs. 230 e–f and 231) consists in a distal avulsion of the LCL and posterior capsule from the fibula and tibia.

There is nearly always a bony avulsion from the tibia in such cases, for three fibers under tension from different directions converge at that location – the posterior fibers of the ALFTL from a proximal direction, the anterior expansion of the arcuate ligament from a posterior direction, and expansions of the biceps tendon from a posterolateral direction. The fragment avulsed by these fibers is named after Segond [316], who described this avulsion in the last century. The fragment is easily reduced and (see also Fig. 231) reattached with screws. *Before refixation*, however, one must check the popliteal hiatus and test the popliteus tendon for strength if it can be seen and reached through the tear. In the anterior joint half the synovial capsule is quite thin and can easily be incised to examine the popliteus tendon for damage.

Even in major injuries of the lateral side, the surgeon must gain a clear idea of the extent of the lesion before starting the repair. It must not be forgotten that, as on the medial

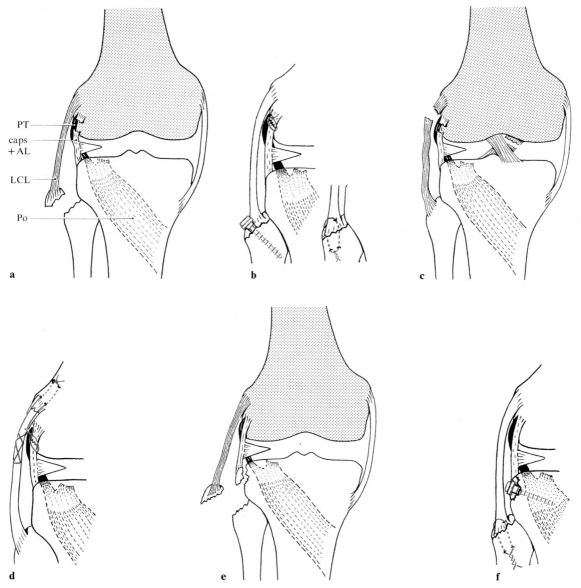

PT
caps
+ AL

LCL

Po

a   b   c

d   e   f

Fig. 230 a–f. Tears of the lateral collateral ligament with associated lesions of the deep capsuloligamentous layers and the corresponding techniques of repair

side, the lesions may lie at multiple levels, i.e., one layer may be torn from the femur while another is torn from the tibia or fibula. All essential structures must be tested for intactness over their entire length. If the varus, valgus or anteroposterior instability permits good access, the cruciate ligaments must be examined first and engaged with sutures that are tied only after the peripheral ligaments have been repaired.

Combined Injuries with Rupture of the Popliteus Tendon

Rupture of the popliteus tendon (Fig. 232 a) represents the next stage in the complex lateral injury.

The popliteus muscle, the most important posterolateral stabilizer, was ruptured in its tendinous portion or at least severely overstretched in the last 2 cm before its anterior

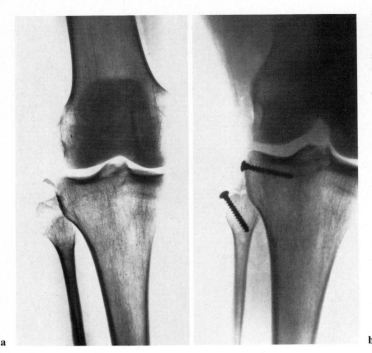

Fig. 231 a, b. X-ray documentation for Fig. 230 e, f. Besides the typical avulsion fracture of the fibular head, note the avulsion fragment of Segond [316], also typical, at the upper border of the tibia. Both fragments are reattached with a screw to effect a ligamentous repair

femoral insertion in over ¾ of the lateral injuries surgically treated by us. In two cases the *muscle belly* was torn from the tendon below the joint line.

The popliteus tendon is subject to a phenomenon similar to that seen in the cruciate ligaments at the joint center. It is possible that the outer sheath will appear intact all the way to the femoral insertion, while in the interior the rigid collagenous fiber mass is so severely traumatized that there is a relative failure of muscular action. The repair of the popliteus tendon, together with its shortening by the Bunnell suturing technique, is the most important step toward restoring posterolateral stability. We devote great care

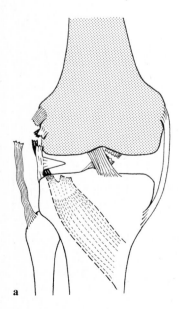

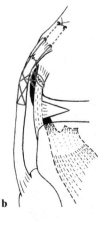

Fig. 232. a Rupture of the lateral collateral ligament and popliteus tendon and **b** the technique of their suture repair

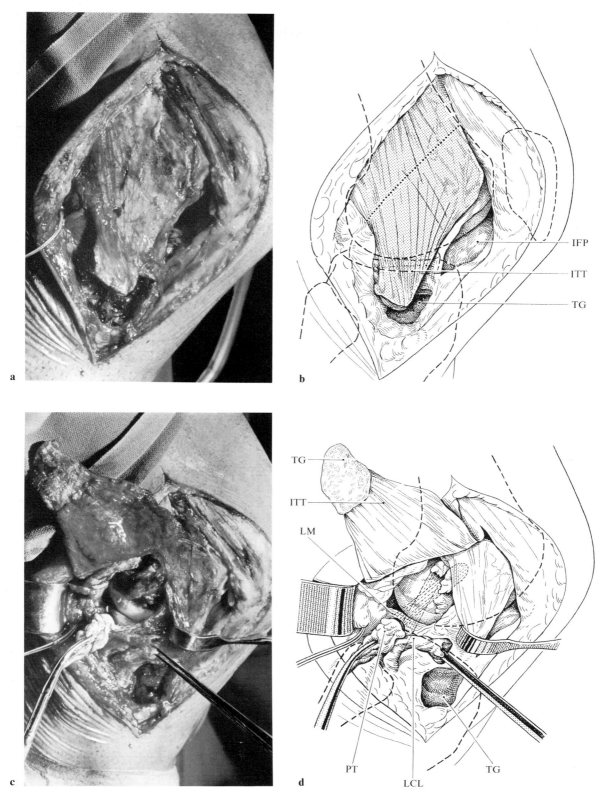

Fig. 233 a–d. Photographs and corresponding positional drawings of the operative findings in a patient with a popliteus tendon rupture. **a, b** The iliotibial tract is detached with the tubercle of Gerdy. **c, d** The tract is reflected upward to afford access to the important deep layers

197

to this procedure and are satisfied with the repair only if we can be certain that it will withstand dynamic loading postoperatively (Fig. 232b).

Figures 233a, b document an operative situation using the recommended approach with detachment of the tubercle of Gerdy and reflection of the iliotibial tract. In Figs. 233c, d the iliotibial tract is reflected upward exposing the ruptured popliteus tendon and collateral ligament. On either side are the torn capsular ligaments and arcuate ligament complex. Repair was carried out according to the principles described.

At this point it should be repeated that the tubercle of Gerdy with the insertion of the iliotibial tract must be detached all the way to the synovial capsule at the border of the cartilage, so that the innermost tract fibers, which are the most effective in terms of femorotibial stabilization, remain attached to the fragment. Later when the fragment is reattached to its bed, normal stability will be restored. It is still necessary in these cases to check whether the connection of the tract to the proximal femoral condyle is intact toward the lateral lip of the linea aspera; otherwise it must be reattached as described under the care of the medial tetrad.

Possible types of popliteus rupture. Most common is a rupture in the femoral course of the tendon; this may occur very close to the bone or may leave a stump. These tears are easily visualized and must be well repaired.

Less favorable and more difficult to recognize are ruptures at the level of the joint space, for they may be hidden behind the popliteal hiatus. Only if the visualized tendon offers normal resistance to traction can it be safely assumed that there is no rupture at a more distal site (Fig. 234).

Most unfavorable are ruptures below the joint line, which also are easily overlooked.

Normally the popliteus tendon has two parts. One is the approximately pencil-thick tendon passing toward the femoral condyle, and the other is a flatter, broader expansion to the arcuate ligament, posterior meniscus horn and posterior capsule. If the muscle belly has been torn from these structures, repair is difficult. In one case we even found a bilevel injury of the popliteus: The tendon was severed at the level of the joint space, and farther distally there was a second rupture in the muscle belly. In another case (the aforementioned runner with the torn peroneal nerve) large parts of the muscle were detached from the tibia and displaced into the joint beneath the lateral meniscus, which was also detached.

Tears such as these in the region of the muscle and its aponeurosis must also be repaired. If the muscle is totally destroyed, a femorotibial tenodesis is still much more valuable than a useless popliteus muscle.

In major complex injuries the outer tear is usually large enough to provide access for placing the sutures. If additional posterolateral exposure is required, the peroneal nerve must first be demonstrated and protected before advancing farther distally to the popliteus muscle.

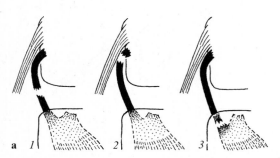 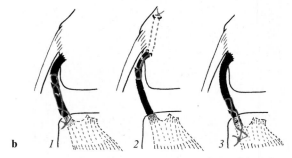

Fig. 234a, b. Sites of predilection for ruptures of the popliteus tendon. **a** The tears shown in drawings *1* and *2* are easily found intra-articularly or at the level of pas-

sage through the meniscus, while tears below the joint line like that shown in drawing *3* are often difficult to locate and repair. **b** The corresponding suture techniques

For refixation to the femur, we freshen the bone somewhat and place the suture transosseously. These transosseous sutures are so important that we use nonabsorbable material (e.g., Polydec 3) or a braided elastic wire, which offers the additional advantage of radiopacity, so that the wire can be checked for damage if postoperative recovery is poor.

As in the suturing of cruciate ligament stumps, it may be easier to pull the suture through the popliteus tendon if a Reverdin needle is used.

If the tendon is ruptured very close to the femur, it can also be fixed with a screw and toothed washer.

Most Severe Lateral Complex Injuries

Maximal injuries of the lateral side, which Trillat [359] calls the "lateral unhappy pentad," actually involve far more than just five injuries. Trillat applies the term "pentad" to injuries in which both cruciate ligaments are ruptured, and "triad" to those in which only one cruciate is torn. However, more recent studies have shown that the concepts of the triad and pentad are insufficient to characterize the potential range of lateral injuries, which can involve any number of lesions from 1 to considerably more than 5 (Fig. 235).

For example, the lesion formerly known as the "lateral unhappy pentad" actually involves tears of the ACL, PCL, LCL, ALFTL, arcuate ligament, popliteus muscle, biceps muscle, possibly the lateral meniscus, and in extreme cases the lateral head of the gastrocnemius and even the peroneal nerve. Thus, a total of 10 structures are injured, 6 of which are passive, 3 active only, and 2 a combination of active and passive, in addition to the peroneal nerve.

In very severe injuries of the lateral side, we must assume that the tear extends through the joint on the posterior side and into the semimembranosus corner, leaving only the MCL intact. Therefore, in extreme cases of this type, when a global posterior instability is demonstrated preoperatively (i.e.,

a posterior drawer sign is present even in IR), the surgeon may find it necessary to make an additional posteromedial incision so that the semimembranosus corner can also be repaired.

In major injuries where only the MCL is left intact, it is a short step to a true dislocation in which the patellar ligament represents the last connection between the tibia and more proximal structures.

Tears of the Quadriceps Extensor Apparatus Associated with Major Ligamentous Injuries

We have seen two cases of patellar ligament rupture, one associated with a medial triad and one with a lateral triad. Direct violence was apparently a factor in each case.

The same applied to a smooth rupture of the vastus medialis muscle from the patella, medial longitudinal retinaculum and fascia of the medial ligament system.

The patellar ligament tears were repaired with approximating sutures reinforced by two wire tension bands through the patella and tibial tuberosity to maintain the desired ligamentous length.

Sites of Predilection for Tears in Major Lateral Complex Injuries

The *cruciate ligaments* may become torn in their proximal, middle or distal portions. Even if both are ruptured, a great variety of combinations are possible. It is even possible for the entire cruciate ligament complex to become torn out the back of the intercondylar fossa during an avulsion of the posterior capsule. In such cases the disinserted "central pivot" may still form a self-contained unit, as it did in the joint, that can be replaced in its entirety and reattached to the avulsion sites. To date we have treated two ruptures of this type; in one the avulsion of the central pivot was complete, while in the other only three of the four attachments had been ruptured.

In Trillat's series [359] of complex lateral injuries, the ACL was ruptured at its distal

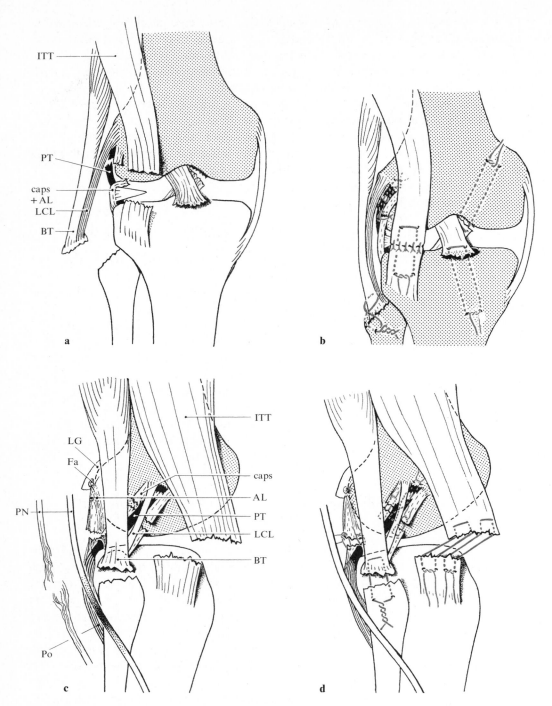

Fig. 235 a, c. Schematic example of a major complex lateral injury with bony avulsion of the biceps and LCL and ruptures of the popliteus tendon, posterior capsule, arcuate ligament, both cruciate ligaments and the iliotibial tract. In reality the arcuate ligament and deep capsule are usually torn below the meniscus, and continuity is almost always preserved in the anterior portion of the iliotibial tract. **b, d** the corresponding techniques of suture repair

200

attachment in 8 cases, at its proximal attachment in 9, and in its midportion in 5; in the same series the PCL was torn at its distal attachment in 6 cases, at its proximal attachment in 9, and in its midportion in 5. The *arcuate ligament* and *posterolateral capsule* were most frequently torn in their distal portions.

In the same series it is reported that the lateral *collateral ligament* may tear at the fibular head, proximally, or in its middle third. Bilevel ruptures can also occur, in which case one end of the ligament hangs from the fibular fragment along with the biceps tendon, while the other end is torn from the femur. This proximal tear is easily overlooked due to the blending of the soft tissues at that level. When the avulsion fragment is reattached to the fibula, the LCL will still be lax on account of the proximal tear.

The lateral *meniscus,* which is directly adherent to the posterolateral capsular ligament and arcuate ligament, is in most cases torn from its peripheral ligamentous anchorage and so can be reintegrated into the capsuloligamentous system during the repair of the popliteus corner.

According to Trillat the *popliteus* may also be torn at the femur, in its midportion, or may be avulsed distally together with its muscle. It is strongly recommended that the popliteus be explored over its entire course.

Tears of the *biceps* always involved an avulsion fracture of the fibular head. In the majority of cases the LCL was also attached to the avulsion fragment.

Injury of the Iliotibial Tract and its Femorotibial Ligamentous Component

Analyses of major ligamentous injuries of the lateral side have provided us with insight into the underlying pathophysiologic mechanisms and have helped us to gain a deeper understanding of post-traumatic instability syndromes.

Trillat et al. [359] report that ruptures of the iliotibial tract occur close to the tibia and may be accompanied by avulsion of the tubercle of Gerdy. We personally have not yet seen a distal avulsion of this type. However, we have found a definite four-fifths rupture at the level of the joint line. The posterior four-fifths of the tract were torn, while the anterior fifth toward the lateral retinaculum was still in place but showed hemorrhagic distension.

The *anterior* half of the iliotibial tract, which Kaplan [165, 168] calls the iliotibial "band," represents a pure iliotibial connection, extending freely past the femur to the hip where it terminates in an elastic muscle belly. The *posterior* half, called the iliotibial "tract," has an attachment with the distal femur and in this way creates a ligamentous connection between the femur and tibia.

This explains why lesions of the iliotibial tract are always located in the posterior half, and why the anterior half can withstand the trauma without tearing.

In the majority of iliotibial tract lesions the tract appears normal when viewed externally, for the injuries are confined to the posterior inner aspect. As in the anteromedial tetrad, there is either a visible avulsion from the femur or an overstretching of the femorotibial fibers. If the tract is still firmly attached to the femur, neither an anterolateral nor posterolateral instability will be present. The importance of the ALFTL in checking anterior tibial displacement has already been discussed, but if its attachments in the femoro-patello-tibial triangle are secure, then it will also be an effective check-rein against posterior displacement of the tibia.

Whenever there is a suspected ligamentous lesion in this region, visual inspection should be supplemented by functional testing of the triangular fiber system. Because the attachments at the tibia and patella are generally intact, particular attention should be given to the femoral attachment, as it is the most probable site of injury.

Injury of the Peroneal Nerve

This nerve is highly prone to injury at the site where it crosses the fibula, for there the bone can act as a fulcrum during a varus trauma. Even in hyperextension injuries, the peroneal nerve is more prone to damage than the popliteal vascular bundles.

If the nerve is divided, it must be accurately repaired using fascicular sutures. If time or technical constraints prohibit a primary nerve suture during the initial operation for repair of the ligaments, the ends of the nerve should at least be reapproximated in preparation for a secondary nerve repair or graft. To make it easier to locate the nerve in the second operation, its course should be marked with a nonabsorbable suture, preferably monofilament, that is attached in such a way that it cannot migrate between operations.

Injuries of the Cruciate Ligaments and Their Repair

The Blood Supply of the Cruciate Ligaments

As described in the chapters on Anatomy and Kinematics, the cruciate ligaments form the nucleus of the functional congruence and stability of the knee. The fact that they extend into the joint yet are extra-articular accounts for the special types of injury to these ligaments as well as for the often severe loss of blood supply to the ruptured segments. Alm and Stromberg [10], Bousquet [33], Dejour and Bousquet [65], Gillquist et al. [105] and Pfab [285] have reviewed the vascular supply of the cruciate ligaments. As they point out, branches from the middle genicular artery enter the cruciate "central pivot" from behind and anastomose with one another. The posterior cruciate ligament is more favorably situated and is supplied by four branches that are distributed fairly evenly over its course. By contrast, only one main branch enters the anterior cruciate at the level where the two ligaments cross and interconnect. Thus, while the posterior cruciate ligament receives its main blood supply at four levels, the anterior cruciate is supplied

by only a single main vessel between its superior and inferior insertions (Fig. 236). In the areas of attachment of the ligaments these vessels enter into small-caliber anastomoses with the subcortical vascular network of the femur and tibia. These anastomoses are too small to supply a ruptured ligament that has lost its main artery; however, these small vessels are extremely important from a surgical standpoint, for their presence at the site of ligament reattachment provides the microcirculation necessary for healing. If they gain attachment with synovial vessels in the suture area, anastomoses will form, thus leading, according to observations by Alm and Gillquist [9] and Clancy et al. [52], to a revascularization not only of reattached ligaments but also of grafts (e.g., a strip from the patellar tendon).

For a revascularization of this type to occur, it is necessary that the site of the ligament reattachment or graft attachment be well covered by synovial membrane. This synovial covering should extend past the rupture site to the bone. A devitalized cruciate ligament that is no longer extra-articular, but is isolated in the joint cavity and surrounded by synovial fluid, will undergo rapid necrosis. On the other hand, even transverse tears and tears difficult to reapproximate have been known to heal with true revascularization if the suture area and the remainder of the ligament could be covered with synovium, and thus successfully extra-arterialized, during surgical repair.

The location of the posterior cruciate ligament makes it less apt to become isolated within the joint cavity. It almost always retains its attachment with the remaining tissues in the popliteal fossa.

Thus, the anterior cruciate ligament is much more vulnerable than the posterior cruciate both in terms of its blood supply and its risk of post-traumatic intra-articular isolation. It is essential that a synovial covering be restored to the ligament, and that its connection with the cruciate ligament complex be maintained.

Some authors claim that the anterior cruciate ligament derives significant nutrition

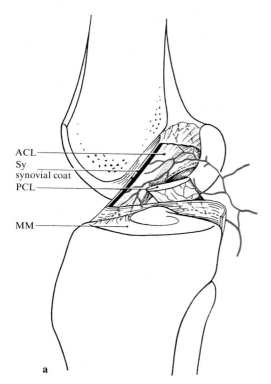

ACL
Sy
synovial coat
PCL

MM

a

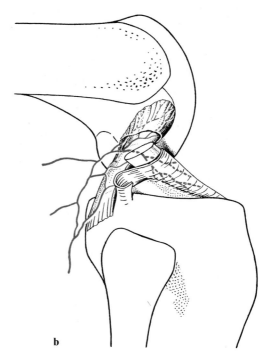

b

Fig. 236a, b. Semischematic representation of the arterial blood supply of the cruciate ligaments. The ligaments lie extra-arterially in a keel-like synovium-lined fold protruding into the joint from behind. The branches of the middle genicular artery also enter the ligaments from the back of the joint. **a** The medial view demonstrates the blood supply of the anterior cruciate liga- ment, which generally is supplied by only one branch which enters the ligament superiorly from behind and anastomoses with the intraosseous vessels in the areas of ligamentous attachment. **b** The lateral view demonstrates the blood supply of the posterior cruciate ligament. It is provided by 3 or 4 arterial branches and so is far superior to that of the anterior cruciate ligament

from the upper tibia, and they describe avascular lesions of the ligament secondary to medial meniscectomy. Supposedly these lesions were caused by removing too much vascularized tissue adjacent to the anterior horn and anterior cruciate ligament during the resection of the meniscus.

The problem of secondary anterior cruciate ligament insufficiency following medial meniscectomy is well known. We see such cases frequently, especially during the course of insurance examinations. It has not been established whether these cases are indeed due to a loss of blood supply to the anterior cruciate, or whether they are more a mechanical result of the meniscectomy itself. Tauber et al. [338] survey the literature on the subject and come to the conclusion that the cause is more mechanical than vascular.

They also speculate that a large number of cruciate ligament lesions were either overlooked during the meniscectomy or were not yet present in manifest form, i.e., the collagen content of the ligament was altered despite a normal outward appearance at the time of the meniscectomy. While we cannot discount the possibility of an avascular disturbance, we believe that the insufficiency is due more to the progressive stretching of a weak or damaged ligament under the increased stress that results from meniscus removal. We know that the semimembranosus corner, with the attached posterior meniscus horn, acts as a synergist of the anterior cruciate ligament. If the mechanical "braking" action of the meniscus is absent, then the anterior cruciate must bear a proportionately greater burden in checking tibial displacement. The larger and more voluminous the resected posterior meniscal horn, the greater the added burden. As long as the semimembranosus corner functions efficiently as a stabilizer, even a weak or damaged cruciate ligament can function in a compensated fashion. But if this stabilizing action is lost, the ACL alone is incapable of compensating and becomes increasingly insufficient.

In the treatment of cruciate ligament ruptures, the restoraton or maintenence of blood supply must be given no less consideration than the mechanical aspects of the repair. Accordingly, sutures must be placed with great care; they must hold the ligament securely without strangulating it. The connections of the anterior cruciate ligament with the posterior cruciate, which are crucial to the nutrition of the ACL, must be maintained or restored if subsequent revascularization is to occur.

Ruptured Anterior Cruciate Ligament with Intact Vascular Pedicle

Ruptures of the ACL at its proximal insertion are often found during operations for chronic knee instabilities. In these cases the inner aspect of the lateral femoral condyle is free of ligament remnants and is covered only with a shiny synovial layer to the posterior edge of the articular cartilage. But the ACL is still present in the central pivot; it rises in normal fashion anterior to the tibial eminence, has a normal synovial covering, and has its usual attachment with the posterior cruciate ligament and nutrient vascular pedicle.

These cases are very favorable for operative repair. In most cases the anterior cruciate has practically a normal length and is entirely viable, being at most somewhat atrophied by disuse. It can be grasped in its proximal portion and carefully separated from the posterior cruciate until it can be resutured to the freshened condyle. The reattached ligament is more valuable than a graft, which is always at least partially devascularized by mobilization and transferrance and so must be revascularized.

A restoration of normal function may be anticipated if stress on the repaired ligament is avoided for a certain period postoperatively, giving the ligament an opportunity to adapt before normal loading is permitted.

Ligamentous tissue has the ability to adapt to stress. For example, ballet dancers or athletes with knee injuries are found at operation to have cruciate and peripheral ligaments of exceptional strength, whereas these ligaments are often very delicate in patients with little physical training who have sustained skiing injuries.

We have observed this adaptation frequently during "second looks" (arthroscopy, removal of metal implants, etc.), finding previously sutured cruciate ligaments to be as healthy-appearing as before the injury. Even a graft could no longer be recognized as such, so normal was its size, course and synovial covering; only its white coloration beneath the synovial membrane was not quite as lustrous as that of a normal ligament.

Unfortunately the results are not always this good. Healing may be poor after a primary repair, and poorly vascularized grafts may rupture from fatigue. Nevertheless, the good outcomes demonstrate that complete healing is possible. Since 1974 our results in the treatment of old and recent injuries have improved substantially, largely because we have recognized the importance of *restoring attachment between the cruciate ligaments* and *covering them with perfused synovium*.

At this point a brief review of the Wittek operation is in order.

Wittek's Use of the "Old Avulsed" Anterior Cruciate Ligament

In 1926 Wittek [394] described a unique technique for the operative treatment of anterior cruciate ligament ruptures. Because the ligament is often short and difficult to reinsert, he drew it as far back as possible and sutured it to the lateral side of the posterior cruciate ligament, more or less opposite to its normal insertion site on the femur. Although the anterior cruciate ligament could not function quite normally in this position, remarkably good results were reported with the technique – so good, apparently, that until recently this method was still practiced by experienced surgeons. Presumably the principle can be explained by drawing an analogy with a swing: It is better for one rope of the swing to be fastened very close to the other rope or even attached to it than for it to hang loose. Or perhaps the tightening of the anterior cruciate ligament by its contact with the posterior cruciate creates proprioceptive input that contributes to stabilization.

The Normal Structure of the Cruciate Ligaments

Anatomic and Functional Aspects That Are Important for Surgical Repair

The cruciate ligaments are intimately connected with each other in the area where they cross; the vascular pedicle forms a part of this connection. They are located behind a common synovial partition in the posterior joint capsule, which extends from the semimembranosus corner to the popliteus corner.

As mentioned earlier in the section on Kinematics (p. 19), the fibers necessary for mechanical strength cannot all fit on the ideal "four-bar linkage." Therefore each cruciate ligament has two parts, allowing each ligament to behave as a separate crossed four-bar linkage. According to Girgis et al. [107], the ACL is comprised of an anteromedial and posterolateral part that can be readily distinguished from each other (Fig. 237). Each part is somewhat specialized and behaves differently in joint movements. According to Smillie [328, 329] the anteromedial fibers of the ACL are taut near extension, the posterolateral are more taut in flexion, and a middle part is more taut in IR.

It is known that the ACL acts with the PCL to check internal rotation of the tibia upon the femur (coiling). According to Furman and Girgis [101], the ACL also stabilizes the extended knee against external rotation! This apparent paradox is explained by the fact that as the knee is extended the ACL is increasingly received into the notch of Grant and Basmajian [113], which has the effect of stabilizing the knee against rotation in both directions.

This notch of Grant is located at the anterior edge of the intercondylar fossa (Figs. 75 and 251 d) and must always be assessed preoperatively. Its size and depth provide important clues concerning the stress to which it is subjected during extension. For example, its width is a measure of how wide the anterior cruciate ligament is or was. In a recent rupture of the ACL, the notch looks as if it has been freshly polished or glazed. In chronic ACL insufficiency, on the other hand, the notch is quite shallow, and in cases of chronic secondary degenerative change, it may even be occupied by an osteophyte which in some circumstances can interfere with the placement of a cruciate ligament graft. This osteophyte may project back into the intercondylar fossa along the bone-cartilage boundary of the lateral condyle and even grow toward the intercondylar eminence, where there is normally no space owing to the presence of the ACL.

If this osteophyte is found in late cases during surgery for degenerative joint disease, it provides important clues as to the cause and pathogenesis of the degenerative change. A knee with well-functioning cruciate ligaments, for example, never exhibits such an osteophyte, because the condyle is continually polished smooth in that area.

The posterior cruciate ligament is also divided into two (or three) parts. In extension the posterior fibers are under maximum tension, while in intermediate and full flexion the middle and anterior portions are taut.

Variations in the cruciate ligaments are also reflected in the width of the intercondylar fossa. It may be very narrow, in which case the cruciate ligaments have very little lateral

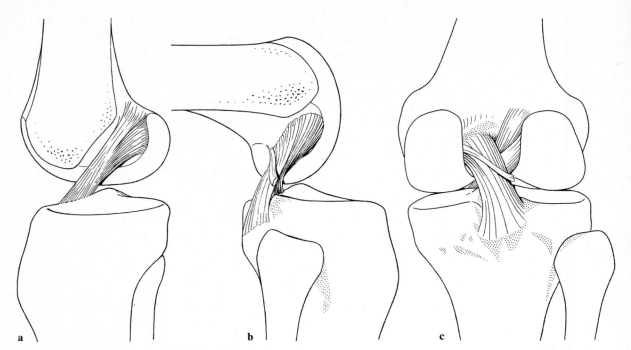

Fig. 237a–c. The areas of insertion of the cruciate ligaments and their relation to one another. **a** The anterior cruciate ligament in extension, showing its typical insertion on the medial surface of the posterior part of the lateral femoral condyle. **b** Course of the far stronger, shorter and more longitudinally-oriented posterior cruciate ligament. **c** Posterior view of both cruciate ligaments in the extended knee

"play" and lie practically on a single plane between the condyles, or it may be wider, allowing the cruciates to fan out more broadly and undergo marked spiralization.

As stated earlier, it is important to allow for individual variations in the form and length ratio of the cruciate ligaments when performing the various repairs. The "fan" principle is yet another mechanism of combining mobility and strength while maintaining fiber isometry.

In conclusion, we should again mention the phenomenon of congenital aplasia of the anterior cruciate ligament. Noble [254] describes this abnormality in connection with the presence of a ring meniscus. We have made no equivalent observation, but we have found an almost complete absence of a true anterior cruciate ligament in three adolescent girls. In each case there was a plica-like anterior extension of the central pivot, which appeared to represent the old phylogenic septum from the patellar apex. We could find no collagenous strands in any of these septa.

Tears of the Anterior Cruciate Ligament and Their Repair

Bony Avulsions

A bony avulsion of the anterior or posterior cruciate ligament is the most favorable type of injury from the standpoint of repair and subsequent healing. As a rule, such lesions are not associated with any internal disruption of ligament integrity (Fig. 238a), and so stability is restored by accurate repositioning and secure reattachment. It matters little whether screw fixation or transosseous suture fixation is the method employed; all that matters is the stability that is achieved.

For avulsions with small fragments, which often show further internal fragmentation,

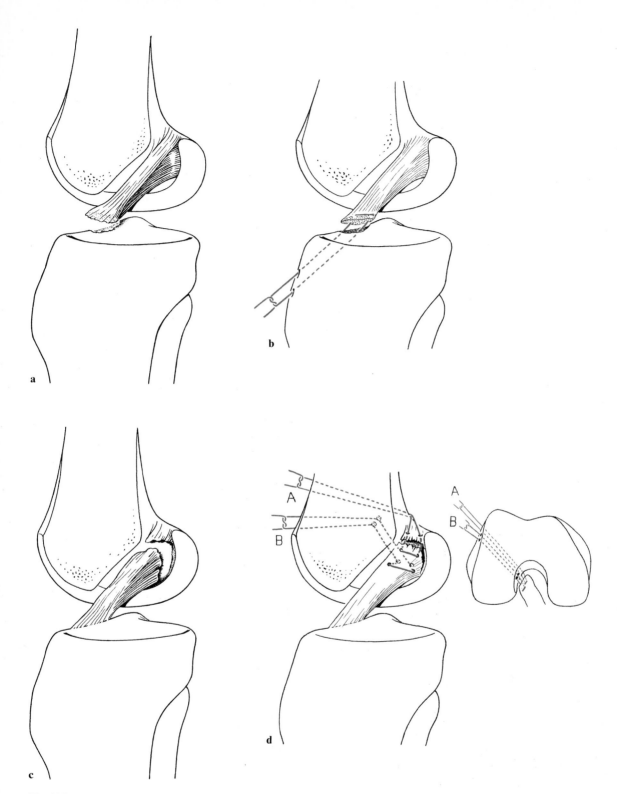

Fig. 238 a–d. Proximal and distal disinsertion of the anterior cruciate ligament and techniques of suture repair (personal technique since 1975). **a** Prognostically favorable distal avulsion with a bone fragment. **b** Transosseous suture repair for an otherwise undamaged ligament.

c Proximal rupture of the anterior cruciate ligament. **d** Repair with an "over-the-top" suture (*A*) and a transcondylar suture (*B*). Suture *A* is used to pull the ligament back into its original position, and suture *B* to fix it to the condyle (see also Figs. 28 and 29) we prefer transosseous suture fixation (Fig. 238 b). Because absorbable sutures do not hold long enough to achieve the desired consolidation, we use nonabsorbable suture material such as Polydec 3 or braided steel wire. But because synthetic, nonabsorbable suture material can be a source of chronic irritation, we make it a rule to avoid the free passage of any type of suture through the joint cavity and bury all threads within the tissues if possible. If passage through the joint is unavoidable, we use the steel wire, for it tends to cause the mildest foreign body reactions.

Pure Ligamentous Ruptures

In the great majority of cases the ligament is torn at its proximal attachment; often it is torn in its midportion, and less frequently at its distal insertion (according to Trillat [359]: 65%, 22% and 14%).

Tears at the Proximal Insertion

As the anatomic specimens in Figs. 78 b, 237 a and 257 a, b show, the anterior cruciate ligament normally inserts on the posterior part of the medial surface of the lateral femoral condyle, just in front of the margin of the condylar cartilage. Some strands even extend to the upper posterior edge of the condyle where they blend with fibers of the posterior capsule (Fig. 78 b).

Because accurate repositioning is essential for the restoration of normal stability, the proximal insertion must be reattached well back on the condyle. The consequences of reinserting the ligament too far anteriorly and proximally are illustrated by the two cases with a visible wire suture that were described in the section on Pathophysiology, p. 21 (Figs. 28 and 29).

Therefore, since 1975 we have repaired proximal ruptures of the anterior cruciate ligament (Fig. 238 c) by an "over-the-top" suturing technique (Fig. 238 c) similar to that described by MacIntosh and Tregonning [216] for cruciate ligament reconstructions.

We pass the first suture (A) through the most posterior fiber bundle of the ACL (Fig. 238 d) and carry it "over the top" of the posterior part of the lateral femoral condyle; this provides a means of pulling the torn ligament as far posteriorly as desired. Then we fix the repositioned ligament to the medial surface of the lateral condyle with a second suture (B) passed through one or two transosseous drill holes. This enables a fast, complete refixation while restoring attachment with the vascular plexus of the femur. As in all primary repairs or plastic reconstructions, we take care that the suture site is extra-articularized and well covered by synovium.

Midsubstance Tears

These tears are the most difficult in terms of primary repair. Often there is no ligament fragment long enough to be fixed directly to the femur or tibia (Fig. 239 a). Nevertheless, the torn stumps must be reapproximated. This requires that sutures be passed in two different directions (Fig. 239 b). Fiber bundles belonging to a distal tear site can be reapproximated with sutures passed through drill holes in the upper tibia. The bundles belonging to a proximal tear site are repaired like other proximal tears: One thread, A, is brought "over the top" to restore approximation, while a second (or possibly third) thread B is passed through one or more drill holes in the femoral condyle to obtain fixation.

Caution is advised during the placement of thread A if the soft tissues of the posterior capsule, PCL and ACL stump are not widely detached. To avoid incidental damage, it is best to develop a suture passageway bluntly with a long, curved, eyed ligature carrier or a Crawford clamp. A passageway must also be carefully developed from the outside back to the intercondylar capsule. This is done by splitting the iliotibial tract and then retracting the vastus lateralis anteriorly until the finger can be passed down over the plantaris and gastrocnemius muscles along the femoral shaft to the posterior capsule; the in-

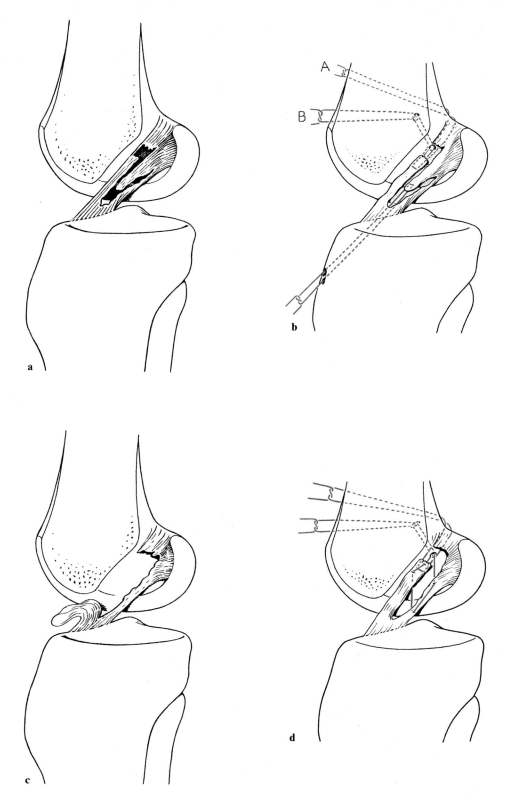

Fig. 239 a–d. Other tears of the anterior cruciate ligament. **a** The two main fiber bundles have sustained different tears. One part is torn in its proximal portion, the other distally. **b** Both components of the tear must be reapproximated by suture. **c** One part of the anterior cruciate ligament is torn and displaced, while the posteroinferior part is only overstretched. **d** Double-suture technique for repairing this special tear

tercondylar fossa is easily palpated. Beforehand, of course, the intermuscular septum must be detached with a periosteal elevator for several centimeters proximal from the lateral lip of the linea aspera. While this is done, care is taken either to avoid detaching the femorotibial tract fibers that are attached to the septum, or to prepare this band for later reattachment.

When the posterolateral passageway has been developed, thread A is carefully passed "over the top" of the lateral femoral condyle from the inside of the joint using the ligature carrier or clamp. From the outside a palpating, protecting finger is held against the site of perforation in the capsule to control the passage of the thread.

With this suturing technique we can obtain good intraoperative stability in all degrees of flexion, thus creating mechanical conditions that are conducive to healing.

Partial Ruptures

Often a tab of ACL tissue will be found on the upper tibia while continuity is apparently preserved in the rest of the ligament (Fig. 239 c). In the past, these tabs were sometimes excised in the belief that the remaining portion could ensure stability. However, this situation frequently led to severe secondary anterior instabilites with global symptoms, in some cases associated with a lateral pivot shift.

In most cases the loose tab represents the anterolateral component of the ACL, the part most important for anterior stabilization. Therefore we make every attempt to repair this lesion, whether by the over-the-top or the transcondylar suturing technique (Fig. 239 d.)

Because knee stability is the sum of a variety of synergistic factors, even a small liga-

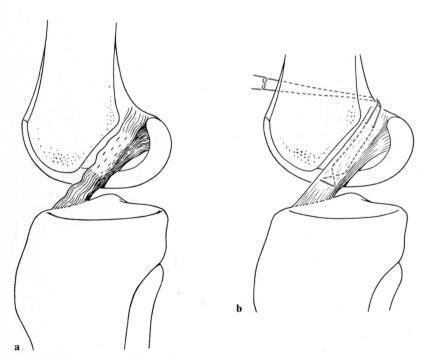

Fig. 240. a The pure "overstretching" lesion of the anterior cruciate ligament with subsynovial disinsertion of the collagenous fibers. **b** This form of proximal disinsertion and overstretching is also treated with an over-the-top suture that is carefully placed to avoid further traumatization. Care is taken not to strangulate the vessels with consequent avascular necrosis when this difficult suture is placed

210

mentous component can make the difference between compensated or decompensated joint function.

Again, it is essential that the synovial covering be restored during the repair.

"Overstretching" or Intraligamentous Ruptures with no Visible Tear

Hidden 1st- to 3rd-degree lesions. Injuries of the ACL like that shown in Fig. 240a are common. But occasionally even a badly damaged ACL will appear normal; in other cases a mild swelling of the ligament or a slight redness of its synovial covering may be the only suspicious signs. When the ligament is tested, however, a marked degree of laxity will be found. If an anterior drawer sign of 5–10 mm or more can be demonstrated intraoperatively, there is no question that the ACL is insufficient. Because the ligament is torn at its proximal attachment in two-thirds of cases, gravity will act as a barrier to spontaneous reapposition and healing. In these cases we carefully incise the synovial tissue over the ligament longitudinally and generally find collagenous fiber bundles that are either ruptured or at least overstretched and swollen. Experience has taught us that unless the ligament is sutured in such cases, it will remain insufficient. James (personal communication), based on similar negative experiences in cases of this type, also recommends repair with a crisscross Bunnell-type suture (Fig. 240b). Care must be taken not to strangulate the ligament when the suture is placed, lest avascular necrosis result. Equal care should be taken when carrying the suture "over the top" of the lateral condyle. We do not drill holes through the condyle in these cases, as this would jeopardize the remainder of the ligament.

It should be noted that these types of ligamentous injury correspond to the "creep" phenomenon described by Kennedy et al. [175]. In this process the ligament becomes gradually elongated, undergoing an irreversible "isoelastic deformation" in response to stress. All ligaments may be subject to this phemonenon.

Recurrent Post-Traumatic Hemarthrosis

The "overstretching" lesions or partial ruptures of the cruciate ligament discussed above can be a source of recurrent post-traumatic hemarthrosis.

According to Trillat et al. [359], when an initial trauma causing a partial tear of the ACL is followed by poor cicatrization, the ligament will remain insufficient. When a second minor trauma occurs, there is further tearing accompanied by bleeding into the joint. This recurrent hemarthrosis is pathognomonic of a "chronic cruciate ligament rupture."

The continuity of the ligament and its synovial covering may well be preserved in such cases, but strength and tension are lacking within its substance. When such a ligament is subjected to excessive stress, it undergoes further interstitial tearing. The vascularized synovium becomes torn, and hemarthrosis recurs. We have repeatedly observed this classic course in our patients and confirmed it at operation.

Compensation Limit and Decompensation Threshold

Nowhere does the question of compensation vs. decompensation arise so frequently and with such urgency as in cases of anterior cruciate ligament insufficiency.

As we have seen, the ACL, semimembranosus corner and ALFTL act in concert to maintain anterior stability.

But in some circumstances a patient with an isolated anterior cruciate ligament rupture can compensate for years with no significant instability, living and working without disability and even engaging in sports. However, even a minor additional injury to the ALFTL or semimembranosus corner may be sufficient to produce a manifest instability with permanent disability; this phenomenon is called "decompensation."

The studies of Butler et al. [42] on primary and secondary passive stabilizers help to clarify this phenomenon. The effectiveness of the secondary stabilizers is not equal in all knees. Thus, a knee with ACL insufficiency, for example, will decompensate sooner than one with strong stabilizers, for the ACL becomes the predominant stabilizer in instances where the secondary stabilizers are weak.

In mathematical terms, we might express the total anterior stabilization by the ACL, semimembranosus corner and ALFTL in NR, ER and IR (not just in NR, as in [42]) for both anterior quadrants as $1 = \frac{3}{3}$. In this hypothetical expression, each element accounts for $\frac{1}{3}$ of the total restraining power and thus has a "stability value" of $\frac{1}{3}$.

The anterior cruciate ligament, representing $\frac{1}{3}$ of the total anterior stabilizing power, may be lost without decompensation as long as the remaining $\frac{2}{3}$ of the stabilizers continue to function adequately. However, if these $\frac{2}{3}$ also become weakened by even a small amount, stability falls below the decompensation threshold. The same applies to any of the three components. In other words, if there is only an isolated lesion of the semimembranosus corner, ALFTL or ACL, $\frac{2}{3}$ of the anterior stabilizing power remains, and the system – *anterior stability* – remains compensated. If two components are damaged, decompensation will result.

The important question remains: How much damage can each of the three components sustain before their total stabilizing power falls below the critical $\frac{2}{3}$ value (Tables 2, 3 and 4)?

We make this calculation for every reconstruction of a recent or old combined injury, for we must recognize the fact that it is impossible to restore torn ligaments to 100% of their pre-injury value.

But if we can restore at least half of the value to each ligament in a duad injury or $\frac{2}{3}$ to each in a triad injury, then in both cases we will achieve $\frac{2}{3}$ of the original functional value and thus reach the necessary "compensation limit" (Table 5).

Table 2. Theoretical calculation of the anterior stability value

ACL	intact	$= 1/3$ anterior stability value
POL	intact	$= 1/3$ anterior stability value
ALFTL	intact	$= 1/3$ anterior stability value
Total		$1/1$ anterior stability value, *normal*
ACL	rupture	$= 0$ anterior stability value
POL	intact	$= 1/3$ anterior stability value
ALFTL	intact	$= 1/3$ anterior stability value
Total		$2/3$ anterior stability value, *still compensated*
ACL	rupture	$= 0$ anterior stability value
POL	rupture	$= 0$ anterior stability value
ALFTL	intact	$= 1/3$ anterior stability value
Total		$1/3$ anterior stability value, *decompensated*

Table 3. Theoretical calculation of the total anterior stability value (TASV) with partial damage in the three components

Normal case	Damage	Residual value	Partial value for anterior stability
ACL	0%	100%	1/3 or 4/12 or 3/9 or 2/6
POL	0%	100%	1/3 or 4/12 or 3/9 or 2/6
ALFTL	0%	100%	1/3 or 4/12 or 3/9 or 2/6
	TASV	100%	1/1 1/1 1/1 1/1 = normal anterior stability

Compensatory Reserve

If we achieve not just the minimum goal of $\frac{2}{3}$ value for each ligament, but manage to obtain a greater stability value of, say, $\frac{4}{5}$, then the prospect for recovery is improved considerably, because the resulting compensatory reserve will guard against setbacks from minor traumata and will enable healing and rehabilitation to progress without incident.

Compensation Limit, Compensatory Reserve and Prognosis for Full Functional Recovery

If, during a primary or secondary repair, we achieve a total anterior stability value

Table 4. Reduced anterior stability value after combined injuries

		Damage	Residual value	Contribution to total anterior stability
Example 1	ACL	25.0%	75.0%	3/12
	POL	25.0%	75.0%	3/12
	ALFTL	0.0%	100.0%	4/12
	TASV	16.7%	83.3%	10/12 = 5/6 = 83.3%
Example 2	ACL	25.0%	75.0%	3/12
	POL	25.0%	75.0%	3/12
	ALFTL	25.0%	75.0%	3/12
	TASV	25.0%	75.0%	9/12 = 3/4 = 75.0%
Example 3	ACL	33.3%	66.7%	2/9
	POL	33.3%	66.7%	2/9
	ALFTL	0.0%	100.0%	3/9
	TASV	23.3%	77.7%	7/9 = 77.7%
Example 4	ACL	33.3%	66.7%	2/9
	POL	33.3%	66.7%	2/9
	ALFTL	33.3%	66.7%	2/9
	TASV	33.3%	66.7%	6/9 = 2/3 = 66.7%
Example 5	ACL	50.0%	50.0%	1/6
	POL	50.0%	50.0%	1/6
	ALFTL	0.0%	100.0%	2/6
	TASV	33.3%	66.7%	4/6 = 2/3 = 66.7%
	Compensation			
	Decompensation			
Example 6	ACL	50.0%	50.0%	1/6
	POL	50.0%	50.0%	1/6
	ALFTL	50.0%	50.0%	1/6
	TASV	50.0%	50.0%	3/6 = 1/2 = 50.0%

(TASV) that is above the compensation limit, then the knee will increasingly restabilize as healing progresses. This means that stability may even improve over a two-year period on the basis of objective evaluations. On the other hand, if this minimum value is not obtained at operation, then the structures available for stabilization will be inadequate. These knee joints become progressively lax during the rehabilitation period and usually develop effusion in response to the excessive loading. In the most favorable case the muscles provide a "second line of defense" that will enable at least a functional stability to be achieved. This, too, is a kind of compensation, but it is different from that which we regard as ligamentous compensation with true restitution.

Our rules governing the interrelationship of stability components also apply to posterior stability, as well as to stability under a varus or valgus stress.

The latter stability values are, of course, secondary problems and are less critical than the anterior and posterior values, for when

Table 5. Theoretical calculation of the minimum operative goal when all three structures are ruptured

Stability value	Pre-injury	Post-injury	Minimum goal for surgical repair
ACL	1/3	0	2/3 of 1/3 = 2/9
POL	1/3	0	2/3 of 1/3 = 2/9
ALFTL	1/3	0	2/3 of 1/3 = 2/9
TASV	1/1	0	6/9 = 2/3 = 66.6%

all the synergistic components necessary for restoring total anterior or posterior stability have been repaired, any varus or valgus instability is automatically relieved.

ciate and has correspondingly larger areas of attachment on the femur and tibia. Therefore, its refixation must also be stronger and more secure and must employ at least two

---

There can be no significant valgus or varus instability without anterior or posterior instability.

When the three components of an anterior or posterior stability have been corrected, the varus-valgus instability is also eliminated.

The correction of a varus or valgus instability does not automatically eliminate an anterior or posterior instability.

Although it may appear initially that an operation for the correction of a varus or valgus laxity has also restored anteroposterior stability, eventually the anteroposterior and then the lateral instability will recur, because the cruciate ligaments, not the collateral ligaments, are the *principal* guide mechanism of the joint.

Tears of the Posterior Cruciate Ligament

Bony Avulsions

According to reports by Trillat et al. [359], ruptures occur with about equal frequency at the femoral and the tibial insertions of the ligament. Our clinical material, though smaller than that of Trillat, shows a clear predominance of distal ruptures. These are undoubtedly more frequent when bony avulsions are also counted (Fig. 241).

These bony avulsions, like those of the ACL, have the best chance of healing if accurately repaired with a screw or nonabsorbable suture.

Pure Ligamentous Ruptures

The posterior cruciate ligament has twice the size and rupture strength of the anterior cru-

sutures. The broad, fan-shaped attachment of the ligament requires that it be reinserted in fan-shaped fashion using several sutures passed through multiple drill holes (Figs. 242–246).

We have rarely observed complete tears through the midsubstance of the posterior cruciate ligament; however, we have found an intermediate form between the middle and distal tear. This tear tends to take a jagged downward course, paralleling the posterior downslope of the tibial plateau. It is usually sufficient to refix the ligament to the tibia in such cases, but if necessary we do not hesitate to suture the ligament to the femur as well (Fig. 247) (cf. ACL, Fig. 239).

In the highly schematic drawings in Figs. 248–250d, the tear of the posterior cruciate ligament is part of a complex injury and may be associated with injuries of the medial or the lateral side. As the drawings show, these PCL tears can be reapproximated and secured transosseously with the same suture used to repair the medial and lateral ligamentous tears, and via the same approach. The more extensive the ligamentous injury, the easier it is to gain access to and repair the posterior cruciate ligament, for broad exposure can be obtained in such cases.

For the situation shown in Figs. 248 and 249, additional exposure via the Trickey approach [345, 346] may prove necessary (Figs. 205 and 206).

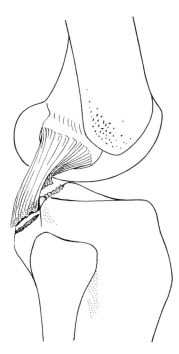

Fig. 241. Proximal and distal disinsertion of the posterior cruciate ligament with corresponding suturing technique. Distal avulsion of the posterior cruciate ligament from the tibia with a bone fragment

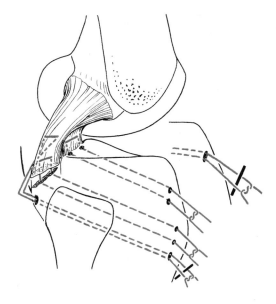

Fig. 242. At least 2 sutures are needed for reattachment of the broad insertion. A "through-the-bottom" tension suture passed through the capsule is excellent for restoring distal tension to the PCL. If the two ends of a suture must be passed through a single drill hole for technical reasons or lack of space, they are tied over a screw head or wire

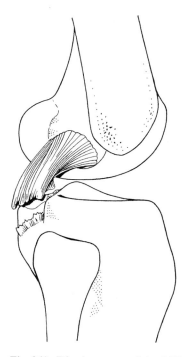

Fig. 243. Distal rupture of the PCL near the bone. The ligament is pulled distally by means of a "through-the-bottom" tension suture. (If the ends of a suture are brought out through a single channel, they must be tied over a firm material)

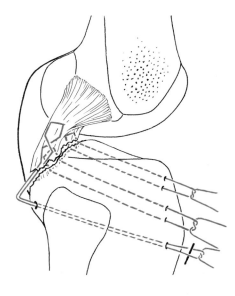

Fig. 244. Suture of the 3 main bundles of the PCL. The dorsodistal bundle is placed under maximum downward tension by a "through-the-bottom" suture

215

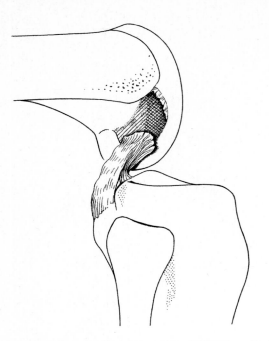

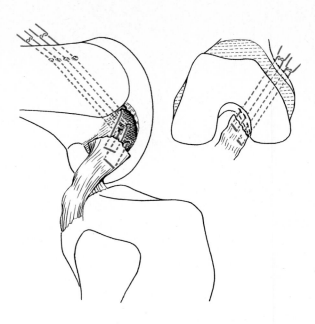

Fig. 245. Proximal rupture of the PCL. The principal zone of attachment is cross-hatched in the drawing (see also Figs. 108, 109 and 112–116)

Fig. 246. Again, at least one double suture is necessary for repair of the proximal PCL rupture to obtain a sufficiently broad area of reattachment. The detail drawing shows the synovial recesses overlying the sides of the condyles proximal to the cartilage surface. These must not be injured during the repair and are easily avoided from a proximal direction by keeping the drill holes outside the suprapatellar pouch. One should not hesitate to place a third pair of sutures through additional drill holes if the three main bundles of the PCL cannot be adequately reattached with the first two. The main drill holes should be placed very close to the condyle-cartilage boundary to optimize the tension on the reattached PCL

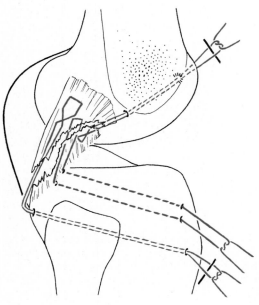

Fig. 247. Further variants of the PCL rupture. Example of sutures placed proximally and distally to repair a midsubstance tear. The distal suture is routed "through the bottom"

216

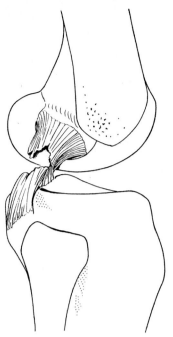

Fig. 248. Midsubstance tear of the PCL

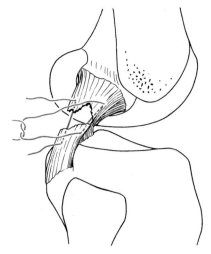

Fig. 249. This type of tear can be repaired through a separate posterior exposure if necessary (Trickey [345]). Often such a tear is also accessible from the side, as shown in Fig. 250a, b

Isolated Cruciate Ligament Tears

Isolated Tear of the Anterior Cruciate Ligament

Mechanism and occurrence. There are circumstances in which the ACL can sustain an isolated rupture, while the synergistic lateral and medial structures may show only 1st-degree spraining or perhaps occult 2nd-degree lesions of the semimembranosus or popliteus corner. These coexisting lesions are all too often neglected and are probably the reason why the prognosis for these "isolated" cruciate ligament tears is often poorer than expected. We have found that knee joints in which the *ACL is the principal anterior stabilizer* are predisposed and tend to become decompensated if ACL insufficiency arises. While an occasional patient will be noted during an operation for other causes to have an old rupture of the ACL but is without symptoms referable to it, in most cases the "isolated ACL rupture" is recognized early, and the secondary increase in instability following operative as well as non-operative treatment is greater than initial findings would indicate. Therefore, it is seldom enough to repair the ACL alone in "sole rupture" cases; the medial and lateral synergists must also be stabilized as needed, even in acute cases.

The acute hyperextension mechanism in the medially rotated knee is capable of rupturing the ACL at the notch of Grant on the roof of the intercondylar fossa (Fig. 251). In most cases the stumps are badly lacerated, and a primary suture may be difficult or impossible (Fig. 252).

Occasionally these forms of cruciate ligament tear are associated with a peripheral detachment of the medial meniscus. In other cases hemorrhagic suffusions occur in the region of the semimembranosus corner. It is also important to check the course and attachments of the synergistic ALFTL. This does not require much dissection, since an

217

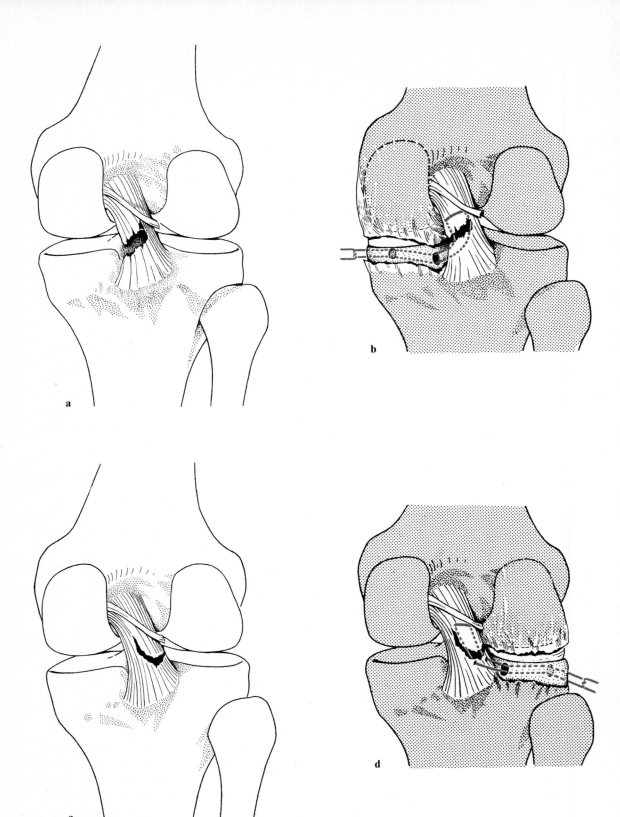

Fig. 250 a–d. In most cases a medial or lateral injury accompanying the posterior cruciate tear obviates a special exposure. The ligamentous lesion can be followed around the posteromedial or posterolateral corner to the PCL, which is engaged with a transtibial suture and reapproximated

218

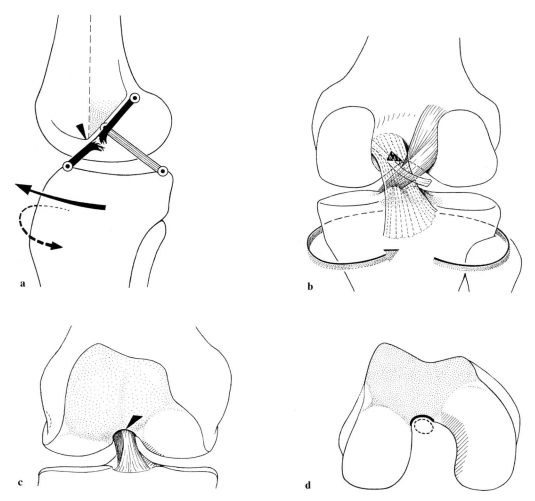

Fig. 251 a–d. The mechanism of the anterior cruciate ligament tear by hyperextension. **a** In IR the tense ACL can be torn at the edge of the intercondylar roof by acute hyperextension. **b** IR and hyperextension cause the ACL to angulate at the anterior osteochondral boundary of the intercondylar tunnel. **c** A fulcrum effect occurs at the notch of Grant which predisposes to a tear. **d** Axial view of the distal femur parallel to the femoral long axis showing the femoropatellar and femorotibial joint surfaces. In the area between the joint surfaces is the well-delineated notch of Grant which receives the ACL. In **c** and **d** note the areas of the medial tibial and femoral joint surfaces *shaded with parallel lines*. These areas, which have a heavy cartilage covering, engage strongly against each other due to the coiling of the cruciate ligaments during IR and so are a frequent site of pathology (e.g., osteochondritis dissecans)

access is created in that region anyway for reattaching the ACL to the femur.

Recently another mechanism has been postulated as a cause of the isolated ACL rupture. It seems that landing with the knee flexed after a long-jump or after a high fall can cause a smooth rupture of the ACL due to the braking action of the quadriceps.

We have observed a similar self-injury mechanism in a skier.

An amateur ski racer skied through the finishing gate in a "layout" position with the upper body horizontal and the knees deeply flexed. On regaining an upright stance with the aid of his quadriceps, he felt something tear in his knee. There was immediate swelling with hemarthrosis. Arthroscopy disclosed a fresh proximal rupture of the ACL. At operation no further joint pathology could be found despite careful exploration.

At first sight such a mechanism seems paradoxical, but the antagonistic relationship of the quadriceps to the ACL has been repeatedly confirmed and has been vividly demonstrated by de Montmollin and le Coeur [230].

The patellar tendon pulls the tibia forward, while the quadriceps simultaneously pushes the femur backward on the tibial plateau via the patella. In cases where large forces are involved, a consequent rupture of the ACL can easily be imagined. It is of interest in this regard that long-jumpers have a high incidence of classic meniscus tears despite an absence of the classic rotational trauma mechanism. We know that the posterior horns of the menisi (see Semimembranosus Corner, Fig. 92 ff.) help to check anterior displacement of the tibia, suggesting a connection with the mechanism of injury described above.

The ever-changing interaction of the synergists and antagonists is ubiquitous and subtle; when the balance is upset by a trauma-producing mechanism, a lesion usually results.

Just as the quadriceps is an antagonist of the ACL, it is an excellent and demonstrable synergist of the PCL. This function is discussed in the section on Examination and in Fig. 161c ff. It also forms the theoretical basis for the palliative operation proposed by Augustine [15] for posterior cruciate insufficiency.

Isolated Tear of the Posterior Cruciate Ligament

Mechanism and occurrence. The circumstances enabling an isolated rupture of the PCL are even easier to grasp. Whereas isolated ACL tears are caused mainly by skiing or soccer injuries, PCL tears are chiefly the result of motor-vehicle accidents, especially falls on motorcycles. In most cases the anterior aspect of the tibial head is struck directly while the knee is flexed. The peripheral ligamentous structures are relatively lax in this position and have a large elastic reserve, while the short PCL is tight and has exhausted its elastic reserve. These circumstances are sufficient to enable an isolated tear. A similar mechanism is involved in "dashboard injuries," in which the knee strikes the dashboard of an automobile directly on the upper tibia.

Treatment of Isolated Cruciate Ligament Tears

As a rule, we feel that the diagnosis of a cruciate ligament rupture constitutes an indication for operative repair. We have found that good to perfect stability can be restored in many cases by the suturing of fresh ligamentous ruptures (see also the section on Results, p. 292).

Of course the indication for surgery also depends in large measure on the condition of the patient, for we are, after all, operating not on isolated ligament lesions, but on patients. In the young and athletic patient, repair or reconstruction should be undertaken. The older the patient is, and the more willing he is to accept a condition that may limit his activities, the greater our hesitancy to operate.

Secondary Repair and Plastic Reconstruction of the Ligaments in Old Injuries

General

In this second main chapter on treatment we find ourselves in a somewhat uncharted area in which there are few recognized points of reference, although progress in this direction is being made.

Now that the nomenclature for instabilities has become standardized to a large degree, efforts are also being made to create a basis for the comparative evaluation of knee joints in terms of their initial status and the results of treatment.

Below we shall present a series of generally valid statements in an attempt to survey the complex problem of the treatment of the acutely and chronically unstable knee.

The results that may be expected vary considerably, depending on whether treatment is *non-operative* or *operative,* and whether the operative treatment is *primary* or *secondary.*

Non-Operative Treatment

– There are by nature favorable injuries which will heal well without fixation.
– There are cases in which immobilization for a limited time will enable scar tissue to bridge the defect and reapproximate the torn ends, resulting in a good restoration of stability and function.
– There are other cases in which conservative treatment will yield a poor result, and the patient will be permanently limited in his ability to work or engage in sports on account of pain, limited motion, decreased endurance and working capacity, and a *feeling of unsteadiness* when walking on uneven ground.

Primary Operative Treatment

– Many times the operative result is perfect, even following a severe injury.
– Very often the result, while not perfect, is good enough to restore the patient to full functional capacity.
– There are fair and poor results with associated degrees of disability. If the patient desires a better result, secondary revision is indicated.

Secondary Operative Treatment

– There are few perfect results with a restoration of normal function.
– There are good results which improve the patient's functional capacity enough to satisfy him.
– All too often the results are unsatisfactory. Even if the patient himself may be satisfied, the objective results are poor when viewed in relation to costs (hospitalization, surgery, loss of wages, etc.).
– There are many chronically unstable knee joints with instability-related cartilage damage that was severe enough to portend the poor late result.
– Unfortunately, there are also cases that are worse after surgery than before.

These facts prompted us to analyze the results of treatment in relation to the patient's initial status. Too often, it appeared to us that too much importance was attached to a single finding, which then became the goal of the reconstructive procedure. None of the operative methods seemed capable of adequately dealing with the problem in its totality.

It was the principles of kinematics and their relation to anatomic form that took us one step further. Through them, we were able to understand why commonly used surgical procedures such as the extra-articular anterior cruciate ligament reconstruction of Cabot et al. [403], Wittek's operation [394–396], Lindemann's reconstruction [200], Augustine's operation [15], Helfet's operation [124], the "pes transfer" of Slocum and Larson [325], O'Donoghue's reconstruction [268], the "five-one" reconstruction of Nicholas [252], the technique of Hughston and Eilers [136], and the "lateral repairs" of McIntosh and Darby [215] and Ellison et al. [76] were unable to restore normal function in every case and had a palliative effect only. This is not to say that these procedures are worthless; on the contrary, good results can still be achieved with many of these techniques, producing satisfaction and even enthusiasm on the part of the patient. We are pointing out only that results of this quality could not be predicted with sufficient regularity. Too many unknown factors and perhaps even chance events were involved.

Often the instabilities could still be demonstrated objectively, but the patient was better able to compensate for them. Secondary exacerbations during subsequent years were all too common. The ratio of good to fair results was low, and perfection was rarely if ever achieved.

These results contrasted sharply with our own parallel experiences in the treatment of fresh ligamentous injuries.

In the light of these observations and experiences, we adopted the practice in 1974 of anatomically repairing every major ligament that was affected with instability. In that year we performed our first "over the top" cruciate ligament reconstructions; before then we had routinely employed the methods of Cabot et al. [403], Lindemann [200], Jones [162, 163] and Augustine [15].

Since 1974 we have no longer repaired a cruciate ligament without also repairing its synergists. In 1976 we recorded our first perfect two-year results, with a restoration of normal function and stability, in a soccer player and a female volleyball player. In both cases we performed an anterior cruciate ligament reconstruction using the technique described below, a repair of the medial side, and a lateral femorotibial ligament reconstruction.

Since then we have not deviated significantly from this line, and only in exceptional cases have we performed one of the simple palliative procedures. Having found a workable approach, we attempted systematically in ensuing years to simplify and expedite the operations without compromising the quality of the results.

Cruciate Ligament Reconstruction and Repair of the Central Pivot

Based on our experiences prior to 1974, we came to the conclusion that only a functionally competent substitute could effectively replace the cruciate ligaments.

Zur Verth [quoted in 396] and later Wittek [396] and Campbell [46] were among the first to use a distal pedicle graft from the patellar ligament as a substitute for the anterior cruciate ligament.

We first used the method of Jones [163] for the replacement of this ligament, but soon found that the transplantation of a patellar bone block greatly limited the possibilities for an anatomic reconstruction. The bone block could seldom be implanted as far back on the femoral condyle as necessary. The transplant was usually too short. Then in 1974 we became acquainted with the method of MacIntosh [215], in which the transplanted strip consisted of a longitudinal central third of the patellar ligament, the associated galea aponeurotica of the patella, and a section of the lower end of the quadriceps tendon. This provided a transplant of ample length. But the real innovation in this technique was the manner in which the transplant was routed through the joint. Instead of pulling it through a tunnel in the femur, which often places the substitute ligament too far anteriorly and invariably subjects it to angulation and to a torsional mechanism during articular movement, MacIntosh [215] brought the transplant out "over the top" of the lateral femoral condyle.

With this technique it became possible to place the transplant under adequate posterior tension without having to stretch it over a sharp bony edge. In addition, the technique provided an almost ideal means of bringing the transplant to the correct anatomic insertion site.

In 1974 we also became familiar with the Eriksson technique [79]; this offered another advantage. To obtain a transplant of sufficient length, Eriksson used the medial third of the patellar ligament as a distal pedicle graft. The strip included a piece of bone from the patella, which formed the strong proximal end of the transplant. The problem was how to anchor this disk of bone to the posterior medial surface of the lateral femoral condyle.

We felt that Eriksson's technique of transosseous suture fixation was somewhat complicated and could not guarantee that the effective posterior insertion site of the substitute ligament would be optimum. Nevertheless, we incorporated some elements of it into the MacIntosh technique.

Our Current Technique of Anterior Cruciate Ligament Reconstruction

First we estimate the necessary length of the transplant on a preoperative lateral x-ray and compare it with the length of patellar ligament available. A high-riding patella is favorable in such cases, while a low-riding patella creates difficulties.

If the patellar ligament is short, we follow the Eriksson method [79] and take the longer medial third. With a longer patellar ligament, we leave the medial border of the ligament in place to help preserve its form and length (Fig. 253). The incision is made upward from the tibial tuberosity and is continued on up into the quadriceps tendon for a distance of 6–10 cm above the patella (5 cm is not enough and 11 cm is too much); over the patella the incision is carried down to the cortex. If the galea aponeurotica is very thin, we flare the strip broadly over the patella, narrowing it again in the quadriceps tendon. This will eliminate a point of least resistance in the mechanically critical area of the transplant, and the transplant as a whole will have a more uniform tensile strength (Kennedy, personal communication). Before the strip is freed from the patella, it is first mobilized from the quadriceps tendon. Whereas the strip of patellar ligament is full-thickness, we take only a superficial layer 2–3 mm thick from the quadriceps tendon. This will provide adequate strength for pull-through and fixation. If this section is made too thick, it will be difficult later to pull it through the joint.

Next the transplant is freed from the anterior patellar surface. We know from the preoperative x-ray how long the segment must be that extends from the tuberosity through the channel in the tibia to the posterior medial surface of the lateral femoral condyle (Fig. 254). We locate the area of the transplant that will be attached to the condyle (Figs. 252–254), and we include a thin layer of patellar bone in the strip at that location. This will mechanically strengthen the critical area of attachment, and fixation of the bone graft to the freshened condyle will result in better healing than a direct ligament-to-bone suture.

Because the correct position of the bone fragment in the transplant cannot be measured with complete accuracy before it is pulled into the joint, we recommend cutting a somewhat oversize lamella and then trimming it to the correct size with bone forceps after the transplant has been positioned in the joint. Using a periosteal elevator and scalpel, the galea is carefully freed until it is adherent only to an area of bone corresponding to the desired size of the lamella. At one time the separation of this lamella was a difficult task. The cortex is hard, and forceful chiseling would traumatize the pa-

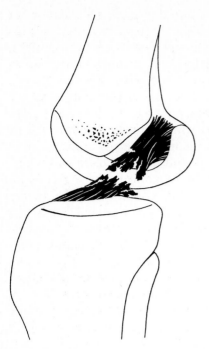

Fig. 252. Laceration of the ACL like that associated with a hyperextension trauma. A primary plastic reconstruction is indicated in such cases

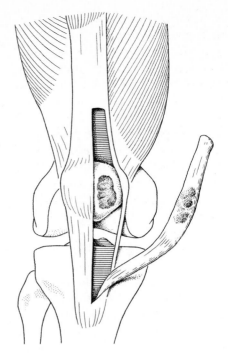

Fig. 253. Reconstruction of the ACL using a strip from the patellar ligament, patellar galea aponeurotica and quadriceps tendon. When cutting the transplant, care is taken to spare vessels coursing upward from the tibial tuberosity. If the galea is very thin the strip should be widened over the patella to obtain more material. The strip includes a thin piece of bone from the anterior patellar surface for a more secure fixation to the femur

tellar and femoral cartilage. Therefore, we now use the AO oscillating mini-saw to make converging cuts into the bone from both sides and use the chisel only as an aid for removing the bony wedge.

Important Note on the Cutting of the Transplant

Before the first incisions are made for cutting the transplant, it is first necessary to study the course of the deep arterial network on the patellar ligament and anterior patellar surface. Usually the incisions can be placed in such a way that a long longitudinal vessel is preserved on the transplant. This is important for its vitality, for we have repeatedly noted the extravasation of blood from branches of the preserved vessel in the new

ligament when the tourniquet is released near the end of the operation.

After the transplant has been developed in its entirety, a No. 3 nylon suture is placed through its proximal end, and it is pulled with the aid of a wire stylet through a Thiemann urethral catheter or an intestinal tube with a *hole at the tip* (Ch 16–20) (see also Fig. 256a); the suture length should be at least twice the catheter length. To make it easier later to pull the transplant through the tibial channel, its broad patellar segment with the bony lamella is rolled up toward the inside, and several turns of thread are made about the roll.

Next the tunnel is drilled through the tibial head. The substitute ligament should undergo as little angulation as possible when entering and emerging from the tunnel, and it should lose none of its length.

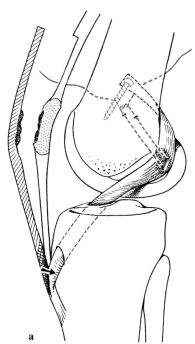

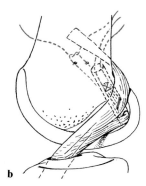

a

b

Fig. 254. a Lateral view of an "over-the-top" ACL reconstruction after the substitute ligament has been pulled through the upper tibia and carried over the lateral femoral condyle to the lateral femoral surface. The piece of bone from the patella is trimmed to size and attached to the freshened condyle with a transcondylar suture. Attention should be given to the blood supply in the region of the tibial head (*arrow*); the incisions must not sever the principal blood vessels, which are easily seen even in a bloodless field. **b** An even truer resto-

ration of normal anatomy can be achieved by splitting off a portion of the transplant in Y-shaped fashion and running it through a 4.5-mm drill hole through the condylar wall behind and below the main strip. This creates a tension like that normally produced by the posterolateral bundle of the ACL. The branched strip should be as short as possible to preserve the integrity and circulation of the transplant, and should be just long enough so that it can be independently anchored in its drill channel

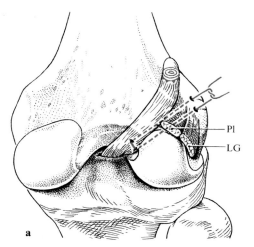

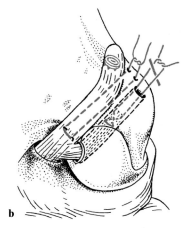

Pl

LG

a

b

Fig. 255. a View of the transplant from behind. The main portion of the transplant passes out of the joint just above the cartilage border and plantaris muscle and is anchored on the lateral side. **b** Carrying the transplant "over-the-top" cannot in itself reproduce the entire normal area of ACL attachment on the posterior

medial surface of the lateral femoral condyle. However, freeing a secondary strip near the proximal end of the transplant and passing it through a transcondylar channel will make it possible to reconstruct the posterolateral bundle of the ACL as well

225

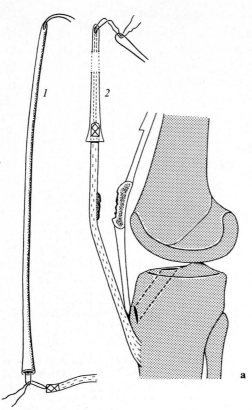

Fig. 256. a Technique for pulling the transplant through the joint in two phases. **a** The free end of the transplant is threaded through a specially prepared urethral catheter with a conical end (*1, 2*). **b** The catheter and transplant together are pulled through the tibia and joint. (*3*) The catheter is pulled through in the direction of the channel axis, as indicated by the arrow. The slightly thinner transplant easily follows. (*4*) The passageway through the joint and "over the top" is easily found with the catheter. (*5*) Before the new ligament is drawn taut and the catheter removed, the intra-articular placement of the transplant is checked, and the piece of patellar bone is trimmed to size so that it can be attached to the ideal site on the freshened femur with a transcondylar suture. (Catheter technique created by us in 1975)

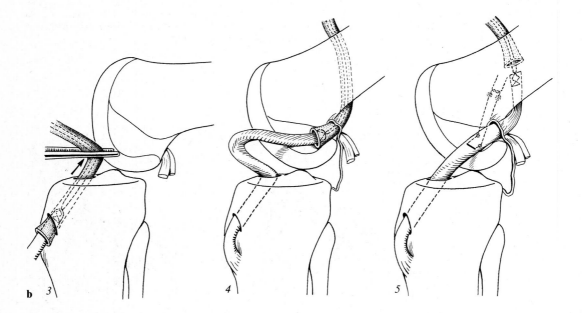

An initial drill hole is made from the outside inward with a 3.2-mm AO drill bit (Figs. 254 and 256a). The drill bit should emerge posterior to the fat pad and anterior to the intercondylar eminence. Then a 2-mm Kirschner wire about 6 cm long is inserted into the hole to serve as a guide for the hollow reaming bit. The AO 6.5-mm hollow reamer, designed for the removal of broken cancellous bone screws, is excellent for drilling over the wire and cutting the tunnel. Care must be taken to cut the tunnel correctly the first time; redrilling will make the channel too large to guide the ligament properly. The tunnel must emerge *in front of* the highest point of the tibial eminence; *otherwise the posterior cruciate ligament,* which attaches directly behind the eminence, may be *severely damaged.* Medially the edge of the tunnel will be close to the anterior meniscus horn but must not damage its anchorage. If the channel is properly drilled, the substitute ligament will pass smoothly from the anteromedial to the posterolateral quadrant with little angulation.

Before it is pulled through, however, the site of attachment on the femoral condyle and the entire passageway "over the top" of the condyle must be thoroughly prepared (see Fig. 238d and discussion of over-the-top ACL suture, p. 208).

The passageway through the posterior joint capsule must be sufficiently enlarged with an elevator or a strong, curved clamp from the joint interior so that the transplant can be pulled through later without difficulty. While the passageway is being bluntly developed, a finger should be inserted from the popliteal side to protect the vessels and nerves from the instrument tip.

A pull-through thread can make it easier to draw the catheter through the joint, provided it is attached to the tip in such a way that the catheter cannot deviate from the intended path.

Because we perform all such operations on the flexed knee, freshening of the medial surface of the lateral femoral condyle should present no difficulties. With the knee flexed to about 130°, the femur is freshened with

the chisel *directly anterior to* the posterior condylar cartilage surface (Figs. 257 and 258a); a shallow groove may even be made with a drill or chisel in the area where the transplant is to be brought over the lateral condyle.

Now at least two transcondylar holes are drilled with the 3.2-mm (or 2.0-mm) drill bit. With the knee flexed to 130°, the drill bit can be applied far back on the condyle in front of the posterior cartilage. With practice (e.g., on model bone), the bit can be directed so as to emerge safely on the lateral metaphysis of the condyle, anterior to the lateral lip of the linea aspera (Fig. 255). When drilling the holes we use an AO tap sleeve with a telescoping sleeve insert (Figs. 258–260); we find that a drill guide is unnecessary when this arrangement is employed. Pull-through threads of various colors are placed through the drill holes for better orientation. Later they will be used to pull through the definitive suture threads.

Before the catheter and transplant are drawn into the joint, the tunnel should be smoothed out with the elevator to prevent snagging on the rough cancellous bone. The catheter and transplant are pulled through slowly along the axis of the tunnel a centimeter at a time (Fig. 256b) to keep from breaking the bony bridge on the anterior tibia. The transplant should be as smooth and cylindrically-shaped as possible. The lumen of the tunnel must be just large enough to allow the new ligament to pass through undamaged, yet small enough to guide the ligament properly. Torsion of the ligament must be avoided due to the consequent circulatory impairment and loss of effective length.

If all preparations have been made on both the tibia and femur, the catheter and transplant can be pulled completely through the joint and brought out "over-the-top" of the femoral condyle.

The pull-through phase having been completed, the transplant can be grasped by the catheter or its free end and pulled back and forth through the joint in order to test it for freedom from torsion and correct placement of the bone fragment.

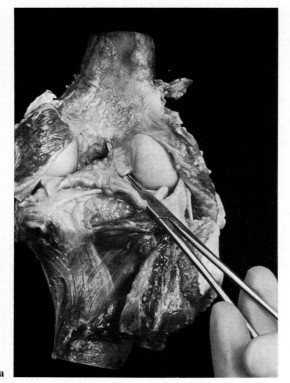

a

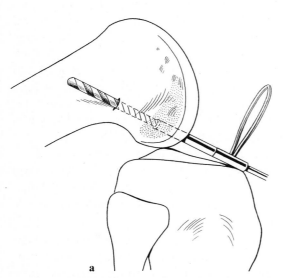

b

Fig. 257. a Anatomic specimen in which the posterior capsule has been detached proximally and reflected downward to demonstrate the joint interior. The *curved clamp* has been passed beneath the ACL at its posterior insertion to demonstrate how far back on the femur this ligament is attached. The "over-the-top" placement of a substitute ligament or repair sutures is best suited to imitate this course. The anatomic repair is improved by placing an extratranscondylar suture far posteriorly to provide additional fixation of the ligament to the femoral condyle near the cartilage border. The specimen and positional drawing **b** show the main posterior semimembranosus attachments from a different aspect (numbers explained in Fig. 97)

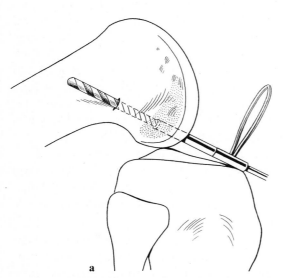

a

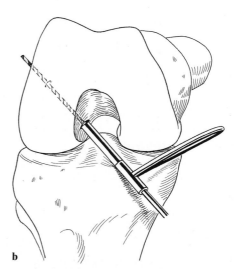

b

Fig. 258a, b. Technique for placing the transcondylar drill hole. **a** With the knee flexed to about 130°, a direct hole can be drilled in the area of attachment of the ACL. At this angle the drill bit automatically emerges proximal and anterior to the intermuscular septum. **b** The guide sleeve is laid directly against the upper tibia for drilling

228

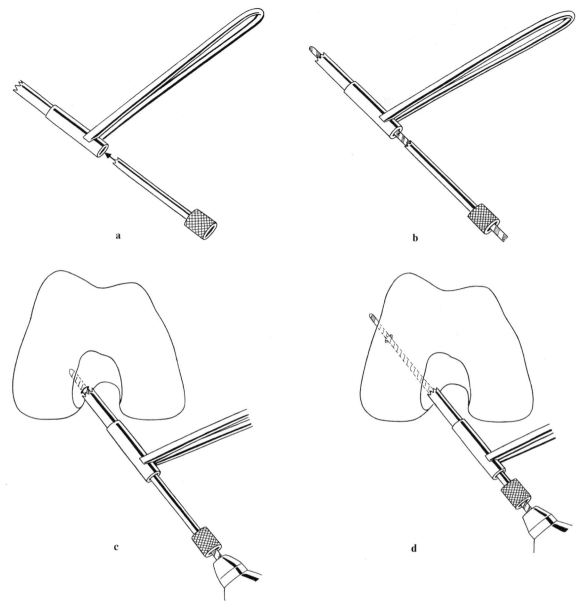

Fig. 259. a Method of using the 4.5-mm AO tap sleeve with the 3.2-mm straight drill sleeve as a "telescoping drill guide." **b** The sleeves are coaxialized with a long 3.2-mm drill bit. **c** As drilling proceeds the 3.2-mm sleeve telescopes into the 4.5-mm tap sleeve, thereby protecting the soft tissues from the portion of the drill bit still outside the tap sleeve. **d** End of the drilling phase with the sleeves fully telescoped

Now the thread is removed from around the rolled portion of the transplant, and the bone lamella is cut to the necessary, minimal size with bone forceps. (This may also be done after the strip is pulled through the tibial tunnel and before it is carried "over the top" if the bone fragment can be placed against its later area of attachment on the femur.)

Next, one or preferably two No. 0–1 nonabsorbable sutures are placed in the transplant at the presumptive fixation site.

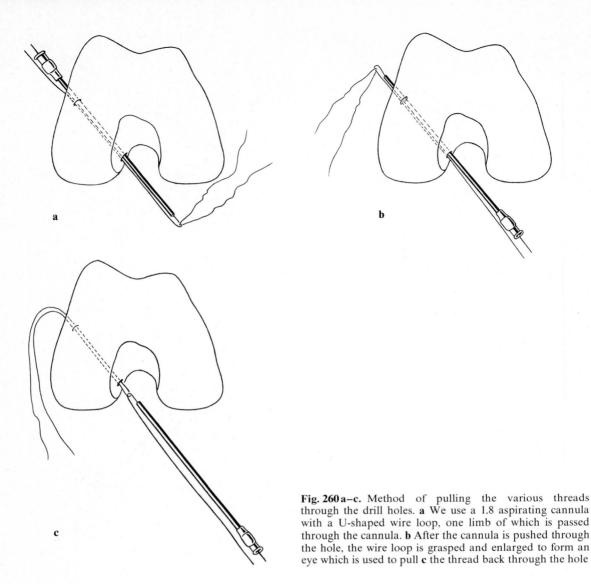

Fig. 260a–c. Method of pulling the various threads through the drill holes. **a** We use a 1.8 aspirating cannula with a U-shaped wire loop, one limb of which is passed through the cannula. **b** After the cannula is pushed through the hole, the wire loop is grasped and enlarged to form an eye which is used to pull **c** the thread back through the hole

This must be done in such a way that:

1. the sutures pass over the bony lamella and do not hamper bone-to-bone contact;
2. they are situated slightly distal to the transcondylar holes so that the new ligament will become tensed when the sutures are drawn tight.

If the transplant is positioned correctly, tension applied to its proximal end by the femoral condyle can be felt at its distal end by the tibial tuberosity.

Now the definitive sutures can be pulled through the condyle with the aid of the different-colored pull-through threads placed earlier (Fig. 260). In addition, a suture should be placed through a flap prepared from the infrapatellar fat pad and synovial fold and pulled through one of the transcondylar holes in order to obtain a synovial covering. This flap must closely invest the new ligament from the tibia to the femur in order to promote vascularization. Usually fine, absorbable stay sutures (0000) must be placed to secure the covering. These, perhaps combined with interligamentous sutures, complete the attachment of the new ligament to the central pivot, which again occupies its normal extra-articular position.

The proximal end of the new ligament is definitively attached to the lateral side of the femur with a small-fragment screw (length 28 mm) and a toothed washer, but only after all repairs to the semimembranosus and ALFTL have been completed. The transcondylar sutures, too, are not definitively tied until all other repairs have been made.

Finally, the joint capsule and donor site for the transplant are closed. Usually a tension-free closure is easily obtained in the region of the patellar and quadriceps tendon. A galeal defect often remains on the anterior surface of the patella, but the layer of superficial fascia can be sutured over this defect without danger of later complications. If now the tightening of the transosseous sutures is observed through the arthrotomy opening, it will be seen that tension is developed in various directions, and that even a fan-shaped ligamentous attachment has been recreated.

With practice, one will even be able to place the sutures in such a way that the anteromedial and posterolateral parts of the original ACL are faithfully reconstructed.

If portions of the original ligament are present, they are *never excised,* but are *reintegrated.* They provide the best means of truly uniting the new ligament with the central pivot.

In our opinion the decisive advantage of this "over-the-top" technique is that it enables the graft to be transposed undamaged by traction along its natural fiber axis (Fig. 253), while the transcondylar sutures serve only to fix the ligament to the condyle and help create a fan-shaped area of attachment.

Recently we have modified the reconstruction somewhat by splitting off a posterolateral portion of the transplanted strip and pulling it out through a 4.5-mm hole drilled in the far posterior part of the condyle (Figs. 254b and 258b). The main anteromedial part of the transplant is still carried "over the top" and is tightened with the transcondylar suture on the medial surface of the condyle as previously described.

Case Reports on the Medium-Term Results of Our Anterior Cruciate Ligament Reconstruction

Three cases from our first series illustrate the excellent functional results that can be obtained with the technique described:

The soccer player in Fig. 261 had sustained a hyperextension-IR injury of the right knee. At operation about 2 weeks later we found a fresh, irreparable mophead tear of the anterior cruciate ligament and a complete peripheral detachment of the medial meniscus with hemorrhagic suffusion of the entire semimembranosus corner. Though we always attempt to save the meniscus, it was not possible in this instance. We performed a primary cruciate ligament replacement by our technique, something we seldom do in acute cases.

In the same year the soccer player was able to return to his former first-string position in the team and resume playing in his usual manner without disability or complaints.

A second soccer player who had undergone a prior meniscectomy presented with a global anterior instability and a 3+ lateral pivot shift. His disability was such that he was no longer able to play soccer. Today, six years after our ACL reconstruction with a medial and lateral repair, the operated knee is as stable as the other one. The patient has been playing soccer regularly for years without complaints and rates the result as "perfect."

The third case involves a female patient who also underwent our ACL reconstruction and six years later is playing volleyball with normal stability in the operated knee and without complaints.

Thoughts on Healing in the Postoperative Period

Because the most critical time for a transplant is that following a period of immobilization, we must add some thoughts on the healing and rehabilitation period: In the absence of function and movement, the zone of attachment to the bone cannot undergo the restructuring necessary for sound healing.

Cooper and Misol [55] investigated the transition from ligament to bone in the normal histologic section and found that the fiber bundles of the ligament blend with a zone of fibrocartilage, which in turn blends with the bone. This zone mediates the transmission of forces and explains why the ligaments do not often "break" smoothly off the bone, in the way that an electric cord breaks at the point where it emerges from the plug unless this junction is covered by a tapered sheath.

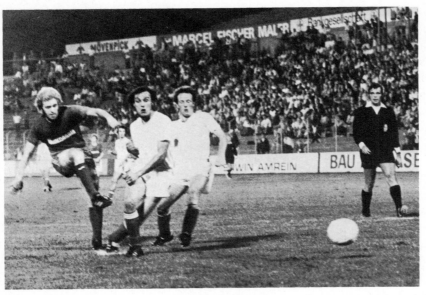

Fig. 261. The soccer player on the left has regained his shooting power following an anterior cruciate ligament reconstruction in the right knee

In most cases of ligamentous avulsion this intermediate fibrocartilage layer remains attached to the bone, forming a small stump. Only in cases where the bone appears completely denuded in the rupture area has the fibrocartilage been avulsed along with the ligament.

When a reconstructive procedure is done or even when an avulsed ligament is repaired, it takes some time before this transition zone is fully restored, for the collagenous fiber bundles, too, can regain their normal architecture only when subjected to loading.

Generally the knee joint treated for such an injury is returned to unprotected loading too abruptly. Even after 6–8 weeks' immobilization, the proprioceptive control mechanisms are not yet ready to reassume their protective role.

By contrast, a fractured bone is allowed weeks or months to remodel before it is expected to bear loads with no danger of refracturing. But because the ligaments are "only soft tissues" that are invisible on an x-ray, too little attention is paid to their healing problems.

Yet ligaments, like bone, must be given sufficient time for internal remodeling before their loading is increased. If excessive loads are applied before the ligaments are "ready" to bear them, there will be a disproportion between stress and stress-bearing ability, and failure will result.

Even flexing the knee to 130° places a tremendous strain on a newly-created ligamentous attachment, and the ligament will be wrenched off the bone unless it has been able to restore the fan-shaped attachment of its fibers under the influence of progressive loading.

To date we have had to reopen the knee on three occasions due to the premature avulsion of transplants from the femur. In each case the transplant looked good and was not devitalized; it had simply parted from its proximal femoral attachment, as in acute injuries. The patients themselves had suffered no new trauma, but had felt "something happen" in the knee during ordinary activities. This was followed by a noticeable deterioration of condition, which prompted each patient to come in for examination of his own volition.

In each case we reattached the substitute ligament by the "over the top" method after first refreshening the condyle. The results since then have been encouraging.

Possible Late Sequelae in the Quadriceps Extensor Apparatus

The x-rays in Fig. 262 show the two-year result for one of our cruciate ligament reconstructions. The outline of the channel is clearly visible, as well as the appositional bony protuberance on the medial surface of the lateral femoral condyle; there is no radiographic sign of irritation from this protuberance.

Initially we had strong reservations about sacrificing a portion of the quadriceps apparatus in patients who were engaged in competetive athletics. Remarkably, however, we have had only one patient, an athletic young man, who had to be treated for secondary complaints in the form of degenerative tendon disease at the patellar apex. He formerly had a severe global anterior instability, and now the operated knee is almost as stable as the other one; there is a residual anteromedial drawer sign of 2–3 mm.

In another patient a tendon ganglion developed outward from the tibial tunnel. He had no pain, and in the three years since excision of the ganglion there has been no recurrence, the knee remains stable, and the patient is able to engage in sports.

Except for one patient from the early series, who had been operated on three times

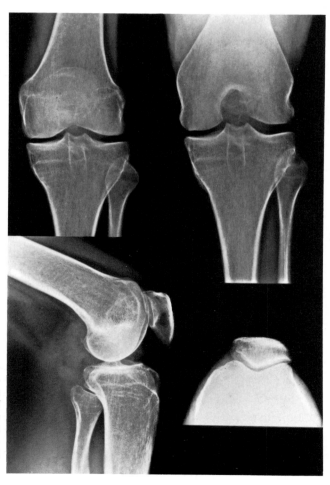

Fig. 262. X-ray status of a knee joint 2 years after a successful anterior cruciate ligament reconstruction. The drill channel is visible in the upper tibia. Also visible (in the *tunnel and lateral views*) is the bony deposit originating from the piece of patellar bone used to fix the transplant to the femur. The patella (*sunrise view*) is positioned normally in the femoral trochlea and shows normal surface form

233

before us und twice by us for severe cartilage pathology and decompensated anterior instability and now must wear a Lennox-Hill brace at all times (muscular insufficiency?), all the patients get along well without mechanical aids or appliances.

Recent Developments in ACL Reconstruction

For the past year we have also been performing ACL reconstructions by the Brueckner principle; but instead of taking a free graft from the patellar ligament, we leave the graft attached to a vascularized pedicle from the infrapatellar fat pad (Noyes, Clancy). This technique can even be used for replacing both cruciate ligaments simultaneously and shows particular promise as a method for reconstruction of the PCL. However, it will be a year or so before we can meaningfully compare the results of this operation with those of other procedures.

Posterior Cruciate Ligament Reconstruction

Generally speaking, the results of reconstructions of the posterior cruciate ligament have been less encouraging than those of anterior cruciate reconstructions.

We have found that the palliative operation of Augustine [15] (Fig. 264) is still of some value in patients with posterior instabilities of moderate severity; this is also confirmed by Anselm [13].

We have not had any experience as yet with the gastrocnemius transplant of Hughston.

In their most recent paper, published in 1980, Hughston et al. [138] confirm the difficulties of posterior cruciate ligament grafts and therefore advocate primary operative repair for all acute tears of the PCL.

Using the technique illustrated in Fig. 263 we obtained fair results in the first two cases. The results could not be called good, but the patients were better off than before the operation.

In another case we followed a good result *for 1½ years,* until a stumble left the patient with a sudden, severe posterior drawer instability. It is apparent that the transplant never underwent adequate revitalization and remodeling, and that this ultimately led to its fatigue failure. Perhaps we did not attach the graft properly to a viable bed, or perhaps we did not cover it adequately with synovial membrane to ensure its extra-articularization.

Nevertheless, we believe that the transplant itself is essentially sound, because the segment of quadriceps tendon above the patella is thick and strong enough to provide a powerful ligament substitute. However, the very thickness of the transplant may account both for its ability to function well for 1½ years and for its failure to become revitalized.

As a result of these experiences, *we have become hesitant* to perform true reconstructions of the PCL and are conducting follow-ups of our later cases, treated with a modified technique, in order to evaluate the long-term results.

Arthroscopy in the Planning of Cruciate Ligament Repairs

Major reparative operations on the ligaments are complicated procedures. The surgeon should never allow them to become "routine"; he must be able to adapt them in accordance with the situation at hand. Many of the newer methods are also very time-consuming and require a trained surgical team.

It is clear that intraoperative "surprises" are unwelcome in such a setting. Fortunately, preoperative planning can be greatly assisted by the use of arthroscopy.

If arthroscopy discloses the presence of cruciate ligament remnants, we make it our goal to utilize them and plan our approach accordingly. In this way we have been able to directly repair the majority of old PCL ruptures, usually obtaining better results than with pure replacement procedures.

234

Fig. 263 a–c. Technique for reconstructing the posterior cruciate ligament. **a** Analogous to the ACL reconstruction, a strip of quadriceps tendon (lateral), patellar bone and one-third of the patellar ligament based on the tibial tuberosity is used to replace the PCL. The strip extends farther above the patella than for the ACL and includes a greater amount of tissue in the region of the quadriceps tendon just above the patella. The proximal part of the strip is kept thinner, for this part is used only to pull the transplant through the medial femoral condyle. Thus, the thick, suprapatellar portion of the transplant serves as the actual ligament substitute. **b** Lateral view of the tendon substitute showing the manner in which it is routed through the joint. To spare nutrient vessels, the patellar ligament should not be split all the way to the tibial tuberosity. Even with the catheter, the piece of patellar bone cannot be pulled entirely through the drill channel in the tibia; this is advantageous for it provides an ideal intratibial anchorage that protects the vascularized portion against excessive tension from the direction of the tuberosity. **c** Anterior view of the reconstruction. The patella has been retracted medially for better visualization. Postscript: To date the results of this transplant have been unsatisfactory

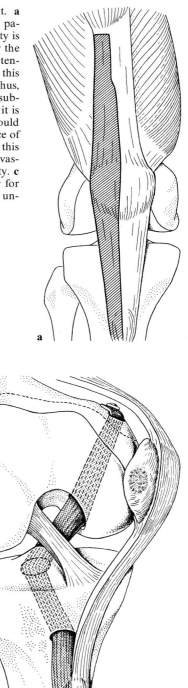

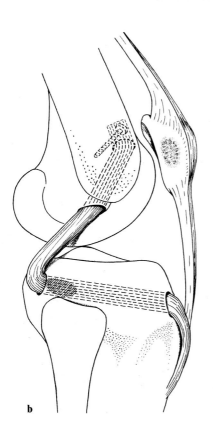

235

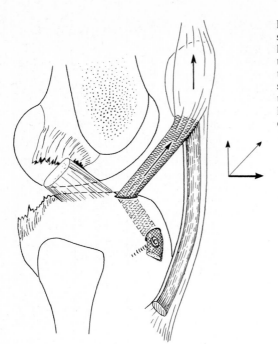

Fig. 264. Augustine's operation [15] for chronic PCL insufficiency. To enhance posterolateral stability we take the lateral third of the patellar ligament, left attached at the patellar apex, carry it laterally in front of the ACL and route it through a 6.5-mm channel drilled in the upper tibia. The strip should be just long enough that its end can be fixed to the upper tibia with a screw and toothed washer. The parallelogram of forces shows the forward-directed force that is exerted on the tibia by quadriceps contraction

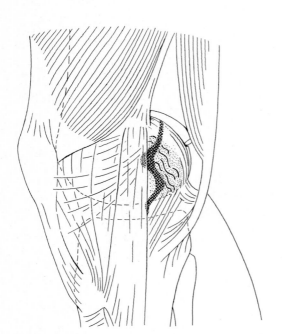

Fig. 265. Old tear of the POL with chronic insufficiency of the semimembranosus corner

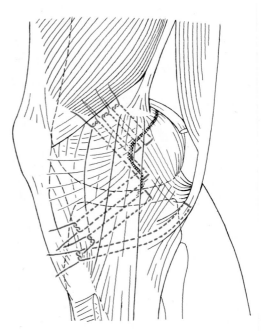

Fig. 266. Suture technique after freshening the femur and if necessary the tibia. If the forward extension of the semimembranosus tendon is lax and stretched, its bed is freshened and it is drawn anteriorly with a nonabsorbable suture

Use of an Existing Cruciate Ligament in Secondary Repairs

Our experiences with total replacements of the PCL and our encouraging results (in suitable cases) with the utilization of old ruptured anterior cruciate ligaments in triple-repair procedures for chronic global anterior instabilities have enabled us to exhaust every possibility in cases where a useful remnant of the PCL is present.

In replacements of the cruciate ligaments, it is advantageous if an existing ligament with its blood vessels and proprioceptive nerves can be utilized in the repair. Even if the ligament is of poor quality at operation, it should develop well with proper trophic conditions and postoperative care.

Old Ruptures of the Posterior Cruciate Ligament at Its Proximal Attachment

A stump is seldom visible in old lesions of this type, owing to the subsynovial location of the tear. But if the surgeon knows how the PCL normally feels on the lateral surface of the medial femoral condyle and how it can be identified with a probe, he will at once notice the absence of substance beneath the synovial membrane. If the rupture is confirmed by eliciting a posterior drawer sign, and the ligament can be pulled forward and upward, the repair can be carried out.

A small, sharp periosteal elevator is used to strip the synovial covering down from the margin of the cartilage until firmer tissue, representing the remnant of the PCL, is reached. One *or two* strong, nonabsorbable sutures (No. 3 nylon) are passed through the ligament and used to draw it forward and upward. If it is still attached to the bone in places but is lax, it is detached from the condyle at those sites along with a small bone fragment and is brought anteriorly and superiorly with sutures as described previously. Owing to the short length of the PCL, an advancement of only 5 mm is a significant distance and may be enough to restore full stability.

The ligament is reattached as in the repair of acute tears (Fig. 246). Two or preferably four drill holes are made through the medial femoral condyle from its medial, proximal, extra-articular surface to the area of insertion of the PCL. The ligament sutures are pulled through the holes by the cannula technique. The PCL can then be repositioned and the sutures temporarily fixed with clamps. If the ligament is correctly positioned, the posterior drawer test will be negative in all degrees of flexion. Care must be taken that the sutures are firmly anchored in the substance of the ligament, for much will depend on these sutures postoperatively.

Note: These sutures are not definitively tied until stress has been relieved by repairing the medial and lateral synergists which help to stabilize the tibia against posterior displacement.

Old Ruptures of the Posterior Cruciate Ligament at Its Distal Attachment

We know from x-ray studies of old PCL ruptures with a bony avulsion fragment that displacement of the fragment by only a few millimeters can cause a 2+ to 3+ posterior drawer instability (5 mm = +25% length of PCL!).

Thus, if we find at arthroscopy or operation that the posterior horn of the meniscus (medial or lateral) is easily lifted from the tibial plateau and that a varus or valgus instability is present with the knee in extension, we are safe in assuming that the PCL has been torn from its attachment.

There should be no difficulty in restoring the tibial attachment of the PCL as long as its more proximal portion is intact. A small periosteal elevator passed behind the intercondylar eminence will encounter little resistance in the area of the insertion of the ligament, indicating that only scar tissue is present there due to a prior avulsion of the PCL. If necessary, portions of the ligament still attached to the bone can even be mobilized along with a small bone fragment by means of an angled chisel or other suitable instrument.

237

The tibial attachment of the PCL is accessible from the medial or lateral side, depending on the location and extent of coexisting peripheral lesions. With sufficient disruption, it is possible to pull the tibia forward into the neutral position, grasp the distal PCL with a curved clamp and push it downward and backward. Three strong, nonabsorbable sutures are placed in the ligament using a special Reverdin needle which has a closable eye 1–2 mm from the point.

Before the first drill holes are made, the PCL attachment is reached through the main posteromedial or posterolateral incision by bluntly dissecting around the posterior border of the upper tibia to the middle of the popliteal fossa. There the depression in which the PCL insertion normally lies is readily palpated through the joint capsule. (We recommend practicing this beforehand on an amputation or cadaver specimen.)

Next, as shown in Fig. 244, four holes are drilled from front to back through the medial or lateral side of the upper tibia to the area of insertion of the PCL.

Two of the sutures are pulled through the drill holes from back to front using the cannula-and-wire-loop technique, with one limb of each suture occupying a hole. The sutures in the ligament must be about 1 cm proximal to (higher than) the posterior openings of the drill holes so that the ligament will be tightened when the sutures are tied.

with the other hand a Crawford clamp is introduced into the joint from the front and advanced gently down along the posterior intercondylar area of the tibia. The finger in the fossa will feel the clamp coming and keep it from straying. Then the clamp is gently pushed through the posterior capsule and used to grasp a pull-through thread that is held ready in the fossa. This thread is pulled back into the joint at its center to form a U-shaped loop with which the third ligament fixation suture can later be snared and pulled out of the joint.

This "through-the-bottom" tension suture must be pulled from the popliteal fossa through one or two drill holes in the upper tibia. The drill holes made earlier, which may already be occupied by sutures, should be marked temporarily with Kirschner wires to keep from drilling into the old holes and destroying the sutures!

The hole for the through-the-bottom suture must emerge about 1 cm below the point where the suture passes out of the joint capsule. Normally this is just below the greatest posterior flare of the tibial plateau (see Figs. 237c and 244), i.e., below the PCL in Fig. 237c.

Only in this way can adequate downward tension be exerted on the PCL. In this region the tibia is free of muscular attachments, and the popliteus muscle courses more distally, just below the point where the tibia starts to taper.

The nerves and vessels of the popliteal fossa must be adequately protected during all drilling maneuvers! The drill bit must never be allowed to plunge through the bone uncontrolled. If necessary, the popliteal structures are protected with a broad or spoonlike spatula.

The third and final suture in the PCL is brought out the back of the joint via the "through-the-bottom" route.

For this the depression marking the tibial attachment of the PCL is first palpated with the index finger in the popliteal fossa, and

Old Multilevel Mid-Third Ruptures of the Posterior Cruciate Ligament

We have not yet seen a ruptured PCL with a smooth transverse tear in the middle third. The tears always extend through multiple levels, resulting in a diagonal or step-shaped tear configuration. Usually tissue continuity is preserved, and the lesion is amenable to secondary repair (cf. multilevel tear of ACL, Fig. 239 a, b).

Even in late repairs it is possible to recognize the old tear site. The scarred area can be bluntly demonstrated with probes, elevators and curved clamps until it is possible to fix the main ligamentous strands to the opposing bone transosseously as in Fig. 205 or by the "through-the-bottom" technique.

Because the proximal and distal stumps of the PCL may retain their vascular pedicle, direct repair with overlapping sutures can restore the ligament to a functional unit, whereas it would not in old tears of the ACL. We have followed a number of remarkably good results with this repair of old PCL injuries – substantially better than the largely unsatisfactory results of plastic reconstructions. In each case we rejoined the cruciate ligaments to form a single "pivot" and restored their synovial covering.

It must be reemphasized, however, that *none* of these repairs were done without also repairing the peripheral synergists, and that in this respect we take particular pride in our results of recent years, as will be pointed out in the next chapter.

An Additional Maneuver to Approach the Posterior Upper Tibia

Starting from a broad anterior or medial approach of the types described earlier, the deep layer of the crural fascia can be reached beneath the medial belly of the gastrocnemius by going below the semimembranosus attachment and around the medial tibial border, 5–10 cm distal to the joint line. This fascia covers and connects the soleus muscle (distal) and popliteus muscle (proximal), which lie in a common layer. By bluntly dissecting along this layer with the finger, one can easily reach the posterior upper tibia and joint capsule and can even get beyond the midline to the lateral side. If the dissect-

ing finger is kept close to the muscle bellies, the layers will separate by themselves in such a way that the entire popliteal neurovascular bundle with the gastrocnemius muscle bellies remains external to the plane of dissection.

If necessary the tendon of the medial gastrocnemius can be incised or temporarily detached at the femoral condyle, even from a medial approach.

With these aids, orientation is easily achieved even in difficult situations, and there should be no obstacle to accurate placement of the sutures for the repair of PCL ruptures.

Old Combined Ruptures of the Anterior and Posterior Cruciate Ligaments

These truly disabling, combined anteroposterior instabilities are among the most serious of knee problems.

In the early years we usually treated such cases with a brace, rather than operatively. In *one* case we performed an arthrodesis at the request of a patient who had significant anteroposterior instability combined with severe valgus laxity. Though a young man, the patient had had a lengthy history of post-traumatic knee trouble. The status of the soft tissues was precarious following a split-thickness skin graft. This patient wanted to be able to work standing in his store without a brace and specifically requested surgical fusion, with which he was very pleased. But arthrodesis is not a procedure which we ordinarily perform.

Arthroscopy is a valuable preoperative aid in combined ruptures of the ACL and PCL. It is possible to determine whether one of the cruciate ligaments can be reinserted or repaired, and to plan accordingly a replacement procedure for the other. So far we have had good results with these tactics.

We do not yet have long-term results on operations for the simultaneous replacement of both cruciate ligaments. Presumably there will be further developments in this area as in others, but the short follow-ups to date for individual cases do not permit a definitive evaluation to be made.

We have not yet implanted artificial ligaments, considering them inferior to autologous transplants on general grounds, although we cannot dispute that they may be valuable as internal splints for a limited period.

The use of carbon fibers as described by Jenkins et al. [157] still awaits evaluation as to its long-term results.

Secondary Repair of the Periphery and Reconstruction of the Five Main Ligaments and Capsule

The Capsule

Vidal et al. [365] emphasized in 1977 the important contribution of the posterior capsule to stability, and Palmer [280] pointed out in 1958 the particular importance of the deep portions of the capsule for the physiology and pathophysiology of proprioceptive stability control. Thus, it is important that lesions of the capsule be repaired, and that the capsule be restored if possible to its normal length. However, the capsule itself, which in many places consists only of thickened synovial membrane, is unable to stabilize the knee joint against mechanical stresses without assistance from other structures. In the posterior region mechanical stability relies essentially on:

1. The semimembranosus muscle and its associated oblique popliteal ligament;
2. the popliteus muscle and its associated arcuate popliteal ligament;
3. the medial gastrocnemius;
4. the lateral gastrocnemius with the fabella-based ligament system.

The capsule which lies between these structures and lines their deep surfaces is so thin that it often cannot be demonstrated as a separate layer. For example, Tabutin [in 359] writes that on the posterolateral side there is no capsule at all between the fabella (or equivalent tissue) and the attachment of the lateral gastrocnemius tendon, but that the gastrocnemius tendon itself forms the "capsule" at this location.

It appears that the capsule "fits in" posteriorly where needed in accordance with the lengths and attachments of the dominant structures (1–4 above).

Vidal et al. [365] state that there are eight elements responsible for passive stability in the knee. Proceeding in a circle around the ACL, these are:

– the lateral collateral ligament
– the posterolateral corner (popliteus corner)
– the lateral condylar plate
– the posterior cruciate ligament
– the medial condylar plate
– the posteromedial corner (semimembranosus corner)
– the medial collateral ligament.

We take exception to this list in several respects. First, it omits the iliotibial tract as a passive element! Second, Vidal [365] places so much importance on the "condylar plate" that he makes its injury a fourth component in his classification of medial lesions. Thus, his "tetrad" encompasses the MCL, ACL, posteromedial corner and medial condylar plate and so is not comparable to the term as we use it. We do not believe that the medial "condylar plate" merits the status of a distinct stabilizing element, for between the firm, well-defined structures of the POL, the semimembranosus with its oblique popliteal ligament, the medial gastrocnemius, and the PCL, which form an integral framework for maintaining form and strength in the posteromedial joint, we find only a thin, synovial capsular lining.

It is acknowledged in the literature that even with sound surgical repair, the prognosis of a complex injury worsens as the number of involved ligaments increases. But in Vidal's tetrad this is not the case, since the results for the triads and tetrads by his classification are similar.

On the lateral side the capsular plate is even more rudimentary, for this region is already densely occupied by the oblique popliteal ligament, the arcuate ligament complex, the lateral gastrocnemius tendon, the fabellofibular ligament, the LCL and the popliteus.

Naturally all these structures must be given close attention when tracing the course of acute as well as chronic tears.

Posterior Capsule

All posterior disinsertions of capsular tissue from the tibia must be located and repaired during the operative treatment of old instabilities. Old proximal tears of the capsule and the gastrocnemius attachments are more easily recognized than lesions in the overstretched, scarred middle third and between the semimembranosus corner and PCL on the upper tibia.

Coronary Ligament

The coronary ligament merits special attention as a component of the fibrous capsule. As mentioned earlier, the "coronary ligament" is a collective term applied to all the meniscotibial fibers surrounding the tibial plateau. It has an important bearing on stability, especially with regard to its anchorage of the middle and posterior portions of the menisci. On the medial side this attachment is strongest at the POL, and on the lateral side it is strongest just in front of the popliteal hiatus, in the area where Segond avulsion fractures can occur.

The meniscotibial connections should be carefully checked in their entirety and securely refixed to the tibia with sutures.

On the *medial* side, restoration of the meniscotibial connection of the semimembranosus corner is the first and most important step of the repair. Next, the meniscotibial connection between the POL and PCL must be checked, and if a rupture is present the outpouching distal fibers may have to be excised before freshening the tibia and re-

attaching the proximal fibers to it; we recommend transosseous sutures for this purpose (Figs. 267 and 268).

On the *lateral* side the meniscotibial attachment just above and anterior to the fibular head is the most important connection.

As on the medial side, no pockets must be left when repairing the posterolateral meniscotibial attachment.

Note: An important part of O'Donoghue's reconstruction [268] is based on the transosseous reattachment of portions of the capsule to the tibia!

The Semimembranosus Corner

Injuries of the semimembranosus corner are usually part of a lesion with anterior instability.

Even in secondary repairs there is generally enough local ligamentous tissue present that an anatomic restoration can be carried out. Often it is still possible to locate the old rupture sites, where the only remaining connection is via thin synovial tissue that cannot assume the stabilizing function. Even a slight elongation of the POL will significantly increase the rotational drawer sign (large relative lengthening of short fibers). In chronically unstable knee joints that are badly "stretched out," the semimembranosus tendon itself is distended in its groove on the tibial head.

The first and most important step of the repair is to reconnect the meniscus with the tibia in the region of the POL. Whenever possible we freshen the tibia superficially in the area of insertion before placing the sutures, which extend to the POL. The sutures are correctly placed if they do not interfere with flexion-extension yet relieve the anteromedial instability.

Next, the meniscofemoral attachment is checked and repaired as needed. The POL must pass deep to the MCL at the femur. (Nicholas' [252] advancement of the POL over the long ligament conflicts with anatomic and kinematic requirements, besides requiring sacrifice of the meniscus.)

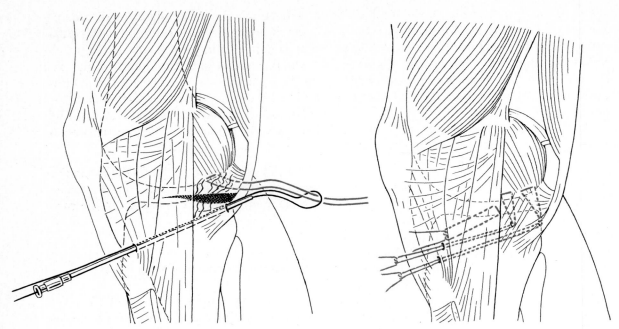

Fig. 267. If the insufficiency or old tear is located in the coronary ligament (the meniscotibial ligamentous attachment), repair is effected with transosseous sutures after freshening the tibial bone beneath the outpouched fibers

Fig. 268. The transosseous sutures extend from the posterior tibia forward, emerging beneath the MCL

Occasionally *cysts* are found in the area of the femoromeniscal fibers at operation. Being localized in the area of ligamentous attachment to the femoral condyle, these cysts can cause stress-dependent complaints. The bone is usually denuded and epithelialized in the region of such cysts. Again, freshening of the bone is important for the anchorage of ligamentous structures that have been sutured to it. If the old tear can still be identified as to type, then the sutures may be placed as shown for acute tears in Fig. 213 b ff. Otherwise we recommend a suturing technique like that illustrated in Figs. 265–268 (or Fig. 220). The technique recommended by Hughston and Eilers [136] is similar.

As in all operations near the proximal attachment of the MCL, the medial articular nerve must be protected!

In some cases it may prove necessary to resect excess, unstructured capsular tissue behind the POL.

Automatic Terminal Rotation and Ligamentous Tension in the Semimembranosus Corner

Before deciding upon the extent of the excision or the placement of the sutures, it is necessary to judge the effect of automatic rotation throughout extension.

Knee joints with much terminal rotation require a greater "ligamentous reserve" than those with little such rotation. If the femoral condylar radii are small, the correct placement of sutures is often a very difficult matter, for small deviations in such cases are much more significant than in knees with large condylar radii.

The Semimembranosus Tendon

At the end of the repair the semimembranosus tendon must be under the correct amount of tension and must be securely reattached to the posterior capsule and the

POL. If the tendon is too lax, we tighten it along its natural axis in the direction of the tibial tuberosity with a strong thread (e.g., Polydec 3) anchored at the insertion of the patellar ligament. In this way the entire five-part foot of the main tendon is again drawn snugly against the tibia.

Reconstruction of the POL

In the rare instances where there is not enough tissue available for repairing the posterior femorotibial connection, a distal pedicle graft may be taken from the semimembranosus tendon and used to replace the POL (Fig. 269).

As the drawing indicates, we cut a thick strip from the posterior part of the tendon. It should be as long as possible and should extend up to the muscle belly; its thickness may be up to half that of the donor tendon. Its distal end remains attached distally at the foot of the main tendon.

The strip is brought forward beneath the limb pointing toward the tibial tuberosity and is securely sutured to both the tibia and the meniscus, reproducing the attachments of the natural POL. The free end of the transplant is then pulled through the capsule below the MCL and sutured or screwed to the site of attachment of the POL to the adductor tubercle.

Sometimes it is not easy to find the best fixation site on the femur, but the behavior of the new ligament during knee movements can be tested by tentatively fixing it to the bone with a Kirschner wire.

Repair of the Semimembranosus Corner in Global Posterior Instability

Very often the only demonstrable lesion in such cases is a stretching of the femoromeniscal fibers as a result of chronic overstressing in a posterior direction. We correct this by chiseling off the femoral at-

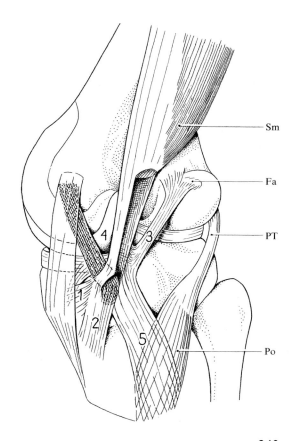

Fig. 269. Reconstruction of the POL using portions of the semimembranosus tendon. The graft is anchored to the freshened tibia below the meniscus; this may also be done with transtibial sutures (not shown here)

243

tachment of the posterior ligamentous fibers together with a bone lamella and advancing it proximally beneath the MCL by a distance of 1–1.5 cm. The ideal refixation site can be located by tentative fixation with a Kirschner wire (1.7 mm). The advancement in this case does not violate the rule of isometry. The part of the ligament overlying the freshened bone site can be reinserted there.

In cases of chronic posterior instability this advancement has a visibly beneficial effect and is also favored because the site of reinsertion corresponds to the site of the fresh rupture. In most cases of this type the tear begins up below the gastrocnemius tendon and extends anteriorally across the femoral condyle to a point beneath the MCL; there is visible denudation in the area of insertion on the femur distal to the adductor tendon.

The Medial Collateral Ligament and Its Secondary Repair

Rarely does the true MCL suffer such severe damage and loss of substance that portions of it cannot be utilized for the repair.

Nearly always, the MCL can be correctly reattached to the femur following repair of the semimembranosus corner. Generally the tibial expansion of the ligament has undergone good scar regeneration and is functionally competent. However, its proximal attachment to the femur is almost always insufficient and must be revised; this has a good prospect of success if the deep short fibers are properly reattached.

Depending on the situation, a periosteal elevator can be inserted beneath the MCL from below and used to mobilize its femoral attachment sufficiently to restore tension to the ligament. We freshen the bone superficially in the area of reinsertion so that the ligament can regain attachment to the bone at the correct location. We attach the superficial layer of the ligament to the posterior border of the longitudinal retinaculum, the fascia of the vastus medialis and the adductor tendon, in this way obtaining a re-

inforcement system that is augmented by active muscular tension.

For clarity, we refer the reader to the drawings and specimen photos presented in earlier sections.

Fig. 211 shows the deep capsular structures; the sites of attachment of the excised MCL are visible as dark areas. Figs. 43, 49–53 show the normal collateral ligament in flexion and extension, demonstrating its position, fiber architecture and relation to the retinaculum and semimembranosus corner. As in the natural ligament, the posterior fiber bundles of the repaired ligament should be able to slip below the anterior fiber bundles in fan-like fashion when the knee is flexed.

All repairs of the capsule and medial ligaments are relatively simple, provided there has been not more than one previous operation in that region. But as the number of prior operations increases, it becomes increasingly difficult to find ligamentous tissue with a normal collagenous fibrous structure. The tissue may be thicker and may appear firm, but it consists of an unstructured scar-tissue plaque that is poorly suited for anatomic repairs. The characteristic parallel fiber arrangement is lost, and the fibers in the plaque form an irregular meshwork. Correspondingly poorer results are obtained in such cases, as is repeatedly confirmed in the literature.

When we find scar-tissue bands of this type, we thin them out and prefer to use only portions of them for the anatomic repair.

In rare cases we have opted for a tendon transfer from the pes anserinus group patterned after Helfet's operation [123, 124]. While in our experience this operation is unable to provide a perfect functional result, we feel that it still has its justification as a palliative procedure, although we have used it on only a few occasions in recent years.

On the Question of Using the Pes Anserinus for Reconstruction of the Medial Ligaments

When we began our intensive use of plastic operations for ligamentous repairs, we performed pes anserinus transplants for a variety of purposes, following the methods of Lindemann [200], Helfet [124] and others. Our results at that time were unsatisfactory compared to what we now know can be achieved. To be sure, the patients were often better off than before the operation, both objectively and subjectively, but their functional capacity was still far below the pre-injury level. It was remarkable, moreover, how often the patients suffered secondary, postoperative injuries from the most trivial causes. For example, a simple stumble was often sufficient to cause a marked deterioration of stability. In our optimistic belief that our transplants were conceptually sound, we naturally assumed that these secondary traumata were to blame for the ultimate failure of the reconstruction.

Today we view things differently. Aside from the fact that stability was never properly restored, these knee joints lacked the essential active protection and perhaps even the fine motor control that is needed when unexpected forces intervene and disrupt consciously controlled activity patterns.

Therefore, with few exceptions, we have abandoned the transplantation and use of the pes anserinus as a ligament substitute. So far we have had good results with preserving the pes while anatomically repairing the deeper, passive ligamentous structures. Because in past years we have introduced other basic innovations of operative technique, we will never be able to objectively assess the pure effect of preserving the pes anserinus. Nevertheless, we can offer the following observations: Now and again we operate on knee joints in which a pes anserinus transplant was done one or more years earlier to stabilize the medial side. In all these cases, which represent poor outcomes, the medial side is indurated and unstructured. Neither the layer of the pes anserinus tendons nor the ligamentous and capsular elements beneath it exhibit anything like a normal structure. In our view this is virtually inevitable when the ligamentous structures are not stressed in conformance with kinematic principles, but are subjected to diffuse, unphysiologic stresses and strains that prevent the band from acquiring a well ordered

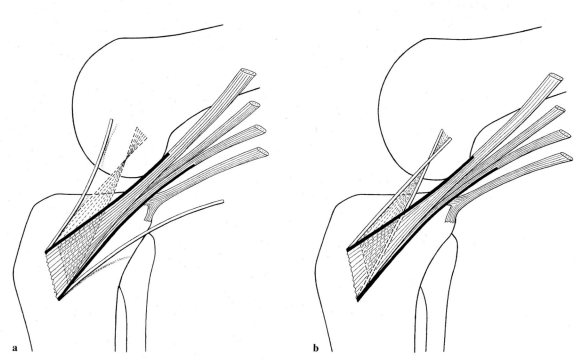

Fig. 270a, b. Reconstruction of the MCL as a means of reinforcing repairs of the cruciate ligaments and semimembranosus corner

245

structure. In contrast, we have reoperated some of our own cases in connection with secondary meniscus operations, over-the-top cruciate ligament reconstructions, etc., and were able to evaluate structures we had previously repaired. It was surprising how easily the joint could be reapproached through the mobile tissue layers, and how the structure of the collagenous tissue was for the most part anatomically normal.

If it should prove necessary in certain situations to reconstruct the MCL using collagenous, structured material, then, aside from a Helfet-type operation, it is better to transfer a portion of a tendon than to incapacitate an entire tendon. This possibility is shown in Fig. 270. The tibial insertion of the pes is already near the ideal distal attachment of the MCL, and the transplants can be sutured or screwed to the femur after slight freshening of the bone. If desired the most proximal fibers can also be attached to the adductor tendon and the vastus medialis muscle and its fascia. As in our repair of the MCL, it is necessary that the short and intermediate-length fibers of the deep layer, which are important for rotatory stability, be well restored, for the long ligament cannot assume this function alone.

Repair of the Popliteus Corner

The Popliteus Tendon

The key structure of this region is the popliteus tendon. It must be assessed both as to its course and its quality. In most cases of posterolateral instability this tendon is strained and is often thinned out in the intra-articular segment just below its femoral insertion. This corresponds to the situation in acute injuries, for hemorrhagic suffusions and strains tend to occur in this preterminal segment.

If the tendon is sound in the hiatus and in its distal portion down to the muscle, we chisel off the femoral attachment of the

strained tendon in the form of a small block 7–10 mm wide and 10–15 mm long. In some cases it is sufficient to flip this block 180°, pull the tendon taut, and reattach the block to its bed over the ligament. This will advance the tendon by a distance of 1.5 cm, which is usually just enough.

In cases where this is not sufficient, the block must be reimplanted farther proximally and anteriorly, and the tendon is attached to the former bed with transosseous sutures.

The LCL can also be tightened by a proximal block advancement of this type. Because the LCL and popliteus tendon course in different directions, we recommend detaching two separate blocks so that each can be reattached in its ideal location.

Transplants for Reinforcing or Replacing the Popliteus Tendon

If the popliteus tendon is badly damaged, we perform a bypass. If the tendon is absent we perform a direct replacement using the same method. Either the iliotibial tract or the biceps tendon may serve as the donor.

If the *iliotibial tract* is fully intact and has not been used as a donor elsewhere, a 1- to 1.5 cm-wide strip is mobilized and left attached to the tubercle of Gerdy. The necessary length of the transplant is determined beforehand by stretching a thread from the tubercle along the upper tibia to the level of the popliteal hiatus, and from there up along the course of the popliteus tendon to its area of attachment on the femur. For safety, the strip is cut 2 cm longer than the measuring thread and is then reflected anteriorly downward. Then a channel for the strip is cut through the tibial head from front to back with a 4.5-mm drill bit. The posterior hole must emerge just below the cartilage of the tibial plateau and should be adjacent to the groove of the popliteus tendon (Fig. 271 a).

Now the strip from the iliotibial tract is drawn through the bony channel *and* through the overlying tissue belonging to the

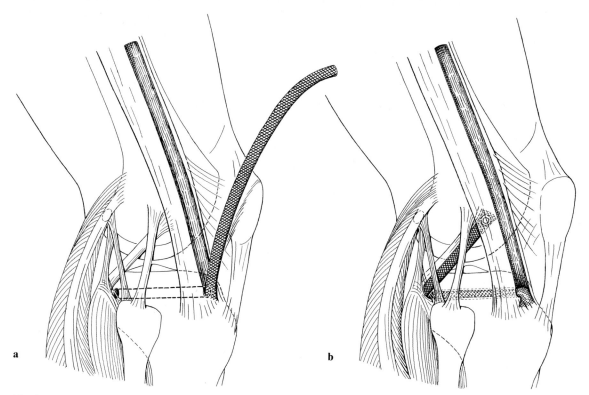

Fig. 271 a, b. Popliteus bypass using a pedicle graft from the anterior portion of the iliotibial tract

arcuate ligament complex, is *woven into the lateral capsule* parallel to the popliteus tendon, and is pulled up to the area of insertion of the popliteus tendon on the femur. There it is secured under tension with a transosseous suture or a bone block and screw as described above, together with any existing tendon remnants (Fig. 271b). With the transplant routed in this way, the lax arcuate ligament is also effectively refixed to the back of the tibia at a favorable site.

The passageway in the capsule is best developed bluntly with a curved clamp passed obliquely downward toward the posterior opening of the channel; the clamp is then used to grasp the transplant strip and pull it upward.

The transplant must be covered for its entire course and should at no time freely enter the intra-articular cavity; this is essential for its revitalization and subsequent remodeling.

The transplant *must* be taken from the freely-coursing *anterior* half of the iliotibial

tract to avoid weakening the normal lateral femorotibial structures. The defect is closed with absorbable sutures combined with a few nonabsorbable sutures.

The biceps tendon. If the tract cannot be used or should not be weakened, a fibula-based strip can be mobilized from the biceps tendon, its length having been determined beforehand with a measuring thread. Its thickness should be one-third that of the biceps tendon. The strip is passed from the fibular head through a bluntly developed passageway to the tibia, to the site below the plateau cartilage directly adjacent to the popliteus tendon groove where the posterior drill hole emerged in the previous technique. (This ensures simultaneous refixation of the arcuate ligament to the tibia.) There the bone is freshened, and the lower portion of the biceps strip is anchored with a transosseous suture or with a screw and toothed washer in such a way that its free

247

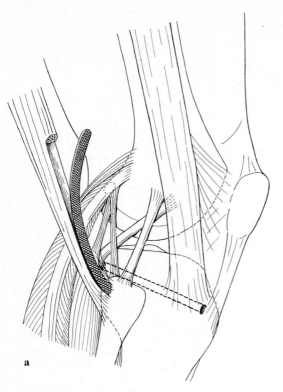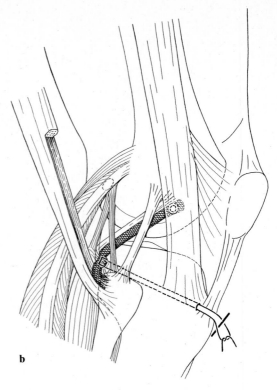

a   b

Fig. 272a, b. Popliteus bypass using a pedicle graft from the biceps tendon. This has the effect of also restoring part of the arcuate ligament connection. In both cases (Figs. 271 and 272) the bypass strip refixes the arcuate ligament to the back of the tibia while simultaneously closing the abnormal meniscotibial recess that forms posterolaterally on anterior dislocation of the tibia

portion can be passed bluntly up through the capsule to the femur, exactly as described above. This end is secured to the femur by transosseous suture or by a screw and bone block. The donor site is repaired with absorbable sutures only (Fig. 272).

The Lateral Coronary Ligament and Lateral Meniscus

Before further closure is undertaken in the region of the popliteus corner, it must be determined whether the tibial attachment of the meniscotibial fibers is still sound. If this attachment is too lax, the area of insertion on the tibia is freshened, and the lateral coronary ligament is reattached, if necessary with transtibial sutures (Fig. 273). These sutures are passed through 2-mm drill holes by the cannula-and-wire technique described earlier and are knotted on the anterior side of the tibial head (Fig. 274).

The Arcuate Ligament

Refixation of the popliteus tendon and meniscus having been completed, the next step is repair of the arcuate ligament complex. This complex is often difficult to identify. Old lesions are most easily found if the typical localizations of acute tears are borne in mind.

1. In acute injuries the arcuate ligament complex is most frequently detached *at the tibia*. It can be reattached to the freshened tibia transosseously just below the plateau cartilage between the posterior cruciate attachment and the fibula; this may be done in primary as well as in secondary repairs.

248

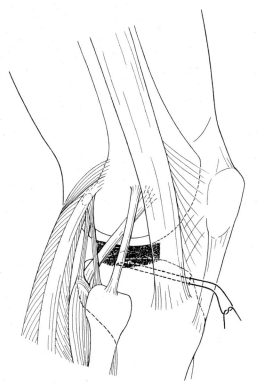

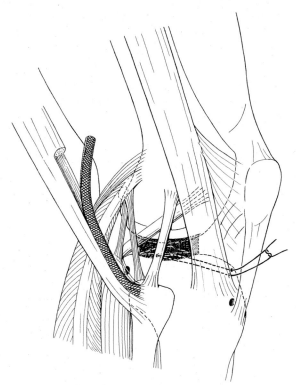

Fig. 273. Repair of the lateral coronary meniscal ligament. If a Segond-type avulsion is present (with or without a bone fragment), the suture should include the arcuate expansions directly below the coronary ligament as well as the posterior iliotibial tract fibers that course to the posterior part of the upper tibia

Fig. 274. In all peripheral repairs and reconstructions, such as the popliteus bypass and the LCL reconstruction, it is essential that the deep layer also be repaired. This includes reattachment of the capsule and the arcuate ligament to the posterior tibia, fiaxation of the lateral meniscus, and fixation of the ligamentous fibers that have sustained a Segond-type avulsion (see Fig. 273). The proximal attachment of the arcuate ligament also must be restored where it passes to the femur together with the lateral gastrocnemius tendon

2. If the ligament has been detached *at the femur* together with the lateral gastrocnemius tendon, it is reattached transosseously after freshening of the femur. If the ligament is badly stretched, its attachment may even be advanced proximally somewhat, but not to the point where it would interfere with extension. In such cases the tendon and capsule pulled proximally over the bony wound bed can reattach to the bone immediately above the cartilage and can thus obtain a greater area of insertion on the femur.

3. If the old tear is located in the *midportion* of the ligament, it is necessary to test

the segment from the fabella (or equivalent tissue) down to the styloid process of the fibula (the "fabellofibular ligament") as well as that from the fabella farther medially to the tendinous expansion of the popliteus. These ligamentous bands combine to form a triangle which stabilizes rotational movements on the lateral side. Tension can be restored to *both* parts of the ligament by lowering the fibular attachment and improving the connection with the broad popliteus tendon.

Major lateral injuries are generally accompanied by damage to the posterior cruciate ligament. Its repair must *precede* that of the periphery. The tibial end of the PCL can

249

be well demonstrated with a suitable approach and reattached by the "through-the-bottom" transosseous suturing technique.

Repair of the popliteus corner is seldom done alone; generally it is done as part of an operation for combined instability (i.e., anteromedial, anterolateral and posterolateral), or as a step in the correction of a global posterior instability, in which case the PCL and POL also must be repaired.

Repair of the Lateral Collateral Ligament

This ligament can be tightened either by the proximal advancement of its bony insertion, as mentioned, or by sinking it distally into the fibula. In rare cases both proximal and distal revision are needed to restore tension (previous "bilevel" tear). If reconstruction is indicated, this may be done with a one-third to one-half thickness strip of biceps tendon, as in the popliteus bypass, that is brought up and attached to the femur along the normal

course of the LCL. Before it is anchored to the bone the transplant must be embedded in vital tissue on all sides (Fig. 275). This technique is also recommended because the biceps, according to Kaplan [170] and others, dynamically stabilizes the LCL. With this method the new ligament remains attached to the biceps, and so this physiologic "dynamization" is preserved.

Repair of the Lateral Femorotibial Ligamentous Attachment

Development of the Technique

This functionally important attachment via the intermuscular septum and posterior portion of the iliotibial tract has long been a problem for us in terms of surgical repair. This structure, given the somewhat obscure term "formations antéro-externes" by French authors, is indeed difficult to comprehend at first glance. Only recently has its

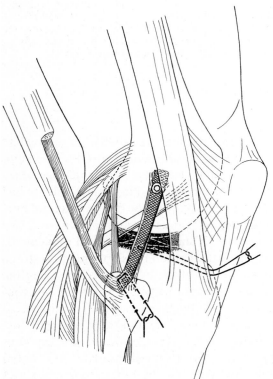

Fig. 275. Reconstruction of the LCL using a pedicle graft from the biceps tendon. Like other transfers, this generally represents only a part of a complex lateral repair that encompasses all deep ligaments from the PCL to the ALFTL, as suggested by the fixation suture in the deep layer

importance become a matter of general awareness.

Kaplan [170], in his description of the connection between the femur, intermuscular septum, iliotibial tract and tibia, was among the first to point out the presence of a ligament-like attachment between the femur and tibia.

For us, the realization that the arrangement of the ALFTL was parallel and symmetrical to the MCL on the medial side was an important step toward the development of stabilizing techniques.

Gradually it became clearer that a stabilizing procedure against "anterior instability" was necessary on the *lateral* side. First the operations were aimed solely at correcting the symptom of "lateral pivot shift." Now they are routinely used as a part of comprehensive reconstructive procedures to correct anterior instability.

The middle capsular ligament on the lateral side could not bear the main responsibility for anterior stability due to the very thin meniscofemoral attachment in the anterior two-thirds of the lateral capsule, although there is a firm meniscotibial connection on this side that is strong enough to produce the Segond avulsion fracture. This site is on the lateral side above the fibular head and anterior to the LCL, where there must be minimal displacement of the lateral meniscus relative to the tibia during rotations and flexion-extension (Figs. 91, 130 and 131).

As Jakob et al. [155] have shown experimentally, the functional importance of this middle capsular ligament is minor compared to that of the ACL and iliotibial tract. Thus, besides repair of the ACL, measures aimed at stabilizing the knee against pathologic anterolateral rotational instability must focus on the layer of the iliotibial tract and intermuscular septum.

We were first confronted with the "lateral repair" of MacIntosh and Darby [215] in 1973. We adopted this original method first as a solitary operation for lateral pivot shift, but in the following year began using it only in combination with repairs of the medial side and simultaneous repair of the ACL. But because this procedure, like other well known reconstructions, did not correspond to physiologic laws, we soon had misgivings about it. We saw how sizable tension differences developed in the transplant during intraoperative flexion and extension, and knew from experience that this sooner or later would lead to stretching. The strip, which was passed beneath the LCL, required a free travel of up to 1.5 cm during flexion-extension if it was to maintain a uniform tension during movements, but the manner in which it was routed prohibited isometry. The operation also caused the LCL to become dynamized in its proximal third by the tensor fasciae latae via the iliotibial tract, which was unphysiologic and predisposed further to secondary insufficiency.

Therefore, we abandoned this technique in favor of the Ellison variation [75, 76], in which the "palliative transfer" is not firmly attached to its passageway and so is able to glide back and forth beneath the LCL, adapting its effective length in response to position changes. However, even this procedure ultimately proved unsatisfactory. Kennedy et al. [176], in their analysis of the results of the Ellison procedure, concluded that when used alone the technique had a disappointing success rate in the correction of anterior instability symptoms.

Time and again we saw patients with severe varus instabilities in both flexion and extension following lateral reconstructions of this type, and some patients who underwent the Ellison procedure were able to demonstrate a significant spontaneous drawer sign at will. Together with the lateral pivot-shift phenomenon, these are among the most serious instabilities of the lateral side, for they are very disabling in the majority of patients.

These experiences taught us that for every active stabilizer there must also be a passive element which, by virtue of its length and position, is able to "sense" tension changes and transmit them to higher centers. Active stabilization cannot exist without passive control, for a coordinated functional sequence is impossible under active control alone.

The mixed results which we obtained in our own early cases and observed later in the course of insurance evaluation caused us to become more hesitant in the use of iliotibial tract transfers of this type.

In no case should a transfer be done that would weaken or destroy the normal anterolateral femorotibial ligamentous structure. Hence, strips of iliotibial tract used for the reconstruction of other ligaments (popliteus bypass, etc.) should be taken only from the *anterior half*, or if necessary the anterior two-thirds, of the tract. The posterior third with the deep layer must remain intact for the preservation or restoration of true femorotibial anterolateral stability.

Thus, our experiences with the various techniques led us in 1974 to adopt a combination of the operations of MacIntosh and Darby [215] and Ellison et al. [76]. The steps in this somewhat complicated procedure are illustrated in Fig. 276.

Two adjacent strips are taken from the iliotibial tract, each about 8 mm wide and thus narrower than in the single-strip technique described earlier. The anterior strip is longer and is left attached distally to the tubercle of Gerdy, while the second strip remains attached to the tract proximally and is mobilized along with a portion of the tubercle as in Ellison's procedure. We take care to leave the posterior portion of the tract intact and develop an aperture for the "Ellison strip" proximally at the lateral lip of the linea aspera (Fig. 276 b) without further damaging and weakening the femorotibial structures still present. The strip is then carried distally beneath the fibular half of the lateral collateral ligament and passed back beneath the main part of the tract to its site of origin on the tubercle of Gerdy, to which it is reattached with a screw.

The second, longer strip is passed back through the arcuate ligament, pulled through the capsule and gastrocnemius tendon close to the femur, and then brought back forward to the tubercle. If a fabella is present, we loop the strip through the capsule and tendon directly adjacent to this structure, bringing the strip back forward in the usual manner. Thus, we may envision the fabella as a link which connects the transplant with the semimembranosus tendon by way of the oblique popliteal ligament. In this way an effective mechanism is provided for dynamic stabilization during rotation. Isometric conditions are remarkably good with this technique, and the LCL is spared because the second strip is routed external to it.

Next, the defect in the iliotibial tract is meticulously closed with a combination of absorbable and nonabsorbable sutures; the portion of the strip passing from the fabella is included in the repair.

If a tension-free suture is not obtained (width of transplant $= 2 \times 8 = 16$ mm), we place several longitudinal relaxing incisions, each 5–10 mm long, in the anterior portion of the tract toward the patella.

This combined procedure has significant advantages over the operation of MacIntosh and Darby [215] or Ellison [75, 76]. These joints can be moved and exercised soon after surgery with no danger of loss of stability. Lateral varus instabilities in flexion and extension are abolished. In addition, we saw no more spontaneous drawer signs with this technique, although we were unable to correct existing drawer signs with it. The disadvantages of this procedure are the considerably longer operating time and the need for a broader field of dissection. Moreover, some of the knee joints showed persistent swelling in the area of the femorofibular ligament which was exacerbated by exercise. Three patients exhibited a kind of audible tendon "jump" which they found annoying but was not disabling.

We do not know which portion of the loops was to blame for this phenomenon. A faulty crossing of the loops could be responsible. The exercise-dependent swelling was a result of friction between the deep mobile strip and the collateral ligament.

But aside from these minor drawbacks, we found this technique to be a definite plus. For the first time it enabled us to restore a stability equal to that of the unaffected side, even in chronic instabilities, and thus to achieve a true "restitutio ad integrum."

In accordance with our concept of the triple repair, however, this lateral reconstruction formed only one part of a combined operation, for these cases involved global anterior instabilities with drawer signs in ER, NR and IR, a positive lateral pivot-shift phenomenon, and valgus instability. We practiced our technique from 1974 to 1978. As our experience grew and the number of operations increased, we perceived a need to simplify the procedure on the lateral side and bring the reconstruction more in line with the normal anatomy of the region. We adopted a new variation, therefore.

A full two years have passed since we began work on this book. Today we can state with some assurance that the results of the transplantation technique described below are at least as good as those of the method we practiced from 1974 to 1978. In addition, the technique is simpler and less time-consuming. Our patients have had no problems with lateral irritation, thereby simplifying their postoperative rehabilitation.

Theoretical Comparison of the Methods of 1974–1978 and 1979–1980

We have seen that when knee joints with a longstanding anterior instability become decompensated, they have deteriorated to the point where the instability has spread from the anteromedial quadrant to the anterolateral and posterolateral quadrants. The posteromedial quadrant with the PCL and semimembranosus corner is always the most stable.

It is clear that chronic, recurrent subluxations of the pivot-shift type will in time lead to stretching of the popliteus corner. The advantage of our 1974–1978 method was that the strip routed through the popliteus corner augmented tension in the posterolateral region.

The less rotational freedom the knee has postoperatively in an anterior or posterior direction, the better the long collateral ligaments and the ACL will be able to recover during this period.

Conversely, the more lax the inner capsule, the greater the rotational freedom, and the poorer the recovery of the long peripheral ligaments and central pivot.

In our method of 1979–1980 there is no such direct action on the popliteus corner. However, the narrowing of the iliotibial tract does have the effect of tightening the posterolateral corner indirectly. If much additional posterolateral rotational laxity is present, we combine the new iliotibial tract transplant with advancement of the popliteus insertion or with a popliteal bypass.

These combinations have proven their worth. For example, an ice hockey player in whom we performed an ACL repair, a through-the-bottom PCL repair and an iliotibial tract transplant by the 1979 method with a popliteal bypass has resumed his athletic career with normal stability in the operated knee. A second patient with a popliteal bypass has returned to his job as a skiing instructor.

We cite these cases not as *proof*, but as important *evidence* of the functional value of these procedures.

Our Current Technique of Anterolateral Femorotibial Reconstruction (1979–1980)

Having progressed through the techniques of 1) MacIntosh and Darby [215], 2) Ellison [75, 76] and 3) our own combination of 1974–1978, we can now present our simplified method of 1979–1980 after two years' experience with more than 150 cases.

In the great majority of cases this procedure represents the third element of a combined repair for global anterior instability (tetrad).

If there is only an anterior drawer sign in NR and IR (anterolateral duad), then we combine repair of the ACL with the lateral reconstruction described below.

If there is only an anterior drawer sign in IR (anterolateral monad), then the ALFTL reconstruction can be done alone or as an adjunct to a lateral meniscectomy. But if a lat-

253

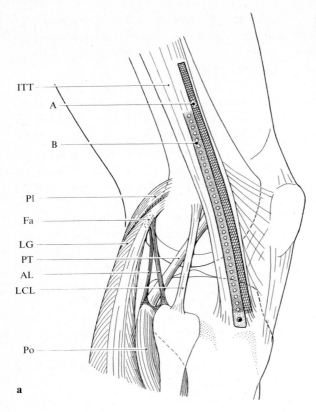

ITT
A
B

Pl
Fa
LG
PT
AL
LCL

Po

a

Fig. 276. a Two strips, each about 8 mm wide, are mobilized from the anterior portion of the iliotibial tract. **b** The anterior strip *A* (length determined with a measuring thread) is left attached to the tubercle of Gerdy, the posterior strip *B* remains attached at its proximal end and is freed from the tubercle together with a block of bone. **c** Strip *B* is passed distally through an aperture in the septum below the iliotibial tract, pulled back forward beneath the LCL and anchored with a screw. **d** Strip *A* is routed below the iliotibial tract and past the LCL to the fabella, then brought back to the donor site in the tract. **e** Fixation of the strips is followed by closure of the tract

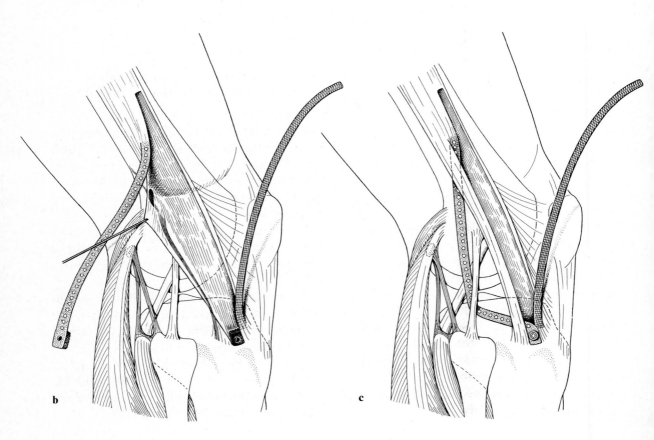

b

c

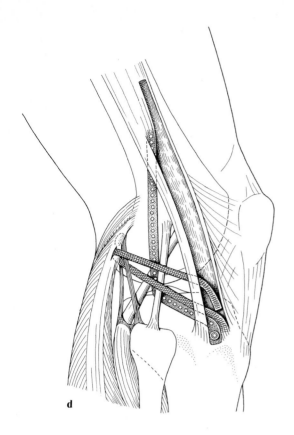

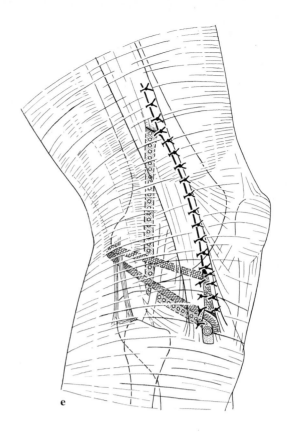

eral pivot-shift phenomenon is demonstrated by the MacIntosh test [in 102, 103], or there is a positive Slocum sign [327], a positive Lachmann test [in 343], a positive Losee test [201], or a positive jerk phenomenon by the test of Hughston et al. [137], then there is no question that the anterior cruciate ligament is insufficient; this has also been confirmed by Galway [102], Jacob et al. [154] and others. The lateral reconstruction alone is inadequate in such cases, for in all probability it will stretch with time; the ACL must also be repaired.

Technique of Operation

The iliotibial tract is longitudinally split between its two main fiber axes as in the approach for an "over-the-top" ACL repair (Fig. 277). The anterior two-thirds with the bifurcation into the patellar retinaculum lies in front of the longitudinal incision and

passes to the front of the tibia, while the posterior portion courses to the tubercle of Gerdy. If femorotibial reconstruction is indicated, we make a second longitudinal incision in the tract about 12–15 mm posterior and parallel to the first, extending down to a point just above the joint line. The strip thus defined remains attached to the tract proximally and distally. The strip is 15–20 cm in length, depending on the size of the joint. It must extend at least 10 cm above the metaphysis of the femur. The proximal part of the strip should be narrowed to about 5 mm and have sufficient proximal extension to minimize the tension exerted upon it by the tensor fasciae latae and gluteus maximus muscles. This will prevent the screw fixation from being torn loose prematurely during postoperative mobilization.

The incisions for the strip having been placed, the rest of the intermuscular septum is demonstrated at the labium laterale of the linea aspera. Somewhat farther proximally

255

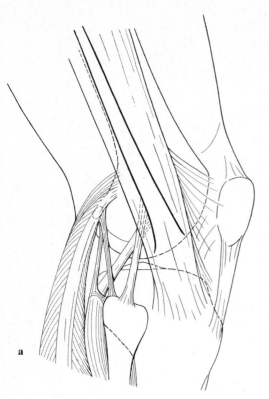

a

Fig. 277 a–f. Our current technique of ALFTL transfer. **a** Two incisions are made in the posterior half of the iliotibial tract parallel to its fibers. They do not extend to the tibia unless special measures (lateral meniscus, etc.) are necessary in that area. **b** The next step is to fix the mobilized strip to the femur. Before it is attached with a screw and toothed washer, it is tentatively fixed to the femur with a 2.0-mm Kirschner wire (which also "predrills" the hole for the small-fragment screw) in order to locate empirically the correct fixation site where the sunken strip will come under *isometric* tension throughout flexion-extension and will prevent anterior drawer laxity in all positions (including Lachmann's position). If the transplant is definitively attached to the freshened femur with a small-fragment screw that does not engage the opposite cortical bone, a second screw with toothed washer must be placed about 1.5 cm *proximal* to it in order to prevent it from turning and loosening postoperatively. The proximal location of this 2nd screw will prevent it from altering the isometric conditions established by the 1st screw. **c** Next the tract is closed over the sunken strip; the sutures include as much of the strip as possible to preserve the structural integrity of the tract and ensure its continued function as a passive and actively dynamized stabilizing system. The mantle of the tract is usually stretched out as a result of the chronic instability, and so closure of the tract usually presents no difficulties despite the absence of the transplanted strip. But if the tension in the lateral patellar retinaculum is too great, it can be relieved by means of longitudinal, fiber-parallel relaxing incisions

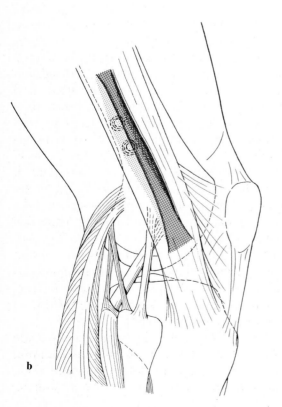

b

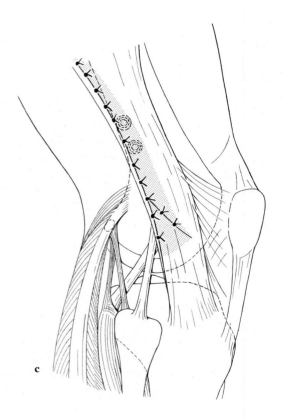

c

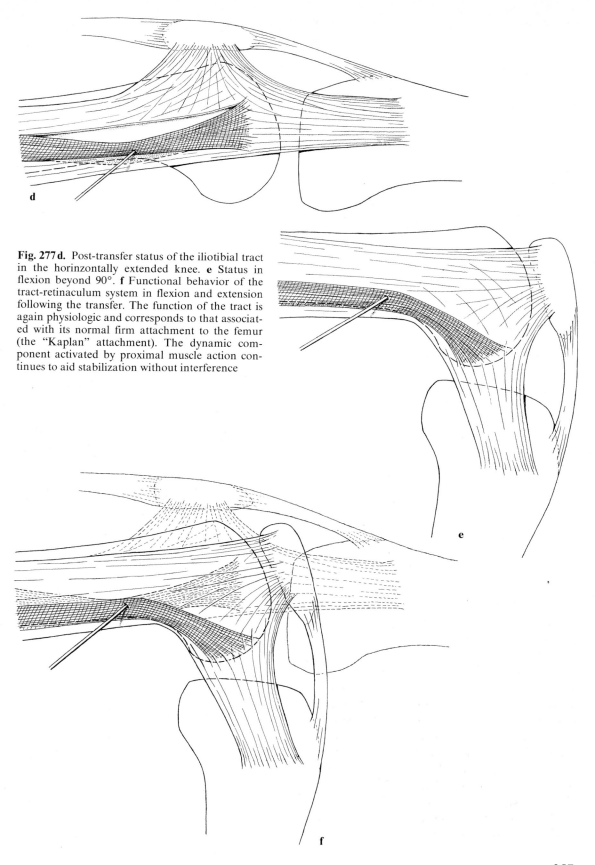

Fig. 277 d. Post-transfer status of the iliotibial tract in the horinzontally extended knee. **e** Status in flexion beyond 90°. **f** Functional behavior of the tract-retinaculum system in flexion and extension following the transfer. The function of the tract is again physiologic and corresponds to that associated with its normal firm attachment to the femur (the "Kaplan" attachment). The dynamic component activated by proximal muscle action continues to aid stabilization without interference

the septum is already detached from the femur over a distance of 3–5 cm in connection with the "over-the-top" approach.

Now the femur is freshened along the septum and the labium; the ever-present epiphyseal vessels are spared if possible. Then the strip cut from the tract is tentatively held against the femur in an attempt to locate the ideal attachment site for isometric loading during movement. Once this site has been ascertained with reasonable certainty, the tract is temporarily fixed to the femur at that point with a 2.0-mm Kirschner wire before again testing the mobility of the knee joint, the behavior of the strip during flexion-extension and its stabilization against anterolateral drawer displacement, which must be prevented at all flexion angles.

Once the ideal point has been located in this way, the Kirschner wire is withdrawn from the femur but is temporarily left in the tract. A tap is twisted into the 2.0-mm hole to prepare it for screw insertion, the Kirschner wire is removed from the strip, and the strip is secured to the femur with an AO small-fragment screw (length 28 mm) and toothed washer.

The screw is not driven home at once. When all but about 1 cm of the screw has been inserted, absorbable sutures are placed in the transplanted strip and in the remnants of the septum to interconnect the two elements. Also, any over-the-top sutures that have been placed are pulled through the strip up near the screw but are not yet tied. Then the transcondylar ACL sutures, which emerge just distal to the screw, are also pulled through this strip. The screw is tightened, and stability is again checked in all joint positions. A second screw placed about 1.5 cm proximal to the first will protect it against premature loosening during postoperative exercise. If an anterior drawer sign can no longer be demonstrated in IR, and if the semimembranosus corner on the medial side has been repaired such that an anterior drawer is absent in ER as well, the cruciate ligament sutures may be tied. The resultant medial and lateral splinting of the anterior cruciate ligament is now so good that even

when the sutures are tied they can no longer come under excessive tension, and so there is no danger that they will tear out.

The strip having been secured, the overlying defect in the tract is closed with simple interrupted sutures of absorbable material interspersed with a few nonabsorbable sutures. The edges of the defect should be smoothly reapposed and should completely cover the transposed strip. Some 2–3 cm proximal to the screw the stitches may be placed so as to include the transplant; in this way the old septum-tract-femur-tibia connection will again form a unit.

As discussed in the section on the development of the new reconstruction (p. 250), the technique must be combined with a popliteal bypass in cases with increased posterolateral rotatory laxity. This bypass must always be done *before* the ALFTL reconstruction.

Of the two variations described earlier for reconstruction of the popliteus corner, we prefer the one involving use of the biceps tendon, for it is not possible to take a second strip from the tract for use as a bypass. In addition, the temporary weakening of the biceps in the postoperative period is not unwelcome, due to its posterolateral pull on the lateral tibial plateau.

On the lateral side it is especially important to avoid adhesions in the area of the popliteus tendon, the lateral surface of the condyle and the suprapatellar pouch that can cause pain and limited motion during the rehabilitation period.

Drill holes and sutures should be placed proximal to and outside the synovial duplication.

Concomitant Traumatic Cartilage Damage and Its Treatment

Fresh Concomitant Cartilage Damage

Frequently we see patients with fresh ligamentous ruptures, usually of the ACL, who also have sustained severe cartilage fractures of the medial or lateral femoral condyle.

In addition to repairing the ligamentous injuries in such cases, we meticulously repair the cartilaginous surface of the condyle. The bed from which the cartilage has broken free is freshened into the cancellous bone with a 1.0–2.0-mm drill bit, and the cartilage fragments are fitted into the defect with acrylic tissue adhesive and fixed with 1.2- or 1.7-mm AO screws whose heads are countersunk below the cartilage surface. They are removed after 2–4 months. Bone that can no longer be covered with cartilage is freshened by forage.

joints exhibit signs of patellar chondromalacia, even in primary operations, it is little wonder that these damaged cartilaginous zones exert a negative influence on one another via the humoral pathway. The enzymes present in the effusion give rise to degenerative chondrolytic processes in the vicious cycle of chondrodetritic synovitis. A ligamentous injury or instability [314] can easily cause mild patellar chondromalacia to become decompensated. Lesions that were painless prior to the injury can later be a major cause of postoperative pain and disability.

Concomitant Cartilage Damage in Chronic Instability

It is impossible to perform repairs in the unstable knee on a regular basis without repeatedly confronting the problem of secondary post-traumatic cartilage damage.

We shall not go into the voluminous literature on this subject, but will mention only the study of Ségal et al. [314], who present an excellent analysis of the relations between knee instability and the localization of cartilage damage. The findings of this study, even as they relate to the patella, coincide closely with our own observations.

There is no doubt that many a poor late result is due not so much to persistent instability as to significant cartilage damage, where the cartilage fails to recover despite improved stability in the joint.

The many types of cartilage damage that can occur underscore the fact that ligamentous instabilities invariably represent a serious problem for the joint.

The development of secondary degenerative changes as a result of combined ligamentous instabilities is easily followed. The cartilage damage may be unifocal or secondary and multifocal in its occurrence. Ordinarily we find it on the femoral condyle on the side with the greatest rotational drawer instability. Slippage of the condyle on the tibial plateau leads to damage to the lamina splendens and to fibrillation of the cartilage. Because almost half of arthrotomized knee

The Treatment of Concomitant Cartilage Damage

As the example in Figs. 278–280 illustrates, we remove loose pieces of cartilage and any floating or fibrillated tissue that otherwise would be abraded or comminuted during movement. In these zones or in areas where raw bone is present, we "resurface" the bone (Pridie [287a]) by drilling into it to a depth of 2–3 mm until bleeding cancellous bone is exposed. This is done so that granulation tissue can fill the defect from below and become converted to fibrous substitute cartilage. The diameter of the drill bit is 2.0–4.5 mm, depending on the size of the defect and its localization; generally we prefer the larger bit sizes.

The success of this resurfacing depends in large measure on the simultaneous restoration of functional congruity in the knee by ligamentous repairs, and on early movement of the articular surfaces in normal relation to each other.

Under favorable circumstances, remarkably good results can be achieved with this method. Radiologic follow-ups demonstrate true quiescence with normal structure in the subchondral joint line and adjacent cancellous bone.

In the case of large defects which mechanically interfere with joint motion, this type of resurfacing is no longer adequate, and repair of the defect with osseous or osteochondral grafts is indicated [369].

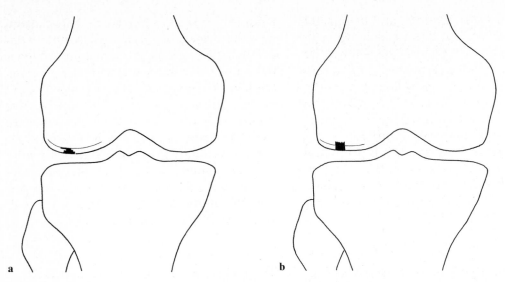

Fig. 278. a Typical cartilage fracture with denudation of the bone. **b** The area of the cartilage defect is freshened by drilling into viable cancellous bone

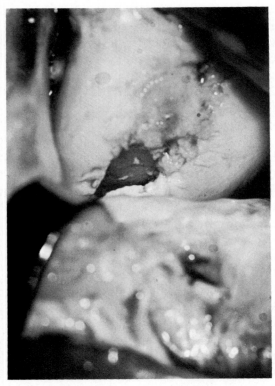

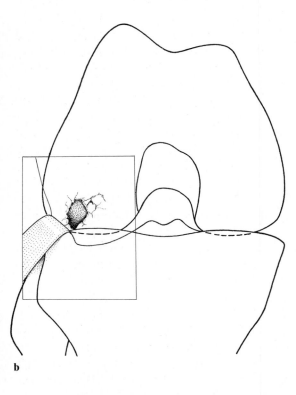

Fig. 279. a Operative photo of a cartilage lesion, **b** with corresponding positional drawing, 11 years after menis-cectomy. The cartilage broke away from the bone in small fragments and a larger undermined lamella

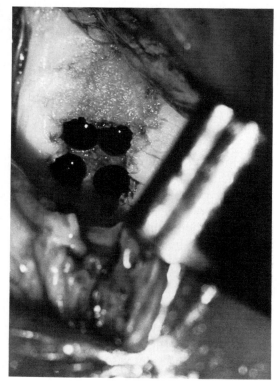

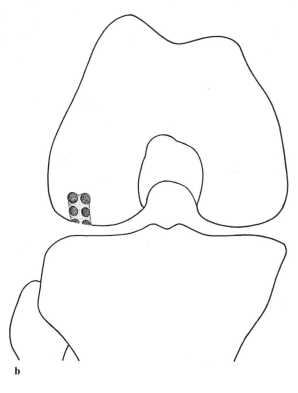

a

b

Fig. 280. a Operative photo and **b** positional drawing for Fig. 279a following removal of the loose cartilage and "resurfacing." The patient returned to competitive soccer and has been playing for 4 years without effusion or complaints

Again, we emphasize the importance of preoperative arthroscopy in order to identify any cruciate ligament tears or significant cartilage pathology *before* the operation so that the procedure can be planned accordingly.

If there has been an initial period of mobilization following the operation, the consequences of any subsequent immobilization will be far less severe. These points are discussed in detail in the section on Rehabilitation (p. 266).

The Effect of Cartilage Damage on Postoperative Care

> The more severe the cartilage damage, the greater the importance of postoperative mobilization.

This rule seems simple enough, but its application is not without compromises.

Complications

An analysis of our results for the period 1971–1977 reveals no serious postoperative complications. There has been no neurovascular damage and no joint stiffness. All knee joints are mobile over a range of 120° and are free of debilitating extension losses (plaster in 5° flexion!). Only in isolated cases were knee joints mobilized under general anesthesia. No infections have been noted in this series.

In all fairness, however, we must mention that in 1979 we recorded two cases of postoperative infection within the space of a few weeks; one involved a recent PCL complex injury, and the other a St. Elsewhere knee that been operated on several times previously.

We were able to avoid more serious complications by opening the knees at once and applying suction irrigation. Both knee joints have good motion ranges of 120 and 130°. The multiply operated knee displays considerable cartilage damage. (The patient has been retrained for a less strenuous occupation and has returned to work.) The other knee has good stability, and the patient has returned to his original job.

Fortunately we have had no other problems with infection before or since, even at the new site, even though we do not administer antibiotics routinely.

General Guidelines for Operative Procedures

Preparing for the Operation

On the evening before the operation, the leg is shaved, painted with Betadine from the proximal thigh down to and including the toes, and wrapped with a sterile dressing. This dressing is not removed until the patient is on the operating table. There the leg is cleansed again with Betadine on a sterile sheet or pad before the patient is positioned for surgery.

Positioning

Most operations are performed with the knee flexed. We position the limb with the aid of a thigh rest that is attached to the side of the operating table, and with which the

flexion angle can be adjusted as desired. Because the rest is small, it is possible to place the leg in three different positions on the operating table (Fig. 281):
1. Off the rest, lying extended on the table parallel to the other leg.
2. Flexed to any angle between 20 and 90° and slightly rotated externally.
3. Flexed beyond 90° with the lower leg hanging over the side of the table.

Care should be taken that the rest does not touch the popliteal fossa or exert pressure there. A great advantage of this positioning method is that under general anesthesia the soft tissues hang away from the joint; i.e., the neurovascular bundle "drops" spontaneously away from the femur and tibia and so is not directly jeopardized by manipulations in the joint area.

The *tourniquet* is placed as far as possible from the knee joint itself. It and the thigh rest should not interfere with each other.

Operative Field

The field must be large enough to satisfy all requirements that may arise intraoperatively. No drapes should be placed closer than 15 cm distal to the tibial plateau or 15 cm proximal to the patella, as they might unduly restrict the area of exposure.

From below, a sterile stocking covered with impermeable plastic is pulled up to the middle of the lower leg. From above, the field is defined by towels wrapped in cuff-like fashion about the thigh. Any gaps in the seal are closed with adhesive plastic film. The actual area of the incision is covered with a transparent plastic sheet that is either self-adhering or secured to the skin with a special adhesive.

Tourniquet

Just before the incision is made, the leg is elevated to reduce the blood volume distal to the tourniquet. Then the pneumatic cuff is inflated. We try to keep the tourniquet pres-

Fig. 281 a–c. Positioning the knee for surgery on the thigh rest of Trillat. **a** Intermediate flexion with the foot resting on the table; **b** large flexion angle with the lower leg hanging free; **c** leg off the rest and extended. The advantage of this rest is that it supports the proximal thigh and exerts no pressure on the popliteal area and its structures. In particular, this allows the neurovascular bundle to drop away from the bones. This advantage is so great that we perform almost all knee operations, including upper tibial osteotomies, in this position

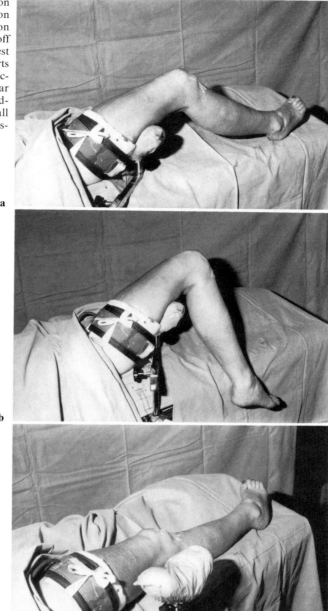

a

b

c

sure in the range of 300–400 mm Hg, and thus as low as possible. A higher pressure must be used in obese patients with a thick layer of subcutaneous fat.

The tourniquet should be inflated with the knee flexed, so that the compressed quadriceps muscle will not hinder additional necessary flexion during the course of the operation. The drapes must also be placed so that they do not limit the desired range of motion.

The tourniquet and the lateral pivot-shift phenomenon: If the pivot-shift phenomenon is elicited under general anesthesia before the pneumatic tourniquet is inflated, it is often more marked than when the patient is awake. In a great many cases the phenomenon can no longer be demonstrated once the tourniquet has been inflated. Presumably this is due to an alteration of the mechanical behavior of the iliotibial tract by the tourniquet pressure.

Duration: Our rule is to maintain tourniquet control for as long as is absolutely necessary to carry out the technical phase of the procedure. This means that once all essential sutures have been placed posteriorly and in the region of the semimembranosus and popliteus corners, and all that remains is closure of the anterior layers, we release the tourniquet, even if 2 hours have not yet elapsed. In this way circulation is restored to transplanted tissues as quickly as possible; visible bleeding vessels can be electrocoagulated or ligated as needed.

During prolonged operations the tourniquet is left inflated for no more than 2 hours. If a bloodless field is still required after that time, the tourniquet may be reinflated for a short time following a 10-minute wait.

Suction Drainage

The formation of hematomas in cavities within the operative area is one of the greatest threats to uneventful postoperative healing. To avoid such hematomas and thus minimize the danger of wound healing disturbances with dehiscence and infection, we place perforated suction drains in all four quadrants. Because watertight closure of the joint cavity is not possible, it is unnecessary to place drains in the joint interior. Paraarticular drainage in the manner described is sufficient to prevent intra-articular hematomas and effusions, provided the ends of the suction drains are in close proximity to the inner capsular sutures or synovial suture. If the subfascial cavities are large, their size can be reduced by placing quilt sutures between the superficial fascia and closed joint so that the flaps are reapproximated to the repaired joint with no intervening pockets or cavities.

264

Instruments

In addition to general surgical instruments, we use the standard drill bits and drilling accessories of the AO. For drilling bone channels for the passage of cruciate ligament transplants, we use the AO hollow reaming bit for broken screw removal.

A rubber catheter (urethral catheter or intestinal tube) with a conical tip is ideal for pulling the transplant through the channel (Fig. 256a, b). Size Ch 16–20 is usually sufficient. To pull sutures and threads through drill holes, we use a cannula through which a wire is passed and looped back to form a snare (see Fig. 260a–c), or a long, eyed ligature carrier with a handle (Fig. 282e). The Reverdin needle in a modification which has a closeable eye situated about 2 mm from the tip is ideal for passing sutures in confined spaces (Fig. 282d).

For retraction, the V-, U- and L-shaped hooks described by Smillie [328] are excellent (Fig. 282).

Suture Material

Wherever possible we use absorbable polyglycolic acid sutures of the Dexon and Vicryl type. The use of different colored threads makes it easier to sort out preplaced sutures and pass them correctly through the corresponding drill holes.

Because these absorbable sutures lose 50% of their tensile strength in 14 days, we use thick No. 0–1 sutures at mechanically critical sites. Where fine approximation is needed, we use sizes 0000, 000, and 00.

Nonabsorbable suture material: For especially critical sutures, such as individual sutures in cruciate ligaments, sutures for reinserting the semimembranosus or popliteus tendon, etc., we use a nonabsorbable nylon material such as Polydec 3. For transosseous sutures, braided wire may also be used.

When suturing the iliotibial tract under tension, we use absorbable sutures interspersed with a few nonabsorbable Mersilene-type sutures, size 0 or 00. We also use

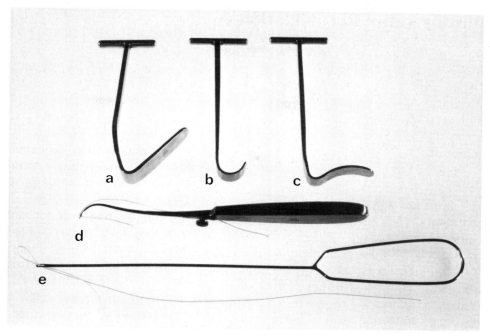

Fig. 282 a–e. Special instruments. **a–c** The retractors introduced by Smillie. **a** V hook for the fat pad and patella. **b** U hook for the capsule. **c** L hook for the outer condylar surface. **d** Reverdin needle with eye situated close to the tip for the placement of cruciate ligament sutures. **e** Eyed ligature carrier of Trillat for passing pullthrough sutures through bone and soft tissues near the bone; it may be bent as needed

one or two such sutures to reinforce the quadriceps tendon between the vastus medialis and patella. Formerly, when we used only absorbable sutures, we occasionally observed postoperative dehiscence in these two areas.

However, it is still our policy to use as much absorbable suture material as possible, for each nonabsorbable foreign body increases the risk of secondary infection and suture fistulas.

Antibiotic Prophylaxis

During the operation great care is taken to prevent exposed tissues from drying out, and dissection is done with a view toward minimizing incidental tissue damage and avoiding the creation of necrosis-prone areas. Tissues are kept moist with Ringer solution containing a broad-spectrum antibiotic.

Aside from these intraoperative antibiotic measures, we have developed no consistent pattern in our use of prophylactic antibiotics over the years and have been unable to arrive at a definite conclusion. Prospective studies are needed in this area before such conclusions can be drawn.

To be safe, however, we administer prophylactic antibiotics in major planned operations if the patient has had prior surgery, if the incisions and soft-tissue status are unfavorable, or if other risk factors are present.

Postoperative Rehabilitation

General

It is widely agreed that postoperative rehabilitation is a key factor in the recovery of function.

Andrews [12], for example, rates the value of rehabilitation as 75% in the overall course of treatment. He further states that a 9-month period is required for ligament healing following the repair or reconstruction of complex injuries.

The crucial importance of rehabilitation following knee injuries is also pointed out by Abbott and Callahan [quoted in 104]. Abbott found that some 80% of knee injuries among the patients at West Point Military Academy represented second or even third injuries of a previously injured knee.

Callahan evaluated knee injuries in 61,000 New York schoolchildren. Even in this youthful population it was found that the probability of a reinjury was more than 15 times greater than that of a primary injury.

Both authors state that the probability of reinjury can be significantly reduced by sound rehabilitation.

Scientific principles of rehabilitation and their practical implications are discussed in detail in the monograph of Simon [320] and the paper of Gerber et al. [104]. Here we shall discuss these principles only as they provide a rationale for the rehabilitative measures and aid in understanding the results obtained.

Uhthoff [360] reports on bone decomposition in dogs following 12 weeks' immobilization in plaster. Even after removal of the cast, the decomposition continued for an additional 12 weeks in younger dogs and for up to 32 weeks altogether in older dogs before new bone formation began.

The severe intra-articular effects of immobilization are clearly demonstrated in the human knee joint sections of Enneking and Horowitz [78].

These observations are consistent with the fact that knee joints subjected to several weeks' plaster fixation experience a trophic crisis for some weeks, during which time they require special protection from excessive mechanical loads. The regeneration of "bradytrophic" tissues (cartilage, fascia, tendons, ligaments) has not yet been adequately researched. Half-regeneration times of 3–4 months have been reported, however.

Noyes et al. [257, 260, 262] have demonstrated in monkeys that the rupture strength of knee ligaments is reduced by immobilization and is slow to recover afterwards. (Noyes' immobilization period was 8 weeks. At this time the rupture strength of the ligaments was 61% of normal; it was 79% after 5 months and 91% after 12 months.)

With regard to the regeneration of skeletal muscle after immobilization, Cooper and Misol [55] found in their studies in the cat a latency of only a few days before new muscle tissue began to form.

All these observations have convinced us of the crucial importance of functional therapy in both operatively and non-operatively managed knee injuries.

However, it is clear that without mechanical protection, functional therapy alone cannot guarantee a stable restoration of the knee joint if the basic kinematic mechanism of the joint has been disrupted by, say, a cruciate ligament injury.

In summary, then, we may describe the goals of rehabilitation as follows:

Goals of Rehabilitation

The goals of rehabilitation after any knee operation are:
- normal active stability with normal working capacity of all extensors, flexors and rotators;
- normal passive stability;
- normal active and passive mobility;
- freedom from complaints, meaning not only a painless joint, but one which "feels" secure to the patient.

The Physiologic and Pathophysiologic Foundations of Postoperative Rehabilitation

The foregoing goals of rehabilitation are more difficult to achieve in the knee than in other joints, for unlike the hip joint or ankle joint, for example, which are guided by bony elements, the knee must derive its active and passive stability from soft tissues. In addition, natural discontinuities exist within these soft tissues that enable them to move relative to one another at numerous locations, with the result that adhesions can severely limit the range of joint motion. What is more, joint pain mainly originates in the soft tissues and can further diminish the working capacity of the muscles through reflex motor inhibition.

General and Patellar Cartilage Problems

Patellar chondromalacia is a very frequent accompaniment of posttraumatic states in the knee. According to Silverskioeld [318] it affects 35% of the population over the age of 30. In fact, some form of malacic change is practically the rule in the patellar cartilage of individuals over 30 [22, 385, 386].

Montmollin [229], among others, found softening of the patellar cartilage as frequently as meniscal lesions. It is not surprising, therefore, that operations for recent and old knee injuries very often disclose a chondromalacia that was clinically silent before surgery. Like other cartilage lesions, however, a clinically latent chondromalacia can be readily activated by a trauma and become painful. It should be noted that the cartilage has no nerve supply, and that the source of the pain in patellar chondromalacia is not yet fully understood. But it is impossible in any case to distinguish painful cartilage lesions from those that produce no symptoms on the basis of morphologic criteria alone.

Certain observations suggest that a correlation exists between the functional state of the muscles and complaints due to chondromalacia. The better the muscular function, the milder the pain symptoms associated with the disease. This may relate to the fact that an intraosseous pressure increase is important in the origin of pain, as Morscher [231] has emphasized, and well-functioning muscles are best able to ensure normal conditions of intraosseous circulation. Conversely, the muscles can function normally only in the absence of severe pain, and so analgesic measures are sometimes unavoidable during the course of rehabilitation (analgesics, anti-inflammatory drugs, diadynamic currents, etc.).

The guidance of the patella in the femoral trochlea is extremely important for the recovery of sound knee joint function. Crucial to this guidance is the distal, transverse portion of the vastus medialis muscle, for only this distal part of the medial quadriceps apparatus can significantly counteract the tendency toward spontaneous lateral patellar dislocation. Isometric exercises are capable of strengthening the muscle, while isotonic exercises mainly promote coordination. It should be borne in mind that the vastus medialis is most effective during terminal extension due to the automatic internal rotation of the femur upon the tibia.

Resistance exercises are not recommended in the early phase of rehabilitation, for they tend to exacerbate complaints (due perhaps to circulatory embarrassment) and thus can initiate a vicious cycle. More general non-resistance exercises are preferred. "Cycling" is especially beneficial, for it produces no sudden peak loads, and the rise and fall of stresses follows a more or less sinusoidal curve. Additionally, there is an ideal phase opposition in the movements of the healthy and affected legs which creates an automatic counterplay that effectively distracts the patient from the injured limb.

Circular walking movements in the water are also favorable, whereas swimming exercises with the customary leg stroke in valgus-flexion-ER are potentially damaging, for the medial ligaments and posterior meniscus horn are subjected to sudden valgus-ER stress with very little muscular protection.

A certain intuitiveness is needed to assess the postoperative stress-bearing ability of the cartilage during bicycle conditioning, for resistance exercises may be started only when the movements are performed with ease and can be maintained at a regular speed.

During the circular walking exercises, the knee joint should move through a range of 100–130° so that the entire cartilaginous surface of the patella will come in contact with the femur (see Fig. 106a). If movements do not go beyond 90° flexion, the medial facet, which is most affected by chondromalacia, will have little contact with the femur, depending on its basic form and whether the patella is high- or low-riding. Only generous flexion combined with active traction from the vastus medialis obliquus can ensure good patellofemoral contact.

If symptoms referable to excessive lateral traction on the patella are present, division of the lateral transverse retinaculum may be necessary to enable the vastus medialis to pull the patella back on the medial side. This problem often arises if a reconstructive operation using elements of the iliotibial tract has resulted in excessive tightening of the lateral retinaculum. However, a well-functioning vastus medialis normally is capable of counteracting postoperative lateralization of the patella.

Muscular Atrophy

As mentioned earlier, the problem of muscular trophism is closely related to the condition of the cartilage and patellar complaints. For a long time the phenomenon of rapid, isolated atrophy of the vastus medialis muscle was a mystery. The study of Cadilhac [43] has shed new light on the problem, however. His histologic investigation showed that the two known types of muscle fiber, I and II, do not occur equally in all portions of the quadriceps. The type-I fibers, which are slow-contracting and are involved mainly in sustained movements, are more abundant in the vastus lateralis, vastus intermedius and rectus muscles, while the type-II fibers, which have a phasic function and are active mainly in rapid movements, are more numerous in the vastus medialis. The type-II fibers are less active during attitudinal reflexes than are the type-I fibers, which work mainly to maintain a position against gravity.

This is consistent with our earlier observation that weightlifters (Fig. 115) develop hypertrophy of the vastus lateralis muscle, whereas bicycle racers and soccer players, for example, always have a well-developed vastus medialis. Thus, evidence indicates that the vastus medialis mainly requires varied or cyclic movements for its development.

Problems of the Suprapatellar Pouch

The suprapatellar pouch (suprapatellar bursa) and associated parapatellar recesses are known to play an important role in the recovery of normal knee mobility (Fig. 283).

As is shown schematically in Figs. 284 and 285, flexion past 90° is impossible if the cavity of the pouch is obliterated by adhesions. Again, this range is subject to individual variation. With a low-riding patella the knee cannot be flexed even to 60–70° unless the pouch is able to unfold; with a high-riding patella, on the other hand, the knee can flex to 90° or more because of the larger fornix

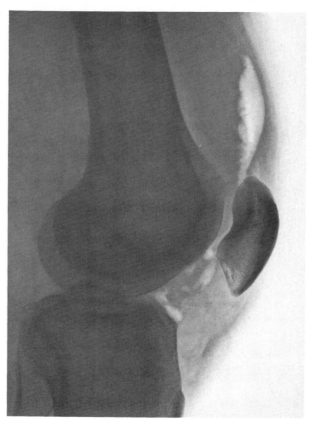

Fig. 283. X-ray of a knee joint demonstrating the cavity system and suprapatellar pouch. Postoperative adhesions of this pouch must be avoided, as they interfere with knee mobility. As a consequence of surgery or trauma, the fatty tissues between the pouch and adjacent femur are often swollen just proximal to the joint cartilage (as seen in the film). The swelling of this tissue, which may look much like the infrapatellar pad, is capable of causing femoropatellar pain resembling that of cartilage pathology

that is formed between the upper border of the patella and proximal margin of the femoral cartilage (see Fig. 285).

The suprapatellar pouch is also important as an "effusion trap." When the knee is extended the posterior portions of the capsule are tight and do not allow fluid to collect behind the femoral condyles. As a result, any excessive fluid accumulation in the knee is forced into the suprapatellar pouch. If the effusion is serous and of low viscosity the danger of adhesions is slight. But if a post-traumatic or postoperative, bloody effusion is present, there is considerable danger that fibrous adhesions will develop between the anterior and femoral layers of the pouch as a result of fibrin deposition.

Ever since the functional importance of the suprapatellar pouch has been recognized, early quadriceps training is routinely prescribed whenever possible following knee operations. An exception occurs in the case of an anterior cruciate ligament repair or reconstruction, where early, complete function of the quadriceps is undesired due to its action as an ACL antagonist in 20–50° flexion. In all other cases early quadriceps training has the effect of transmitting pressure changes postoperatively to the fluid-filled pouch while enabling an early return of good resting tone to the quadriceps. This resting tension exerts a compressive force upon the pouch which creates a kind of "pump" mechanism that aids in ridding the

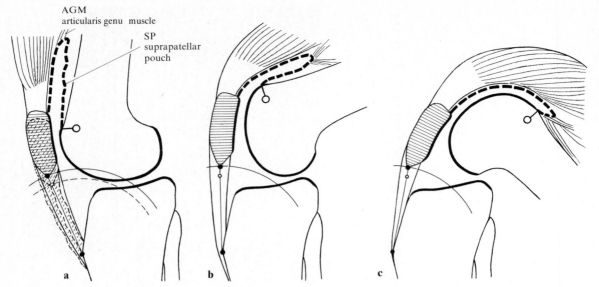

AGM
articularis genu muscle

SP
suprapatellar
pouch

a   b   c

Fig. 284a–c. The function of the suprapatellar pouch, shown schematically for 3 positions of the knee joint. **a** In extension the quadriceps is relaxed, the patellar ligament is lax, and the patella is low (– – –). Contraction of the quadriceps raises the patella, and the mark (♂) at the cartilage boundary on the femoral condyle lies opposite the proximal third of the patella. **b** During about the first 80° of flexion the mark moves only a short distance from the upper border of the patella, and there is little unpleating of the suprapatellar pouch. **c** When flexion is continued past 90° to 135°, the distance between the mark and proximal patellar border is increased several-fold, and the suprapatellar pouch becomes fully unpleated. The patella moves posteriorly on a circular path during flexion due to the backward shift of the femorotibial contact point and so comes to occupy a relatively lower position. The variation of patellar position with the state of quadriceps contraction (a) is often the cause of an iatrogenic low-lying patella following a Roux-Hauser operation or the repair of a torn patellar ligament. The intraoperative loss of quadriceps tone misleads the surgeon into reattaching the tuberosity too far distally

pouch of excess fluid (Figs. 286 and 287). Without this counterpressure fluid fills the pouch rapidly, as occurs in the vicious cycle of chronic knee irritation with quadriceps weakness.

Because intra-articular fluid tends to accumulate on the posterior side of the flexed knee, we avoid flexion during the initial phase of rehabilitation (Fig. 288). Graduated flexion is started only when the quadriceps has effusion production sufficiently under control in the extended knee.

The function of the quadriceps, which sustains the suprapatellar pouch with its articularis genu muscle, is crucial both for the prevention of chronic effusion and for the restoration of normal joint mobility. For this reason patients scheduled for a "simple" arthrotomy (e.g., meniscectomy) are taught leg-raising exercises on the day before the operation. We instruct the patient also to raise the big toe and dorsiflex the foot during the leg raises, for this enables the quadriceps to be innervated with a minimum of force. As the leg is lowered toward the bed, the muscular tone increases steadily with the length of the lever arm. We find that over 90% of patients are able to perform this exercise on the evening after the operation, given proper prior instruction and the postoperative assistance of a nurse or therapist.

The sooner the patient has developed a good sustained quadriceps tone, the fewer problems he should have with postoperative effusion (Figs. 289 and 290). In fact, our experience indicates that at least in the case of simple operations, for each day that the return of good quadriceps tone can be ad-

270

Fig. 285 a, b. Loss of function associated with the development of post-traumatic or postoperative adhesions in the suprapatellar pouch. The small portion of the pouch that remains between the patella and upper edge of the femoral articular surface still allows flexion to about 80° (**a**); only if further flexion is attempted will the loss of the pouch function cause a restriction of motion (**b**)

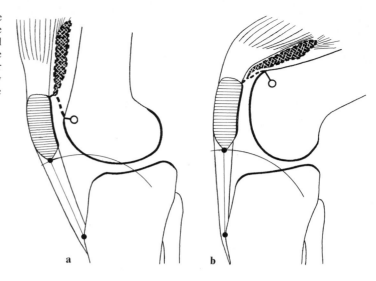

Fig. 286. The quadriceps exerts a direct action on the suprapatellar pouch. The anterior border of the pouch is in direct apposition to the quadriceps tendon, so that movements of the tendon also displace the anterior pouch wall. Early postoperative quadriceps exercises provide a means of preventing or retarding the development of adhesions between the anterior and posterior pouch walls. The pouch has its own tensor, the articularis genu muscle, whose fibers insert on the uppermost fornix of the pouch and sustain it during extension

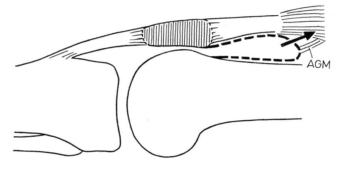

Fig. 287. Early postoperative quadriceps exercises produce a tensile force T that exerts a compressive force P on any effusion that is present in the suprapatellar pouch. Intermittent contractions of the muscles create an alternating compression that "pumps" the fluid out of the pouch into the loose surrounding tissues, resulting in a more rapid reabsorption of the effusion. This is accompanied by a steady improvement of quadriceps function with a tone increase that further inhibits fluid accumulation

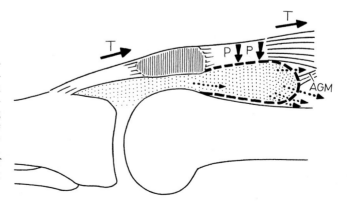

271

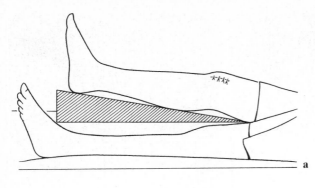

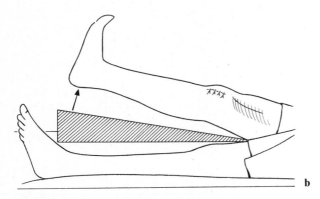

Fig. 288. a Postoperative positioning after arthrotomies for the rapid recovery of quadriceps function with a good sustained tone. **b** The patient is taught leg-raising exercises on the first postoperative day. Extension eliminates almost all the residual volume in the posterior portion of the knee, with the result that no effusions can accumulate there. In addition, the early quadriceps exercises serve to prevent any progressive effusion formation (contraindicated after ACL repairs)

vanced, one week of subsequent rehabilitative effort is saved. Thus, quadriceps training of this type is very effective in shortening the convalescent period and returning the patient quickly to occupational and athletic activity.

As demonstrated in the works of Puhl [288], Dustmann [74] and others, the health of the *cartilage* also depends in large part on the rapid elimination of effusions and the prompt restoration of a normal intra-articular synovial fluid milieu.

The longer the cartilage is exposed to an abnormal milieu, the longer normal loading of the joint must be deferred.

Thus, the schedule for postoperative mobilization and weight-bearing is by no means rigid, but is guided essentially by the functional status of the knee joint.

If no more appreciable effusion is present during the first postoperative days, then at 2 weeks it is safe to allow the patient to walk normally, and at 4 weeks stresses may be increased until full loading is resumed, provid-

ed the condition of the cartilage and ligamentous stability permit it.

Loss of Active Extension and the Suprapatellar Pouch

The development of adhesions within the suprapatellar pouch and parapatellar recesses are an impediment not only to flexion but also to active extension.

In Fig. 291 there is a loss of flexion *and* of active extension as a result of adhesions following a comminuted fracture of the distal femur. The extension loss occurs because the quadriceps is unable to pull the patella a normal distance proximally, and so the muscular action cannot be freely transmitted from the quadriceps tendon across the patella to the tibial tuberosity.

The active range of motion is from 100° flexion to 10–0° extension, but passively the leg can be extended to 0–5° (Fig. 291).

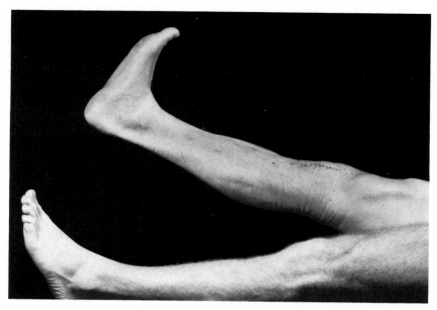

Fig. 289. Postoperative status with leg raised by active quadriceps function. The inhibition of muscular function is overcome by simultaneously dorsiflexing the foot and raising the big toe. This innervates the quadriceps together with other muscles within the "closed motor chain"

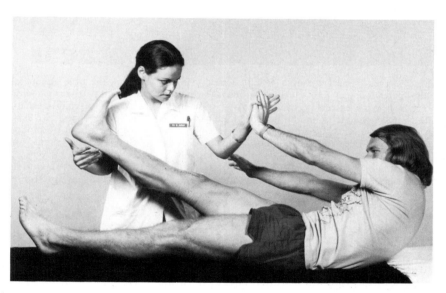

Fig. 290. The reflex activation of the functional chain in Fig. 289 is reinforced by having the patient flex the trunk and twist toward the operated side against a resistance

When this loss of active extension occurs after a ligament operation, for example, it interferes with the patient's ability to actively stabilize the knee. The patient will walk with the knee in slight flexion, thus leaving it to the freshly sutured ligaments to stabilize the knee without muscular protection. Therefore, after ligament operations we wait until the patient can perform full, active extension of the knee, and thus until the

273

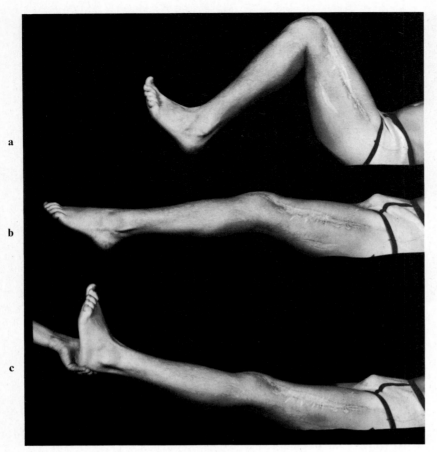

Fig. 291 a–c. Typical example of function loss in the suprapatellar pouch. **a** Flexion is blocked at 100° flexion. **b** *Active* extension is also decreased. **c** When the heel is raised by the examiner, the knee joint can be fully extended without difficulty. Thus, the cause of the extension loss (**b**) lies not in a shrinkage or adhesion of the posterior capsular and ligamentous structures, but in the fact that suprapatellar pouch adhesions do not give the quadriceps extensor apparatus the mobility needed to pull the tibia adequately into extension via the patella and patellar ligament. In all operations care should be taken to avoid traumatizing any of the synovial gliding surfaces about the femur, including the parapatellar recesses, so that no motion-limiting adhesions will develop. The knee should not be subjected to full stresses postoperatively as long as an active extension loss of this type is present. During this period the healing ligaments lack active protection by the muscles

muscles have resumed their protective function, before allowing weight-bearing without a cane.

The situation is different in the mechanically secure knee with stable ligaments (e.g., following an arthrolysis, etc.). In such cases early weight-bearing without a cane can hasten the recovery of full active extension.

The aforementioned second and third injuries following the premature resumption of athletic activity are, according to the observations of various sports traumatologists, generally more severe than the initial injury despite an apparently good primary result. Presumably the coordination between active and passive stabilizing elements was still not adequate at the time the reinjury occurred.

General Pathophysiologic Considerations

Sound rehabilitation begins with an accurate, atraumatic suturing technique at operation. This will allow the bandages to be removed after 48 hours, provided wound healing is progressing well, and early active physiotherapy can be instituted under direct visual control of the wound area.

Next, it is important to avoid hematoma formation by the placement of a Redon suction drain in all critical dead spaces.

Third, wound edema is avoided by elevating the operated limb. According to Allgöwer [5], edemas create conditions which promote cellular swelling and mitosis, thus predisposing to later fibrosis in the joints and muscles.

Fourth, the principle of avoiding prolonged immobilization should be observed. Again according to Allgöwer [5], wound healing is not an end in itself, but is a necessary step toward achieving a recovery. Atraumatic surgical technique affords rapid wound healing and thus enables active mobilization to be started within 24–48 hours after closure.

It is of utmost importance that attention be given intraoperatively to preserving the blood supply of all tissues (except the cartilage). Only tissues that have not been excluded from the circulation can survive and contribute to a functional recovery.

Tools of Rehabilitation

Postoperative Positioning

As illustrated in Fig. 288, elevation of the limb on a wedge (inclined plane) is suitable following simple operations when it is desirable to rehabilitate the leg *from an extended position*. The patient can perform his quadriceps exercises independently by raising the leg from the wedge.

If the leg must be placed in *slight flexion* postoperatively (e.g., after ligament surgery), we utilize a Braun splint for this purpose. The knee can easily be positioned in about 30–40° flexion on this device.

Right-angle positioning (Fig. 292) is necessary in situations where the mobile tissue layers at the distal end of the femur have been traumatized, or if considerable muscle stripping was necessary in the distal femoral region. Flexing the knee to 90° prevents adhesions from forming in the suprapatellar pouch, for it is largely unpleated in this position. This position should not be maintained too long, however. After 4 days at the earliest or 7 days at the latest, a program of reg-

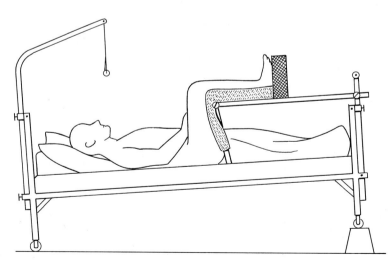

Fig. 292. Postoperative positioning after arthrolyses or distal femoral fractures with injury of the tissues in the suprapatellar pouch and parapatellar recesses. In this position the pouch is for the most part unpleated and is less susceptible to adhesions. Later quadriceps exercises will pull it back in a proximal direction (see Fig. 286).

In this position the peroneal nerve is vulnerable in the immediate postoperative period and so must be protected with special foam padding. The same splint can be used to set a flexion angle of 40 or 10° for positioning with a plaster cast after ligament operations

275

ular, intensive, active mobilization should be instituted, for prolonged 90° immobilization of the knee can lead to serious adhesions and greatly hinder the recovery of full flexion and extension.

Right-Angle Positioning on the Motion Splint

This offers another means of right-angle positioning with a rigid frame. It should be incorporated into the rehabilitation plan if prolonged bed rest and limb elevation is anticipated, due, for example, to concomitant injuries. These motion splints (Fig. 293) can be suspended in such a way that the patient himself can manually control and assist flexion-extension exercises. This permits early mobilization of the suspended leg with almost ideal support.

This is a good alternative in cases where extenuating factors preclude a comprehensive operative management.

The motion splint must be carefully adapted to the individual patient so that the desired movements will be axially correct and will provide proper guidance for the healing soft tissues. During subsequent days the apparatus should be continually checked to make sure the traction is balanced and that the suspension and line of traction are suited to the patient's arm strength. If proper attention is paid to this somewhat difficult point, these splints are a valuable aid to rehabilitation following arthrolyses or severe knee joint injuries.

Automatic Motion Splints

Electric "Kinetec" motion splints have been available since 1980. They replace the suspended splints for many indications and are much easier to monitor. Their major advantage is that they can be set to adjust the positioning angle automatically (e.g., from 10 to 80°) in very slow cycles of up to several hours. For example, in the knee with ligamentous injuries and associated cartilage damage, this apparatus permits very gentle, passive mobilization. According to the most

recent study of Salter [307] in experimental animals, this form of mobilization is effective in promoting optimum cartilage regeneration. The only advantage of the "manual" motion splint over the automatic splint is that it enables better exercise of the knee in 90° flexion or greater.

Postoperative Immobilization

Just as the advantages of the early postoperative mobilization of fractures without external fixation have been recognized, efforts have also been made to eliminate immobilization following operations on the knee joint and other ligamentous surgery.

The advantages of mobilization, or "functional therapy," are great: rapid reduction of edematous swelling, restoration of normal mobility between soft tissue layers, minimal loss of motion range, a reduced rate of algodystrophic complications, and better muscular function with a correspondingly better blood flow through the tissues.

It is generally known that under functional conditions scar tissue is able from the very start to align itself structurally in accordance with stress lines and is able to strengthen in this state. This does not occur in the immobilized joint; the collagen fibrils of the scar tissue acquire a random orientation and later require a period of non-weight-bearing so that the cells and fibers can become ordered and adequately strengthened. Moreover, the muscles undergo atrophy during the immobilization period, and when the plaster is removed the poorly-structured, healing ligaments are subjected to undue stress owing to a deficiency of muscular protection.

There are cases in which very good ligament strength is noted after 4–6 weeks' immobilization in a plaster cast. However, due to the disuse atrophy of the muscles and the incomplete recovery of the proprioceptive reflex control mechanisms that protect the ligaments, a progressive laxity often develops in subsequent weeks, and the instability recurs. We have seen this mainly in

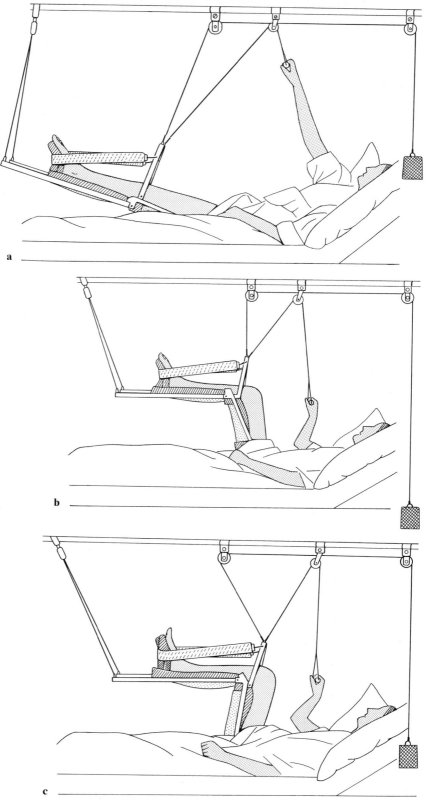

Fig. 293a–c. In injuries that require prolonged flexion with assisted exercises, the *motion splint* provides an important therapeutic aid. The leg is suspended in 90° flexion with a balanced-traction system (**b**) that enables the patient to perform assisted flexion and extension exercises by pulling on a line attached to the splint via a pulley

patients who regained a large range of motion very quickly after surgery, before the recovery of muscular function had progressed to an adequate degree. Typically these patients also exhibit a mild to moderate effusion as a sign of the disproportion between stress and stress-bearing ability, or in this case between range of motion and stabilizing muscle power. Too-rapid mobilization puts an especially severe strain on the healing ligament-to-bone attachments. When the ACL is refixed to the femur, for example, several weeks are needed for the ligamentous attachment to regain an adequately strong fan-shaped structure. Precipitous mobilization will forcibly twist the ligament from its attachment.

As in fracture healing, some degree of rest is necessary to enable adequate fusion of the ligament ends.

In bone, insufficient healing due to excessive movement leads to the development of a pseudarthrosis. On the other hand, immobilization in plaster enables the bone to consolidate over the fixation callus, and stable internal fixation enables primary bone healing to occur.

In ligament healing as well, healing processes vary with the type of fixation employed. The equivalent of a pseudarthrosis is insufficient ligament healing with an overstretched scar that lacks a directional fibrous structure, i.e., a scar plaque with poor stabilizing value.

It seems almost contradictory for us to advocate early mobilization on the one hand while immobilizing knee joints for several weeks on the other. The ideal solution would be to produce an individual orthotic device for each knee joint. It would allow the knee a normal mobility with accurate maintenance of the shifting axes of flexion and rotation, yet would protect the healing ligaments from excessive stress in any form.

At present there is no apparatus that can satisfy these requirements. Simple uniaxial mobility subjects the knee joint to an unphysiologic restraint in several planes. No hinge mechanism can follow the increasing valgus angulation of the tibia and allow the associated rotation through 0–90° flexion. Even the limited-motion cast violates these kinematic laws, although the range of motion it allows does not entail a very great axial deviation. Despite the use of limited-motion casts, however, we have found serious suprapatellar pouch adhesions (!) requiring mobilization under general anesthesia, and so we are not convinced of their value. Moreover, these devices are quite difficult to apply, and a hinge that is not located in the ideal axial position does more harm than good. Frankel and Burstein [98] also stress the importance of maintaining a correct axis of flexion and rotation during all knee movements. If the axis is incorrectly placed, the individual points on the articular cartilage surface lose their normal paths of motion and angular accelerations. As a result, the paths of adjacent points on both articular surfaces no longer just come into contact with each other, but they actually intersect, leading to a "collision" of the points during joint motion. This results either in an overstretching of the soft tissue structures, enabling the articular surfaces to escape damage, or in damage to the cartilage surface with the development of secondary degenerative change.

Because there is still no ideal means of managing the postoperative knee with an orthotic device, the only recourse is to rely on protective fixations for temporary immobilization. Because we base our suturing technique on the principle of fiber isometry, however, we have been able in many cases to dispense with complete immobilization in favor of partial immobilization, which begins with the application of a prefabricated plaster splint in the immediate postoperative period.

Our fixation technique is described below.

Postoperative Fixation

On the day before the operation a posterior plaster splint is molded to the patient's leg, which is flexed 45° for an ACL repair and 10–25° for a PCL repair. This splint surrounds the posterior aspect of the leg like a

U, covering slightly more than half the limb circumference, and extends from the ankle to the thigh. We exclude the foot, because the muscular activity of the calf during foot movements is only beneficial, and because the slight free rotation of the lower leg does not jeopardize the stability of the knee joint.

After the operation this prefabricated plaster splint is applied over the dressing, and the leg is elevated on a frame. The plaster, owing to its U shape, fixes the knee against valgus and varus angulation while prohibiting flexion-extension. Limited mobilization is begun on the 1st postoperative day under the direction of a physical therapist (since 1980 we have used the "Kinetec" motion splint for this purpose).

The therapist *neutralizes gravity forces* and by supporting the leg in neutral rotation ensures that the permissible range of 30–70° flexion for the ACL and 10–40° for the PCL is not exceeded.

In this postoperative phase of rehabilitation, extension to the point of automatic rotation is not desirable due to the associated stress on the ACL and semimembranosus corner. Similarly, a repaired femoral cruciate ligament attachment in particular would be twisted and unduly stressed by movement from 50 to more than 90° flexion and might be torn from the bone before a "broad-based" and tear-resistant cicatrix has formed.

If wound healing is confirmed, a circular plaster cast is applied for discharge following 1 or preferably 2 weeks' early partial mobilization.

Immobilization Following an Anterior Cruciate Ligament Repair

Because the knee ligaments are under the least tension at a flexion angle of 40°, we begin with a partial immobilization phase in 40° flexion on a splint for approximately 2 weeks.

In a second phase we straighten the leg to 20° flexion and fix it in the first closed plaster (for 2–3 weeks). There is still no terminal automatic rotation at this flexion angle.

In the third phase we try to extend the leg to about 5° and allow full weight-bearing in this plaster.

Immobilization Following a Posterior Cruciate Ligament Repair

In the first phase the leg is partially immobilized in 10–15° flexion, i.e., much closer to extension; were the flexion to be greater than 20°, the full weight of the lower leg would be transmitted to the sutured or reconstructed PCL.

In the second phase we immobilize the leg in 10–15° extension, and in the third phase in 5° extension. With peripheral lesions of the medial or lateral side, the position of fixation is guided by the accompanying cruciate ligament injury. If both cruciates are injured, the more important posterior cruciate is the guide.

We intentionally immobilize the leg in 5° rather than 0° extension in order to prevent recurvatum in the plaster, for a tendency toward hyperextension-recurvatum exists in all serious injuries of the central pivot.

"Dynatronic" Therapy in Plaster

"Dynatronic" training offers a means of utilizing the period of plaster immobilization for activation of the muscles [315].

We began using this therapy systematically about 5 years ago. It involves cutting a window about 6 cm square in the plaster 2–3 cm proximal and medial to the patella, through which daily electrical stimulation is applied to the muscle. In this way muscular conditioning is possible even in the immobilized limb. The resulting tension minimizes or prevents the development of adhesions in the suprapatellar pouch, and there is an earlier restoration of mobility between the fascial and ligamentous layers.

Interestingly, this therapy is highly rated subjectively by the patients, for the activity apparently has the effect of stimulating blood flow, which produces a pleasant sensation and often has a pain-alleviating effect.

The disadvantage of this therapy is its cost. The patients must come in daily for treatment, and the apparatus has to be applied and maintained by trained personnel.

Another Means of Early Muscular Activation

Another, less costly means of muscular training in plaster is by employing a fixation that allows better muscular activity.

If the patient can actively extend the lower leg to 20° or less with his quadriceps, we apply a circular plaster cast with the knee in 20° flexion.

A second circular cast is applied with the knee in 5° extension, and full weight-bearing is allowed. This reflexly activates the extensor muscles and the flexor-rotators, so that an active stabilization function is achieved by the time the cast is finally removed.

Immobilization Time

The immobilization time depends on the complexity of the injury and on the mechanical stability of the surgical ligament reattachment. In ideal cases, such as bony avulsions that can be securely reattached with a wire suture or screw, 3–4 weeks' fixation is adequate, whereas in difficult suturing situations and delicate complex injuries 7–8 weeks may be required.

Sometimes we allow the patient to exercise for a week or so without plaster but then reapply the cast temporarily if laxity develops (if the knee feels "rubbery"). This can occur as late as the 3rd or 4th month after surgery.

When we compare our immobilization times with those of experienced U. S. surgeons, we find that theirs are appreciably longer.

For example, James [in 312] reports that he puts the limb in a closed cast from thigh to toes for the first 5 weeks, applies a hinged motion cast with a 30-to-60° flexion range for the next 3 weeks, and finally prescribes a "derotation brace" for 4 months. This is accompanied by several months of physiotherapy, cycling and swimming.

These numbers were not selected at random. They correspond by and large to the recommendations of other symposium participants [in 312], although there is no consensus regarding the optimum flexion angles at which the knee should be immobilized.

Unfortunately the level of the desired stress that leads to a rapid functional incorporation of the scar tissue into the existing system is only slightly below a level that must be deemed "excessive" and will result in the formation of an overstretched scar.

Formerly we attempted to solve the dilemma of mobilization vs. immobilization by prescribing in a selected, reliable patient group a removable splint that was worn at home. Each day the patients came in for active physiotherapy, at which time the splint was removed. The results were very encouraging.

Recent Developments in Postoperative Mobilization

Since the end of 1980 we seldom place an operated limb in a circular plaster cast. Instead, we have been testing a removable plastic cast that fits as well as a plaster cast but is provided with a zip fastener that allows it to be opened far enough (2–3 cm) that the leg can be withdrawn for daily exercises under the guidance of a physiotherapist.

Initially motion between 20 and 50° is allowed. After 3–4 weeks this range is increased by 5° per day. Full extension and especially hyperextension are avoided, for automatic terminal rotation places undue stress on the posteromedial corner and the cruciate ligaments. Full extension is not attempted until about 6 weeks postoperatively. If active stabilization is found to be satisfactory at that time, full-motion-range exercises may be performed.

Following repairs or reconstructions of the posterior cruciate ligament, motion should be kept within the range of 10 to 30 or at most 40° during the first 3–4 weeks, as the PCL is unprotected by peripheral synergists as flexion increases.

To date the results of this graduated mobilization program have been so encouraging that after the forthcoming evaluation we plan to pursue the technique further. One thing must be remembered, however: As in the internal fixation of fractures, an ambitious program of functional therapy is impossible unless it has been preceded by a correspondingly accurate and refined operative technique.

Active Mobilization

Current techniques of active physiotherapy make it possible to reflexly innervate, strengthen and restore function to individual muscle groups within specific "motor chains." With proper application of this principle, it is possible to overcome functional inhibitions stemming from the lesion while demonstrating to the patient that he can regain the use of muscles he considered unresponsive to voluntary contraction. A classic example of this is the patient who cannot raise his extended leg in recumbency even weeks after the knee operation and complains that his quadriceps seems "paralyzed." If such a patient is placed in the prone position and asked to raise the affected leg from the table, he can do so without difficulty. He is then asked to roll onto his back over the healthy side, still keeping the leg in the raised position. Thus, the leg is first extended behind the body, then to the side of the body and finally, when the patient is on his back, the leg is raised in front of the body, held in place by the reflexly-activated quadriceps. The gravity-controlled postural reflexes that are evoked by this sequence of movements maintain leg elevation first with the gluteus muscles and lower leg flexors, then with the tensor fasciae latae and vastus lateralis muscles, and finally with the entire quadriceps. Through this recruitment of muscular function it is possible to circumvent disruptions of voluntary motion

patterns. Klein-Vogelbach [181] states that the principle of "proprioceptive neuromuscular facilitation" is a basic element of physiotherapy. The composite movement (Figs. 289 and 290) is subject to similar reflex controls. Raising the leg after first dorsiflexing the foot and raising the big toe automatically produces an active extension of the knee joint, accompanied by good innervation of the vastus medialis. The strengthening effect of the exercise can be enhanced by extending the motor chain past the diagonal.

The exercises may train muscular strength or promote endurance, depending on the way they are performed. Exercises against a large resistance with a low rate of repetition increase strength, whereas exercises done against a small resistance at rapid intervals promote endurance.

The buoyancy of a water milieu offers additional possibilities for exercising against a small resistance.

Weight-Bearing During Rehabilitation

In discussing the question of weight-bearing during rehabilitation, a clear distinction must be made between the ability simply to bear the body weight and the ability to bear stresses produced by the action of additional forces.

It is one thing for a patient to walk safely without crutches 6 weeks after a patellar fracture, bearing the full weight of the body, but it is quite another for him to jump and land on the affected limb, subjecting the patella to additional stresses that may be sufficient to cause reinjury. While full weight-bearing in the strict sense is possible in this case, the knee has not yet regained a full stress-bearing capability in a broader sense.

Therefore, when evaluating the weight- and stress-bearing capability of the postoperative knee, we must bear the following five questions in mind:

1. How far has consolidation progressed in the bony structures that were divided or repaired during the operation?

2. How stable is the repair or re-attachment of the capsule and ligaments, and how far has their healing progressed?

3. What progress has there been toward the recovery of active muscular stabilization of the knee joint? Have the reflexly controlled protective and stabilizing mechanisms recovered to the extent that the ligaments can withstand full stresses?

4. What is the condition of the cartilage, and is additional time needed for cartilage healing? It must be considered that immobilization is invariably associated with cartilage damage, and that a program of graduated weight-bearing followed by a period of modified-stress activity is important for cartilage healing.

5. Is effusion present as a sign of irritation or poorly compensated function?

After these questions are settled, a decision may be made regarding the permissible degree of weight-bearing and the extent to which stress-producing activities may be resumed.

Physical Therapy

Physical therapy offers an additional, non-active means of alleviating pain and improving joint function. It is particularly useful if certain problems cannot be overcome by early, active mobilization alone. Aside from cryotherapy, the measures discussed below do not constitute a routine part of postoperative management.

Cryotherapy

This form of therapy is easily combined with active mobilization. If effusion or local pain is present, we first cool the joint with small ice pellets to the point where pain sensation is lost before proceeding with active functional therapy. Because the pain impulses in the sensitive tissue are no longer perceived by the patient, they no longer inhibit mobility, and functional rehabilitation is made easier.

In most cases this also produces a state of general relaxation by reducing the tension response in patients with painful knee irritation. The cryotherapy is followed by heat application to induce a prolonged hyperemia which is beneficial for subsequent healing.

Electrotherapy

Electrotherapy involves the use of diadynamic currents, iontophoresis and short waves for pain alleviation. These agents may be employed in the early postoperative phase or in an intermediate- to long-term rehabilitative program to facilitate mobilization.

Heat

Heat is usually unsuitable in the early postoperative period, but later it is beneficial in relieving chronic pain and trophic disturbances owing to the absorption-promoting hyperemia that is produced. It may be administered in a great many forms, such as infrared light, packs, fomentations, baths and peloids.

Ultrasound

Ultrasound may be used to treat indurated scar areas or secondary, tendomyotic changes with associated abnormalities of muscle tension and contractures. Such contractures can easily result from holding the limb in a "favored" position and from abnormal motor sequences based on disturbances of motion patterns; they are a common source of local and distant pains in the functional chains.

Hydrotherapy

For our purposes hydrotherapy refers mainly to the use of water as an environment for performing active postoperative exercises and thus falls under the heading of active physiotherapy, although baths may also serve as a medium for heat application.

Syncardial Therapy

This therapy is indicated for longstanding, obstinate swellings and especially for trophic disturbances of the lower extremities associated with primary circulatory complications, general hydrodynamic difficulties or algodystrophy.

Syncardial massage may be either monophasic or biphasic. In the biphasic form the arterial flow to the tissues is reinforced by a pumping cuff, while the venous return is strengthened with a pneumatic cushion that envelops the entire leg and applies compression after each pulse wave.

As our operating techniques improved and our postoperative mobilization became more efficient, we found less and less use for this type of therapy and have not used it at all in recent years.

Massage of the Soft Tissues and Muscles

Soft-tissue massage is rarely prescribed, for when instituted early it causes the patient to rely too heavily on passive rehabilitative measures. Experience has shown that the best end results are obtained in patients who approach their rehabilitation with a positive, active attitude and do not expect others to "cure" them.

Nevertheless, we do not categorically reject such massage, and we acknowledge its value in the prevention of soft-tissue contractures. In such cases the massage is not limited to the muscles but encompasses all the tissues in the form of a connective-tissue stroke massage.

Manual Therapy

Two types of mobility are present in every joint: the *working or functional mobility* and the *passive, translational mobility*, called also "joint play."

The functional mobility is that which the active muscles can normally exhaust according to the principles of joint kinematics.

Joint play, on the other hand, is the mobility accessible only to passive manipulation; it cannot be utilized by the muscles. This joint play consists of the short translational movements that the bony members can make parallel to the articular surfaces.

In cases of reversible hypomobility, manual therapy utilizes this translational mobility to restore joint play before the cartilage comes under excessive pressure between the long lever arms from purely passive movements of the joint in the usual functional directions. The joint play that is regained through manual therapy serves in turn as a starting point for the restoration of active functional mobility.

Pharmacotherapy

As described in the previous sections, pain, inflammatory irritation and edema represent obstacles to active mobilization. For this reason we do not hesitate to administer drugs as needed during the postoperative period for the relief of these symptoms. Our main object is to blunt the internal defense response of the patient and minimize his distrust of the freshly operated knee, which could interfere with early mobilization and make the entire rehabilitative process more difficult.

Analgesics, Anti-Inflammatory Drugs

Most patients perceive the ability to move the leg early as an alleviation of postoperative complaints, for patients often find the immobilization of a limb in a fixed position to be very distressful. Therefore, we administer the usual analgesics and anti-inflammatory drugs before pain becomes severe. Often we observe marked individual differences in the response to certain drugs, sometimes requiring the rapid change from one medication to another.

In obstinate chondromalacia where long-term management is required, we plan a correspondingly longer course of analgesic and anti-inflammatory therapy.

Diuretics

If troublesome edemas develop despite preventative positioning, we administer diuretics for a period of 1–2 days. A prolonged course of diuretics is ill-advised due to its adverse effect on potassium metabolism and consequent spasmogenic effect on the muscles.

Steroids

Restraint is advised in the use of steroid medications. They may be useful in inflammatory rheumatism or occasionally in other inflammatory irritative conditions of a diffuse nature.

Muscle Relaxants

States of abnormal muscular tension that interfere with function and may be intensely painful respond well to the temporary use of muscle relaxants. Diazepam is effective and often aids the patient in getting to sleep.

Combination products containing a muscle relaxant and an analgesic may also be prescribed.

In situations where it is difficult to find a suitable pain-relieving drug, the necessary effect can sometimes be achieved with *psychoanaleptics* such as clomipramine. By blunting the psychic response to pain, these agents reduce the need for analgesics in the management of such patients.

If the pain is persistent and if symptoms of Sudeck's dystrophy arise, we administer the triple drug combination tested by Bircher [24], which consists of diazepam, hydergine and oxyphenbutazone (or ibuprofen).

Again, we recommend that this treatment be instituted early, for in this way a faster response is obtained and the course of medical therapy is shortened accordingly.

Local Anesthesia

Local intra-articular or regional anesthesia sometimes has a surprisingly beneficial effect. Often a chronically tender or mildly irritated knee joint is in noticeably better condition after a single intra-articular anesthesia, as the basic pain level and irritation may be significantly reduced.

Painful limitations of motion during the course of rehabilitation which impede progress toward the recovery of function and strength are a good indication for the use of local or regional anesthesia. The epidural form is a particularly good indication for the use of local or regional anesthesia. The epidural form is excellent following arthrolyses, because additional anesthetic can be injected as needed via an indwelling catheter in the spinal canal over a period of hours or even days, thus enabling the patient to perform the necessary exercises without pain.

Examination and Mobilization Under General Anesthesia

"Forcible passive mobilization," called also "brisement forcé," can have severe effects, including cartilage avulsions from the condylar surfaces.

The best means of preventing stiffness is to perform regular re-examinations with the consent of the physiotherapist and, based on mobility findings, give orders regarding further treatment. Serious limitations of motion can be almost completely avoided in this manner. However, if problems of this type arise due, for example, to intercurrent disease requiring an interruption or discontinuance of planned postoperative care, we feel it is best to examine the limb under general anesthesia.

The patient's consent is obtained before the anesthesia is administered. If the knee joint cannot be moved under anesthesia past the point of obstruction with ease, then the adhesions in the region of the suprapatellar pouch and parapatellar recesses are freed sharply as in an arthrolysis, and aftercare is started with the knee flexed 90° on the motion splint. A major arthrolytic procedure such as Judet's operation involving distal advancement of the quadriceps need be performed only in patients with motion limitations of long standing. Many months of postoperative rehabilitation are needed in such cases before good active compensation can be achieved.

Therefore, as long as an intraoperative flexion of 110° can be obtained with a simple arthrolysis performed close to the joint, the need for major surgery should be slight. Similarly, it is sufficient to achieve a flexion angle of somewhat more than 90° under general anesthesia without arthrolysis, for once this initial mobility is established most patients can progress well beyond that point during subsequent weeks and months.

Psychological Guidance

In the knee as in no other joint, rehabilitation demands a firm commitment on the part of the patient, the physiotherapist and the surgeon. Poorly-informed and poorly-guided patients do not have a good prospect for recovery. Ignorance and fear lead to non-compliance and mistrust.

It pays to formulate a clear rehabilitation plan that is understood by the patient, that is strictly adhered to, and whose progress is monitored on a regular basis, for an error born of neglect can cause permanent harm. Proper guidance of the patient will spare all parties much trouble and can reduce the need for analgesics and other drugs – not to mention the high costs of avoidable physiotherapeutic measures and months of lost wages and disability compensation.

Clinical Material and Results

General

In order for results to be compared, comparable parameters are necessary.

As Lerat [in 359] points out, however, there is as yet no common, generally accepted scheme for the analysis of therapeutic results.

Therefore, our retrospective study with an interim result for 1977 was conducted according to a scheme that first addressed questions pertaining to our own future goals.

This initial study was to be followed by a prospective analysis of operatively and non-operatively managed cases based on criteria common to both groups, thus enabling a common evaluation of therapeutic results according to the nature of the injury and the method of management.

However, this project had to be postponed when in mid-1978 the author was transferred to a new hospital and given the task of setting up an orthopedic department.

At this hospital we have kept accurate records of pre- and postoperative findings over the past 3 years and have investigated the response of all patients to postoperative care, including 1- and 2-year follow-ups.

During this period (1979–1980) we performed 1013 procedures on the knee, including arthroscopies, at the Department of Orthopedic Surgery of the Bruderholz District Hospital (Table 6).

The 279 ligament operations and the data presented below on our results at the Department of Orthopedic Surgery of the Basel University Hospital during the period 1971–1977 form the practical basis for the present study.

Our scheme for evaluating results prior to 1978 was devised before publication of the evaluation methods of Kettelkamp and Thompson [178], Marshall et al. [210, 211] and Lerat [in 359].

Table 6. Statistical survey of operations performed from 1978 to 1980

	1978	1979	1980
Non-Ligamentous Operations			
Arthroscopies incl. arthroscopic operations	17	208	235
Arthrotomies incl. meniscectomies	17	46	86
Patellar operations	3	19	28
Operations for gonarthrosis incl. prostheses, osteotomies near the knee and arthrodeses	3	34	38
Operations on the Ligaments			
Fresh ligamentous ruptures	17	37	38
Old ligamentous ruptures	13	83	91

Operative vs. Non-Operative Treatment

Godshall and Hansen [208] reported very good results with non-operative treatment if the instability did not exceed 3 mm. For greater instabilities they recommended operative management. In a third, intermediate group, operative treatment was also elected in most cases.

Ellsasser et al. [77] compared the results of the operative and non-operative treatment of ligamentous injuries in professional football players. However, the validity of their comparison is compromised by the fact that mild instabilities were treated conservatively while severe instabilities were treated operatively. Under these circumstances it is inevitable that non-operative treatment will yield better results, for, as mentioned earlier, the prognosis worsens as the complexity of the injury increases. This has also been confirmed by Lemaire [198] and Vidal [364].

Several points in the Ellsasser study [77] merit further discussion.

First, he used the following criteria in selecting patients for non-operative treatment:

1. The knee must be stable in extension whether the injury is on the lateral or the medial side.
2. The ligamentous laxity in 30° flexion should not be more than 10° greater than the preinjury knee laxity (sic!) or than the laxity of the uninjured knee. The limit of laxity should feel firm rather than mushy.
3. Significantly increased rotatory or anteroposterior play should not be present.
4. Tenderness should be localized to the proximal or distal end of the ligament, not diffusely distributed over the ligament.
5. A small effusion is not a contraindication.
6. Limitation of the range of motion is not a contraindication.
7. Roentgenograms should show no signs of acute bone injury.
8. No stability changes should arise during the period of 24 hours after the injury, i.e., the patient's progress should conform to expectations and should show no secondary exacerbations.

Patient with well-developed muscles underwent functional rehabilitation without immobilization in plaster, while a plaster cast was prescribed for patients with inadequate muscles.

Second, it is interesting to note that despite the better than 90% success rate in 74 conservatively managed knee injuries that occurred in 52 players, *15 players injured the same knee more than once,* and 7 of the reinjuries were severe enough to necessitate surgical repair.

Whereas almost all the players that received non-operative treatment returned to the game in the same season, only one of the patients treated surgically returned to play in the same season the surgery was done.

None of the four players with posterolateral lesions (all of whom were treated surgically) and neither of the patients with a medial triad injury returned to play.

Simmons [319] conducted follow-ups in a series of 333 surgically-treated knee injuries in 189 patients and 206 knees. His findings are as follows:

- Repairs of the MCL, ACL and POL:
  within 10 days   70% success rate
  within 14 days to 3 months
                            50% success rate
  late repairs   62% success rate
- Lindemann reconstruction [200] for the ACL: successful in 5 of 7 cases.
- Pes anserinus transfer: successful in 10 of 21 cases.
- In repairs of ACL lesions, $1/3$ of the poor results showed pivot-shift symptoms and an abnormal range of tibial rotation.
- In 8 isolated ACL ruptures treated non-operatively, results were poor in 5 cases.
- Results were best in the 20–30 age group.
- Results were poorest in the 30–40 age group.
- In a series of Workmen's Compensation cases, the failure rate was 65%.
- Peripheral meniscus reattachment yielded good results.

Wirth [388] reported in 1976 on a study of patients in whom partial ruptures were treated non-operatively and complete ruptures were surgically repaired. In the latter series of 15 knees (14 patients), 2 were excellent, 12 good and 1 acceptable after 2–10 years.

Wirth et al. [330] also reported in 1974 on the results of 29 reconstructions by the technique of Brückner and Brückner [37]. Fourteen of these were satisfactory, 3 fair and 12 unsatisfactory.

The possible influence of cartilage derangements on therapeutic results is demonstrated by Franke [95], who found the presence of chondromalacia in 54% of ligamentous injuries.

Ségal et al. [314] view progressive cartilage damage as a direct result of progressive anteromedial instability. According to their observations, an uncompensated anteromedial instability from a initial trauma progresses from a typical triad to the development of secondary osteochondral lesions between the femur and tibia on the medial side, to an increasing detachment of capsular fibers from the tibia in the semimembranosus corner, and then to a femoropatellar "instability" with subsequent femoropatellar cartilage lesions, until finally a full-blown global anterior instability is present.

On the other hand, Burri and Helbing [38] report very encouraging results with a 90% "good" subjective rating in 80 acute ligamentous injuries, 69 of which were fully stable on examination. These authors and O'Donoghue [266] state that a recent injury should be surgically treated as soon as possible, for each day gained improves the outcome. The influence of the motion cast on these good results is unclear, for 24 of the 80 cases in this series (30%) did not involve cruciate ligament injuries.

Lerat et al. [199] report on the results of 31 surgically-treated lateral ligamentous injuries. Partial lateral ruptures were managed non-operatively, and each of the 31 operated cases involved the rupture of at least one cruciate ligament (ACL rupture in 11, PCL rupture in 8, combined rupture in 12).

In addition, there were 7 cases of peroneal nerve paralysis, 4 of which have not recovered. The results were rated unsatisfactory or disappointing. The combined cruciate ligament injury was particularly unfavorable, while the ACL rupture had a better prognosis.

Ginsberg and Ellsasser [106] report similar experiences.

Indication for Operative or Non-Operative Treatment

Our clinical experience from 1971 to 1977 confirms that the primary repair of acute injuries generally produces far better results than secondary operations for old injuries with chronic instability. In addition, the fact that we had to perform many secondary repairs and reconstructions on knee joints with disabling instabilities that had previously undergone a primary program of conservative therapy strongly suggests that surgical treatment is necessary for certain ligamentous injuries of the knee.

Surgery is necessary or justified if it is known that the nature of the lesion makes spontaneous recovery impossible. An example is a cruciate ligament that is torn from its femoral attachment and "floating" on the tibial plateau. Cruciate ligament injuries in general have the most severe consequences of any ligamentous injury, and we feel that they are a definite indication for surgery.

On the other hand, the injury of one or two peripheral ligaments (a monad or duad) without associated cruciate ligament damage has a chance of healing well without operative treatment. In our view the non-operative management of the knee with an uniaxial instability like that occurring in a monad should consist of functional treatment in an elastic bandage reinforced with foam rubber. The peripheral duad may also be managed in this way, but the triad, if not treated surgically, requires true plaster fixation.

For its part, operative treatment will be successful only if all the ligamentous structures for which damage has been presumed on the basis of instability findings have been adequately repaired.

This attitude toward surgical indications is widely prevalent and is expressed by Fetto and Marshall [84] as well as many other authors.

In doubtful situations arthroscopy can provide much information on the status of the ACL and lateral meniscus, while the PCL and medial posterior horn may be quite difficult to visualize if stability is good.

Arthrography is justified only as an adjunctive measure to settle specific questions that remain following a careful clinical examination.

If surgery is indicated it should be performed as early as possible, although operating under unfavorable conditions (emergency surgery at night, etc.) is not recommended.

An old lesion is difficult to recognize and may be likened to an avalanche covered by new-fallen snow. Just as one can recognize the avalanche beneath the snow only if he is familiar with its features, the surgeon can recognize a ligament beneath the scar tissue only if he is familiar with its anatomy.

Our Results for the Period 1971–1977

Clinical Material

During the period from 1/1/71 to 9/30/77, 879 knee operations were performed at the Department of Orthopedic Traumatology of the Basel University Hospital (Orthopedic Clinic of the Surgical Department of the University of Basel). Of these, 182 were ligament operations. Ninety-five of these operations were for acute injuries, 87 were for chronic instabilities.

All surgical procedures and follow-ups were carried out by a small, closed working team under the direction of a single team head in accordance with specified principles.

In addition to the 182 first operations performed by us (several patients with chronic instabilities had undergone 1 to 3 prior operations), there were 16 reoperations of patients that had been operated on previously in our department. Four of these reoperations were on a single patient who was referred to us for treatment early in our practice with prior operations and cartilage damage. In the light of later experience, we now know that these repeat operations were avoidable. Besides this case and a similar one, the remaining reoperations consisted mostly of revisions of irritating fixation screws or secondary cruciate ligament reconstructions with improved technique.

Of the 182 patients, 128 (70%) presented personally for follow-ups during 1976/77, and an additional 48 (26%) were reviewed at home by means of questionnaires and the assistance of their family physicians using our earlier outpatient protocol (Köppel [402]). A total of 176 patients (96%) were included in the review (90 of 95, or 94%, of the acute injuries and 86 of 87, or 99%, of the old instabilities).

Distribution of Recent and Old Injuries

In the population reviewed, 51% had fresh injuries and 49% had chronic instabilites (Fig. 294). Recent or fresh injuries included those up to 3 weeks old, and up to 4 weeks old in a few cases.

Side distribution

Eighty-one injuries (46%) affected the right knee, 93 (53%) the left knee, and 2 (1%) affected both knees.

Sex Distribution

Women	43	= 24.5%
Men	133	= 75.5%

Age

The youngest patient was 16, the oldest 68. The average age was 34; 58% of the patients were below the average age.

The question of whether there is an "age limit" for the operative treatment of ligamentous injuries is of interest in this regard.

Nature usually solves the problem, for ligament ruptures tend to occur in young, athletic patients whose activity level predisposes them to ligamentous injury, whereas older patients are more susceptible to fractures of the tibial plateau and femoral condyles.

If serious ligamentous injuries are present, however, they should be treated operatively even in the older, physically active patient; age in itself is not a contraindication.

Types of Injury

Athletic injuries	116 = 66%
Traffic injuries	89 = 22%
On-the-job injuries	21 = 12%

289

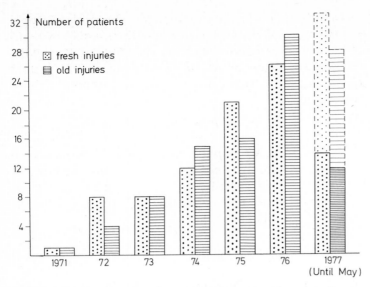

Fig. 294. Total number of fresh and old ligamentous knee injuries treated operatively from 1971 to 1977. – – – in 1977 represents an extrapolation for the whole year

Among the athletic injuries (n = 116), 46 (40%) were skiing-related, 33 (28%) were soccer-related, and 37 (32%) related to other types of sport, mainly handball and tennis.

The traffic injuries resulted mainly from motorcycle and motorbike accidents.

Results

The known differences between the operative results in acute and chronic instabilities prompted us to analyze these differences in the most straightforward yet informative manner possible.

We wanted to know whether a complete functional recovery can indeed be achieved, and how much our treatment can accomplish in the most objective terms possible.

Therefore, we did not rely primarily on the subjective assessment of the patient, although this would have increased considerably the number of "good" and "excellent" results.

The classification should also be simple so that a meaningful comparison can be obtained without the necessity of making over-subtle distinctions. Of course stress x-rays

under general anesthesia would be required for a truly objective assessment, but this is hardly practical.

At present technical means are available which allow comparable stress films to be made without the need for general anesthesia, but such means were not yet available at the time of our review.

We divided the instabilities into 3 degrees of severity:

3–5 mm	= 1 +
5–10 mm	= 2 +
10 mm or more	= 3 +

Thus, for example, an 1 + instability means that the joint surfaces can be separated by a distance of 3–5 mm.

We chose four categories for our result rating

1. "Excellent" denotes a complete recovery with
   – equal stability on both sides and
   – freedom from complaints and
   – ability to engage in all activities without limitation.
2. "Good" denotes
   – instability no greater than 1 + or
   – only sporadic complaints (following extreme activity or during weather changes) or

290

– little reduction in performance ability (no job change, still able to engage in sports).
3. "Fair" denotes
   – improvement over prior status for old instabilities,
   – instability up to 2 + or
   – reduced performance ability due to functional uncertainty compared to pre-injury status for recent injuries.
4. "Poor" denotes
   – no improvement over prior status or
   – instability up to 3 + or
   – recurrence of chronic complaints, or
   – severely reduced performance ability due to functional uncertainty.

Knee joints assigned to the "excellent" category may be regarded as normal for all practical purposes.

Patients with mild instabilities were assigned to the "good" category, even if they were free from other complaints and had no apparent loss of performance ability. This category also includes patients with normal stability but with intermittent stress-dependent complaints or limited mobility.

The result was rated "fair" if a 2 + instability was demonstrated, even if the patient had no complaints or disability and was completely satisfied with the result.

The "poor" category includes all cases that were not improved by the operation or in which performance ability was significantly impaired due to pain or functional uncertainty despite improved stability.

Results for Fresh Injuries, N = 90 (Fig. 295)
   86 medial ligament repairs
   4 lateral ligament repairs
   42 ACL repairs
   6 PCL repairs
   7 primary ACL reconstructions

Sole Medial Lesion, N = 26
   Excellent   8 = 31%
   Good   17 = 65%
   Fair   1 = 4%
   Poor   0

Note: Based on later experience, we must assume that mild unrecognized cruciate ligament lesions were present in this group.

Medial Lesion with ACL, N = 47
   Excellent   8 = 17%
   Good   34 = 72%
   Fair   5 = 11%
   Poor   0

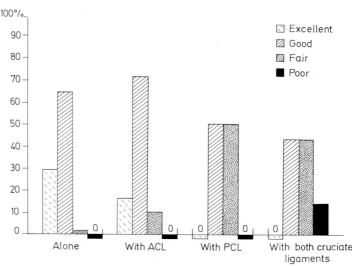

Fig. 295. The results of fresh medial injuries as a function of cruciate ligament involvement

Medial Lesion with PCL, N = 6

Excellent	0
Good	3 = 50%
Fair	3 = 50%
Poor	0

Medial Lesion with ACL and PCL, N = 7

Excellent	0
Good	3 = 43%
Fair	3 = 43%
Poor	1 = 14%

Lateral Lesions

There were only 4 cases of lateral lesions in the series.

Two cases involved injury of the LCL, arcuate ligament and popliteus tendon unaccompanied by cruciate lesions.

In 2 cases there was an associated tear of the PCL.

The result ratings were as follows: 2 excellent, 1 good and 1 fair. The case number is too small for conclusions to be drawn, but generally speaking, and based on our most recent series, our results with lateral injuries have been better than a literature comparison would suggest (see p. 190, 191).

Overall we may say that our results in acute injuries have improved from year to year as the number of operations performed has increased (Fig. 296).

The collective results for all fresh lesions (N = 90) were as follows:

Excellent	17 = 19%
Good	60 = 67%
Fair	12 = 13%
Poor	1 = 1%

The general distribution of all fresh ligamentous lesions is demonstrated in Fig. 299, the results in Fig. 296.

Results for Old Lesions with Chronic Instabilities

Many patients had undergone previous operations and some had a long history of knee problems. Many had had to quit work, had been retrained for a new occupation, or had been forced to take a sedentary job. The reasons for reoperation were varied, but the indication was always definite.

The sum of these results presents a quite different picture. However, one must remember that the first results from the early 1970s are included and that the results from the past 5 years would look much better.

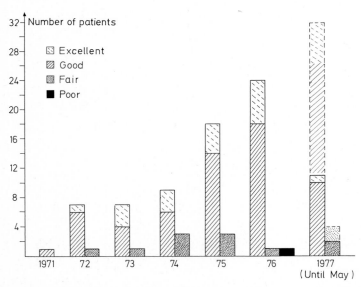

Fig. 296. Collective long-term results for all fresh ligamentous injuries from 1971 to 1977. – – – in 1977 represents an extrapolation for the whole year

292

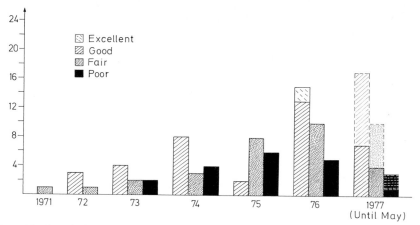

Fig. 297. Results for old injuries with chronic instabilities for the period 1971–1977. – – – in 1977 represents an extrapolation for the whole year

Old Ligamentous Lesions with Chronic In-stabilities, N = 86

Excellent	2 = 2%
Good	37 = 43%
Fair	29 = 34%
Poor	18 = 21% (Fig. 297).

A further analysis of the results according to lesion types and operative techniques is not strictly possible on a comparative basis, for we often combined techniques with one another (e.g., O'Donoghue's medial reconstruction [268] with or without one of two types of cruciate ligament graft, depending on the technique currently favored for the individual ligamentous elements).

Nevertheless, a cautious comparison of the results of individual operative procedures does provide some useful insight into the problem.

As time passed, ongoing follow-ups for the purpose of quality control demonstrated that the results of our late repairs were seriously lacking in regularity. Thus, while in some cases relatively minor instabilities could not be corrected with one type of operation, the same procedure produced a good result in other cases during the same period.

This was the reason, during our ongoing comparison with the improving and more or less predictable results of acute repairs, that we came to recognize the importance of reconstructing natural form and function if we were to achieve predictably better results in a given situation.

Bearing in mind the limitations mentioned above, we may rate our results with specific standard procedures as follows:

O'Donoghue's Operation [268], Type II, N = 20

Excellent	2 = 10%
Good	10 = 50%
Fair	4 = 20%
Poor	4 = 20%

Trillat's Fibular Head Transplant [in 354], N = 13

Excellent	0
Good	4 = 31%
Fair	4 = 31%
Poor	5 = 38%

Augustine's Palliative Operation [15] for the PCL, N = 4

Excellent	0
Good	0
Fair	2 = 50%
Poor	2 = 50%

Modified Lindemann Technique [200] for Replacement of the PCL by the Gracilis and Semitendinosus Tendons, N = 2

Fair	2 = 100%

293

Pes Anserinus Transfer of Slocum and Larson [325] for the Period 1971–1974 as a Sole Measure for Correcting Anteromedial Instability, N = 7

Four cases have since been reoperated using other techniques. Of the remaining 3, 2 are good and 1 is poor.

Lateral Ligament Reconstruction of MacIntosh and Darby [215], N = 10

Excellent	0
Good	5 = 50%
Fair	3 = 30%
Poor	2 = 20%

Operation of Ellison et al. [76], N = 6

Excellent	0
Good	3 = 50%
Fair	3 = 50%
Poor	0

MacIntosh-Ellison Operation, N = 4

Excellent	0
Good	4 = 100%
Fair	0
Poor	0

Helfet's Operation [124], N = 2

Excellent	0
Good	1 = 50%
Fair	0
Poor	1 = 50%

Various Techniques and Later Developments, N = 18

Excellent	0
Good	15 = 83%
Fair	1 = 6%
Poor	2 = 11%

Anterior Cruciate Ligament Reconstruction (All Techniques Combined), N = 35

By the time of our review 40 operations had been performed, but 5 of these were not yet 1 year old and so were not included in the study.

Excellent	2 = 6%
Good	22 = 63%
Fair	6 = 17%
Poor	5 = 14%

Individual Results for Three Different Methods of ACL Reconstruction (Fig. 298)

	1. Jones method [162, 163] up to 1974	2. Over-the-top method of MacIntosh [216] up to 1975	3. Our own modification since 1975
	N = 4	N = 9	N = 22
Excellent	0	0	2 = 9%
Good	2 = 50%	4 = 44%	16 = 72%
Fair	1 = 25%	4 = 44%	1 = 5%
Poor	1 = 25%	1 = 12%	3 = 14%

Assessment of Results

For now our analysis of results must end at this point, but already it is possible to draw several important conclusions with regard to further development.

The last results compare very favorably with results reported by the following experienced authors:

Blazina [in 312] states that a success rate of 70% is very good in the operative treatment of chronic instabilities.

Losee et al. [201] report 41 good results in 50 operations with their "sling and reef" technique, although it is questionable whether a 1-year result is adequate for a definitive assessment.

Kennedy et al. [176] report a 46% rate of good and excellent results with the Ellison procedure [76] alone, but they also state that the results of the procedure are unpredictable in any given case.

Ireland and Trickey [145] describe 14 excellent and 23 good results following a lateral MacIntosh tenodesis [207] in 50 patients, but fewer than half the patients returned to their sport. Twelve patients suffered reinjuries, 4 of which led to a recurrence of instability.

With regard to the pes transfer of Slocum and Larson [325], we have seen several cases that exhibited a gradually progressive valgus laxity after surgery. The obvious conclusion is that the reduced muscular capability for

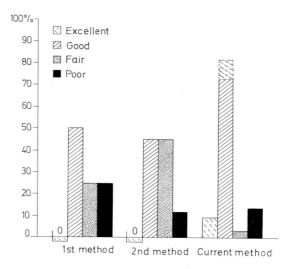

Fig. 298. Results for anterior cruciate ligament reconstructions by three different methods: *1* method up to 1974; *2* method up to 1975; *3* method since 1975

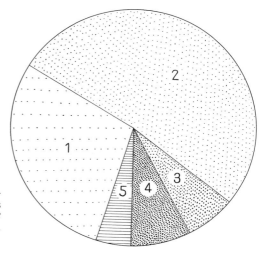

Fig. 299. Circle graph showing relative frequency of involvement of various structures in all freshly operated ligamentous injuries: *1* medial side alone (?); *2* medial side with ACL; *3* medial side with PCL; *4* medial side with ACL and PCL; *5* lateral side

stabilizing the knee against valgus angulation (see also p. 90) is no longer sufficient to protect the MCL from chronic overstretching in the long term. Clinically these knees bear a close resemblance to the postpoliomyelitic flail joint.

Del Pizzo et al. [66] have analyzed 100 consecutive cases of anterolateral rotatory instability. Their findings are of interest in this context, for they show that operations aimed at the correction of individual symptoms seldom produce a good end result.

Each of the 100 patients had undergone an average of 1.23 prior operations when examined, and 84 were reoperated.

These 123 prior operations included the following 182 procedures:

– medial meniscectomy	65
– lateral meniscectomy	14
– pes anserinus transfer	33 (!)
– medial capsule	33 (!)
– medial collateral ligament	30 (!)
– anterior cruciate ligament	5
– posterior cruciate ligament	1
– lateral collateral ligament	1
	182

Of these 100 patients, 16 showed only anterolateral rotatory instability at examination, and of the remaining 84 patients:

– 76 had anteromedial + anterolateral rotatory instability,
– 5 had anteromedial + anterolateral + posterolateral rotatory instability,
– 3 had anterolateral + posterolateral rotatory instability.

Two conclusions may be drawn from this:

1. Operations that do not address the entire problem, including the instability, have no prospect of long-term success.
2. Rotatory instabilities tend to spread to other quadrants through progressive stretching.

Our results made us realize that failures depend ultimately upon cruciate ligament injuries and their consequences, and that long-term success is possible only if we can at least restore the compensatory ability of the knee, taking into account the interaction of *all* functions.

For example, Ellison [in 12] reports the following based on his analysis of synergisms in the knee:

– In NR the ACL accounts for 85% of anterior stability, and the periphery for 15%.
– In ER the ACL accounts for 35–50% of anterior stability and the periphery for 40–60%.
– Under a valgus stress the ACL accounts for 14% of anterior stability and the periphery for 86%.

In their study of primary and secondary passive stabilizers, Butler et al. [42] calculated a similar percentage distribution of restraining functions with regard to straight anterior and posterior drawer displacements.

Experience has shown [42, 75, 76] that when the primary passive stabilizers are lost, the secondary stabilizers can maintain stability for a certain period of time but will eventually become incompetent as a result of gradual elongation.

Butler et al. [42] also measured large individual differences in the percentage functional value of the secondary stabilizers.

Perhaps it will be possible one day to measure the relative restraining value of the primary and secondary passive stabilizers in the various rotational positions under an axial load and under a valgus-varus stress, and to analyze the manner in which these stabilizers "trade roles" as the stress vector changes (e.g., under a valgus stress the MCL becomes a primary stabilizer and the cruciate ligaments become secondary stabilizers). Then we may be able to calculate compensation limits with precision and will no longer have to rely on the somewhat crude assignment of a ⅓ stabilizing value to each of the major elements.

The tension curves of Hertel [126] shed some light on the roles of the major ligaments as passive primary and secondary stabilizers for various functional positions, although these data cannot confirm all clinical observations.

Thus, guided by clinical experience, we must continue to take a broad approach so that we can be sure of achieving a stability that falls within the compensatory range. Above all, we must accurately repair the cruciate "central pivot." We have achieved an 80% success rate in repairs of the ACL, and even this can be improved upon by systematically repairing the secondary stabilizers in all surrounding quadrants.

In the treatment of acute as well as chronic instabilities, evidence indicates that only an individualized anatomic repair offers a prospect of success with a complete, lasting functional recovery.

The various reparative and reconstructive techniques are numerous, and their results are equally varied. The analogy with the game of golf, proposed by Blazina, seems appropriate:

The beginner must start with at least three clubs, while an expert needs 14 clubs to achieve an optimum result.

No beginner can succeed right away with 14 clubs!

List of Sources

Figs. 9–12: Photo C. Baur, Basel

Figs. 17, 25a, 31, 43, 49, 50, 51, 52, 54b, 55, 56, 72, 74, 75, 78, 80, 81, 82, 83, 84, 85, 99, 100, 126a, 129, 211: With the kind permission of A. v. Hochstetter.

Fig. 19a, b: With the kind permission of P. Boehnel.

Fig. 20a, b: B. Tillmann, Kiel, from *Orthop. Praxis* (1974) *12*, 691–697.

Fig. 33: With the kind permission of D. L. MacIntosh.

Figs. 53b, 86, 87, 88, 132: Anatomical Institute of the University of Basel.

Fig. 102b: *Schweizer Illustrierte* (1974).

Fig. 102c, d: from *World Cup 1974*, Pro Sport, Munich.

Figs. 104a, b, 112, 113, 123b, 124: Foto-Archiv K. Baumli, Hirzbodenweg 10, 4052 Basel.

Fig. 118: Photo F. Grossenbacher, Sternengasse 6, Basel.

Figs. 114, 115, 116: from *Montreal 1976*, Schweizer Sporthilfe, Olympische Sportbibliothek, Genf.

References

1. Abbott LC, Carpenter WF (1945) Surgical approaches to the knee joint. J Bone Joint Surg [Am] 27:277–310
2. Abbott LC, Saunders JB, Bost FC, Anderson CE (1944) Injuries to the ligaments of the knee joint. J Bone Joint Surg [Am] 26:503–521
3. Abernethy PJ, Townsend PR, Rose RM, Radin EL (1978) Is chondromalacia patellae a separate clinical entity? J Bone Joint Surg [Br] 60:205–210
4. Aleshin A (1975) Intraoperative ligamentography of the cruciate ligaments of the knee joint (Russian). Vestn Rentgenol Radiol 50/3:42–44
5. Allgöwer M (1969) Biologische Grundlagen zur Wundbehandlung. Langenbecks Arch Chir 325:22–29
6. Alm A (1973) Survival of part of patellar tendon transposed for reconstruction of anterior cruciate ligament. Acta Chir Scand 139:443–447
7. Alm A (1974) On the anterior cruciate ligament. Medical dissertation, Lingköping University
8. Alm A (1974) Old injuries of the ligament of the knee joint. Acta Chir Scand 140:283–288
9. Alm A, Gillquist J (1974) Reconstruction of the anterior cruciate ligament by using the medial third of the patellar ligament. Acta Chir Scand 140:289–296
10. Alm A, Strömberg B (1974) Vascular anatomy of the patellar and cruciate ligaments. Acta Chir Scand [Suppl] 445:25–35
11. Alm A, Ekström H, Gillquist J, Strömberg B (1974) The anterior cruciate ligament. Acta Chir Scand [Suppl] 445:3–49
12. American Academy of Orthopaedic Surgeons (1979) Symposium: Identification and treatment of combined instability of the knee. 46. Annual Meeting (Cassette)
13. Anselm Y (1978) Etudes critiques de l'intervention d'Augustine dans le traitement des ruptures anciennes du ligament croisé postérieur du genou (A propos de 19 cas). Thèse Université de Strasbourg
14. Artmann M, Wirth CJ (1974) Untersuchung über den funktionsgerechten Verlauf der vorderen Kreuzbandplastik. Z Orthop 112:160–165
15. Augustine RW (1956) The unstable knee. Am J Surg 92:380–388
16. Babin-Chevaye J (1968) Réparations ligamentaires du genou. Encycl Med Chir 44790:1–8
17. Bandi W (1972) Chondromalacia patellae und femoro-patellare Arthrose. Helv Chir Acta [Suppl] 11:1–70
18. Barfod B (1971) Posterior cruciate ligament-reconstruction by transposition of the popliteal tendon. Acta Orthop Scand 42:438
19. Barham JN, Thomas WL (1971) Anatomical kinesiology. Collier-Macmillan, Toronto
20. Bartel DL, Marshall JL, Schieck RA, Wang JB (1977) Surgical repositioning of the medial collateral ligament. J Bone Joint Surg [AM] 59:107–116
21. Basmajian JV, Lovejoy JF (1971) Function of the popliteus muscle in man. J Bone Joint Surg [Am] 53:557–562
22. Baumgartl F (1964) Das Kniegelenk. Springer, Berlin Göttingen Heidelberg
23. Beauchamp P, Laurin CA, Bailon JP (1979) Etudes des propriétés mécaniques des ligaments croisés en vue de leur remplacement prothétique. Rev Chir Orthop 65:197–207
24. Bircher J (1971) Klinische Sudeck-Prophylaxe und Therapie (Tierexperimentelle Grundlagen). Springer, Berlin Heidelberg New York
25. Blaimont P, Burnotte J, Halleux P (1975) Rôle des ménisques du genou dans la transmission des contraintes articulaires. Acta Orthop Belg [Suppl 1] 41:143–152
26. Blazina ME (1978) Prosthetic ligaments-indications. In: Schulitz KP, Krahl H, Stein WH (eds) Late reconstructions of injured ligaments of the knee. Springer, Berlin Heidelberg New York, pp 109–114
27. Blumensaat C (1938) Die Lageabweichungen und Verrenkungen der Kniescheibe. Ergeb Chir Orthop 31:149–223
28. Böhler J (1953) Die operative Behandlung der frischen Seitenbandrisse des Kniegelenks. Arch Orthop Unfallchir 102:93–102
29. Bordier G (1975) Anatomie appliquée à la danse. Amphora, Paris
30. Bosworth DM (1952) Transplantation of the semitendineus for repair of laceration of medial collateral ligament of the knee. J Bone Joint Surg [Am] 34:196–202
31. Bousquet G (1972) Les lésions graves récentes du genou. Rev Chir Orthop 58:49–56
32. Bousquet G (1972) Le diagnostic des laxités chroniques du genou. Rev Chir Orthop 58:71–77
33. Bousquet G (1975) Anatomie et physiologie chirurgicale du genou. In: Cahiers d'enseignement de la SOFCOT No 1: Les fractures du genou. Expansion scientifique française, Paris p. 9–23
34. Brantigan OC, Voshell AF (1941) The mechanics of the ligaments and menisci of the knee joint. J Bone Joint Surg [Am] 23:44–66
35. Brantigan OC, Voshell AF (1943) The tibial collateral ligament: Its function, its bursae and its relation to the medial meniscus. J Bone Joint Surg [Am] 25:121–131
36. Braune W, Fischer O (1891) Bewegungen des Kniegelenks nach einer neuen Methode an lebenden Menschen gemessen. Abhandl Math-Phys Cl Koenigl Saechs Ges Wiss 17:75–150

37. Brückner H, Brückner H (1972) Bandplastiken im Kniebereich nach dem „Baukastenprinzip". Zentralbl Chir 97:65–77

38. Burri C, Helbing G (1977) Therapie und Ergebnisse nach frischen Verletzungen des Kniebandapparates. Langenbecks Arch Chir 345:451–457

39. Burri C, Pässler HH, Radde J (1973) Experimentelle Grundlagen zur funktionellen Behandlung nach Bandnaht und -plastik am Kniegelenk. Z Orthop 111:378–379

40. Burri C, Helbing G, Rüter A (1974) Die Behandlung der posttraumatischen Bandinstabilität am Kniegelenk. Orthopaede 3:184–192

41. Burri C, Hutzschenreuter P, Pässler HH, Radde J (1974) Functional postoperative care after reconstruction of knee ligaments. An experimental study. In: Ingwersen OS (ed) The knee joint. Excerpta Medica, Amsterdam, pp 108–112

42. Butler DL, Noyes FR, Grood ES (1980) Ligamentous restraints to anterior-posterior drawer in the human knee. J Bone Joint Surg [Am] 62:259–270

43. Cadilhac J, Georgesco M, Carne P (1978) L'amyotrophie d'immobilisation du quadriceps. In: Simon L (ed) Genou et médecine de rééducation. Masson, Paris, pp 33–37

44. Cameron HU, Macnab I (1972) The structure of the meniscus of the human knee joint. Clin Orthop 89:215–219

45. Campbell WC (1936) Repair of the ligaments of the knee. Surg Gynecol Obstet 62:964–968

46. Campbell WC (1939) Reconstruction of the ligaments of the knee. Am J Surg 43:473–480

47. Castaing J, Burding P, Mougin M (1972) Les conditions de la stabilité passive du genou. Rev Chir Orthop 58:34–48

48. Chalandre P (1977) Le remplacement du ligament croisé antérieur du genou par le procédé de Lindemann. Mémoire du C.E.S. de Biologie et de Médecine du Sport, Université de Grenoble

49. Chapchal G (ed) (1977) Injuries of the ligaments and their repair. Thieme, Stuttgart

50. Chiroff RT (1975) Experimental replacement of the anterior cruciate ligament. J Bone Joint Surg [Am] 57:1124–1127

51. Cho KO (1975) Reconstruction of the anterior cruciate ligament by semitendinosus tenodesis. J Bone Surg [Am] 57:608–612

52. Clancy WG, Rosenberg T, Gmeiner J, Narechania RG, Wisnestke D (1979) Anterior cruciate ligament reconstruction in primates and man: A biomechanical and microangiographic evaluation of patellar tendon substitution. 1st Congress of the International Society of the Knee, Lyon (Communication)

53. Collins HR, Hughston JC, Dehaven KE, Bergfeld JA, Evarts CM (1974) The meniscus as a cruciate ligament substitute. J Sports Med Phys Fitness 2:11–21

54. Cooper RR (1972) Alternations during immobilization and regeneration of skeletal muscle in cats. J Bone Joint Surg [Am] 54:919–951

55. Cooper RR, Misol S (1970) Tendon and ligament insertion. J Bone Joint Surg [Am] 52:1–20

56. Cossa JF, Evrard C, Poilleux F (1968) Un des inconvénients du judo: luxation isolée de l'articulation péronéo-tibiale supérieure. Rev Chir Orthop 54:373–378

57. Cotta H, Puhl W (1976) Pathophysiologie des Knorpelschadens. Unfallheilkunde 127:1–22

58. Courvoisier E (1979) La réfection active du croisé postérieur dans la laxité chronique du genou. Rev Chir Orthop [Suppl 2] 65:51–53

59. Cox JS, Nye CE, Schaefer WW, Woodstein IJ (1975) The degenerative effects of partial and total resection of the medial meniscus in dog's knees. Clin Orthop 109:178–183

60. Dandy DJ, Jackson RW (1975) Meniscectomy and chondromalacia of the femoral condyle. J Bone Joint Surg [Am] 57:1116–1119

61. Davies DV, Edwards DAW (1948) The blood supply of the synovial membrane and intra-articular structures. Ann Coll Surg 142–156

62. Decoulx J (1971) L'instabilité en rotation du genou. Rev Chir Orthop 57:253

63. Dejour H (1972) Physiopathologie des laxités chroniques du genou. Rev Chir Orthop 58:61–70

64. Dejour H (1972) Méthodes thérapeutiques et résultats dans les laxités anciennes. Rev. Chir Orthop 58:100–110

65. Dejour H, Bousquet G (1975) Ruptures ligamentaires du genou. Encycl Med Chir 14092:1–12

66. Del Pizzo W, Norwood LA, Kerlan RK, Jobe FW, Carter VS, Blazina ME, Shields Jr Cl, Lombardo SJ (1977) Analysis of 100 patients with anterolateral rotatory instability of the knee. Clin Orthop 122:178–180

67. Despontin J, Thomas P (1978) Réflexion sur l'étude de l'articulation fémoro-rotulienne par la méthode des tomographies axiales transverses computérisées. Acta Orthop Belg 44:857–870

68. Dexel M (1977) Diagnostik beim instabilen Kniegelenk. Orthop Prax 7/13:500–503

69. Dexel M (1979) Die Klassifikation der chronischen Knieinstabilitäten. In: Morscher E (Hrsg) Funktionelle Diagnostik in der Orthopädie. Enke, Stuttgart, S 20–25

70. DiStefano V, O'Neil R, Nixon JE, Davis O (1976) Pes anserinus transfer: An in vivo biomechanical analysis. J Bone Joint Surg [Am] 58:285

71. Donskoi DD (1975) Grundlagen der Biomechanik. Sportverlag, Berlin

72. Drez D Jr (1978) Modified Eriksson procedure for chronic anterior cruciate instability. Orthopedies 1:30–36

73. Duparc J (1975) Les fractures du genou. In: Cahiers d'enseignement de la SOFCOT, No 1 Expansion scientifique française, Paris

74. Dustmann HO, Puhl W, Schultz KP (1971) Knorpelveränderungen beim Hämarthros unter besonderer Berücksichtigung der Ruhigstellung. Arch Orthop Unfallchir 71:148–159

75. Ellison AE (1977) Skiing injuries. Clin Symp Ciba 29:2–40

76. Ellison AE, Wieneke K, Benton LJ, White ES (1976) Preliminary report: Results of extra-articular anterior cruciate replacement. J Bone Joint Surg [Am] 58:736

77. Ellsasser JC, Reynolds FC, Omohundro JR (1974) The non-operative treatment of collateral ligament injuries of the knee in professional football players. J Bone Joint Surg [Am] 56:1185–1190

78. Enneking WF, Horowitz M (1972) The intraarticular effects of immobilization on the human knee. J Bone Joint Surg [Am] 54:973–985

79. Eriksson E (1976) Reconstruction of the anterior cruciate ligament. Orthop Clin North Am 7:167–179

80. Eriksson E (1976) Sport injuries of the knee ligaments: their diagnosis, treatment, rehabilitation and prevention. Med Sci Sports 8:133–144

81. Eriksson E (1979) Comparison of isometric muscle training and electrical stimulation supplementing isometric training in the recovery after major knee ligament surgery. Am J Sports Med 7:169–171

82. Fairen MF, Banus J, Figueras J, Cabot JR, Vila R (1976) Modelé arthrosique du genou après meniscectomie. Acta Orthop Belg 42:459–470

83. Ferguson AB, Brown TD, Fu FH, Rutkowski R (1979) Relief of patellofemoral contact stress by anterior displacement of the tibial tubercule. J Bone Joint Surg [Am] 61:159–166

84. Fetto JF, Marshall JL (1978) Medial collateral ligament injuries of the knee. Clin Orthop 132:206–218

85. Ficat P (1962) Pathologie des ménisques et des ligaments du genou. Masson, Paris

86. Ficat P (1970) Pathologie fémoro-patellaire. Masson, Paris

87. Ficat P (1972) Reconstruction du ligament croisé antérieur. Rev Chir Orthop [Suppl 1] 58:85–92

88. Ficat P (1973) Les déséquilibres rotuliens, de l'hyperpression à l'arthrose. Masson, Paris

89. Ficat P (1978) Rééducation fonctionelle et articulation fémoro-patellaire. In: Simon L (ed) Genou et médecine de rééducation. Masson, Paris, pp 110–119

90. Ficat P, Couzacq JP, Ricci A (1975) Chirurgie réparatrice des laxités chroniques des ligaments croisés du genou. Rev Chir Orthop 61:89–100

91. Fick R (1904) Anatomie der Gelenke. In: Bardeleben K von (Hrsg) Handbuch der Anatomie des Menschen, Bd 2. S. 367 Fischer, Jena

92. Finochietto R (1930) El signo del salto. Press Med Argent

93. Fischer LP, Guyot J, Gonon GP, Carret JP, Courcelles P, Dahhan P (1978) The role of the muscles and ligaments in stabilization of the knee joint. Anat Clin 1:43–53

94. Forward AD, Cowan RJ (1963) Tendon suture to bone. J Bone Joint Surg [Am] 45:807–823

95. Franke K (1974) Zur Behandlung von Kreuzbandverletzungen des Kniegelenkes. Med Sport 14:342–345

96. Franke K (1979) Erfahrungen mit 200 Operationen zum Kreuzband-Ersatz. 1st Congress of the International Society of the Knee, Lyon

97. Frankel VH (1971) Biomechanics of the knee. Orthop Clin North Am 2:175–190

98. Frankel VH, Burstein AH (1971) Orthopaedic biomechanics. Lea & Febinger, Philadelphia

99. Frankel VH, Burstein AH, Brooks DB (1971) Biomechanics of internal derangement of the knee. J Bone Joint Surg [Am] 53:945–962

100. Freemann MAR, Wyke B (1967) The innervation of the knee joint. An anatomical and histological study in the cat. J Anat 101:505–532

101. Furman W, Marshall JL, Girgis FG (1976) The anterior cruciate ligament. J Bone Joint Surg [Am] 58:179–185

102. Galway R (1972) Pivot-shift syndrom. J Bone Joint Surg [Br] 54:558

103. Galway R, Beaupré A, McIntosh DL (1972) Pivot-shift: A clinical sign of symptomatic anterior cruciate insufficiency. J Bone Joint Surg [Br] 54:763

104. Gerber C, Matter P, Chrisman OD, Langhans M (1980) Funktionelle Rehabilitation nach komplexen Knieverletzungen. Schweiz Z Sportmed 28:37–56

105. Gillquist J, Liljedahl SO, Lindvall H (1971) Reconstruction for old rupture of the anterior cruciate ligament. Injury 2:271–278

106. Ginsburg JH, Ellsasser JC (1978) Problem areas in the diagnosis and treatment of ligament injuries of the knee. Clin Orthop 132:201–205

107. Girgis FG, Marshall JL, Monajem ARS (1975) The cruciate ligaments of the knee joint. Clin Orthop 106:216–231

108. Godshall RW, Hansen CA (1974) The classification, treatment and follow-up evaluation of medial collateral ligament injuries of the knee. J Bone Joint Surg [Am] 56:1316

109. Goodfellow J, O'Connor J (1978) The mechanics of the knee and prosthesis design. J Bone Joint Surg [Br] 60:358–369

110. Goodfellow J, Hungerford DS, Zindel M (1976) Patello-femoral joint mechanics and pathology. 1. Functional anatomy of the patello-femoral joint. J Bone Joint Surg [Br] 58:287–290

111. Goodfellow J, Hungerford DS, Woods C (1976) Patello-femoral joint mechanics and pathology. 2. Chondromalacia patellae. J Bone Joint Surg [Br] 58:291–299

112. Goutailler D, Bernageau J, Lecudonnec B (1978) Mesure de l'écart tuberosité tibiale antérieure-gorge de la trochlée (T.A.-G.T.). Rev Chir Orthop 64:423–428

113. Grant JCB, Basmajian JV (1965) Grant's method of anatomy. Williams & Wilkins, Baltimore

114. Greene RB (1977) Dislocation of the proximal tibiofibular joint. Orthop Rev 6:63–66

115. Gregg JR, Nixon JE, DiStefano V (1978) Neutral fat globules in traumatized knees. Clin Orthop 132:219–224

116. Groh W (1955) Kinematische Untersuchungen des menschlichen Kniegelenkes und einige Prothesen-Kniekonstruktionen, die als „physiologische" Kniegelenke bezeichnet werden. Arch Orthop Unfallchir 47:637–645

117. Groves R, Camaione DN (1977) Bewegungslehre in Krankengymnastik und Sport. Fischer, Stuttgart New York

118. Gschwend N, Bischofsberger RJ (1971) Die Chondropathia patellae. Praxis 60:562–571

119. Gudde P, Wagenknecht R (1973) Untersuchungsergebnisse bei 50 Patienten 10–12 Jahre nach der Innenmeniskusoperation bei gleichzeitig vorliegender Ruptur des vorderen Kreuzbandes. Z Orthop 111:369–372

120. Haeggmark T (1979) Cylinder or mobile cast brace after knee ligament surgery. Am J Sports Med 7:48–56

121. Harty M, Joyce JJ (1977) Synovial folds in the knee joint. Orthop Rev 6:91–92

122. Helbing G, Burri C (1977) Kniebandverletzungen – Operation und funktionelle Nachbehandlung. Zentrabl Chir 102:787–793

123. Helfet AJ (1963) The management of internal derangements of the knee. Pitman, London; Lippincott, Philadelphia

124. Helfet AJ (1974) Disorders of the knee. Lippincott, Philadelphia Toronto

125. Henkemeyer H, Burri C (1973) Klinisches Vorgehen und Ergebnisse bei der funktionellen Nachbehandlung von Bandnähten und -plastiken am Kniegelenk. Z Orthop 111:379–381

126. Hertel P (1980) Verletzung und Spannung von Kniebändern. Hefte Unfallheilkd 142:1–94

127. Hertel P, Schweiberer L (1975) Biomechanik und Pathophysiologie des Kniebandapparates. Hefte Unfallheilkd 125:1–16

128. Heyermann WB, Hoyt WA (1978) Anterolateral rotary instability associated with chronic anterior cruciate insufficiency. Clin Orthop 134:144–148

129. Hollinshead WH (1969) Functional anatomy of the limbs and back. Saunders, Philadelphia London Toronto

130. Holz U, Weller S (1977) Diagnostik und Therapie frischer und veralteter Bandverletzungen am Kniegelenk. Chirurg 48:749–755

131. Honnart F (1978) Voie d'abord en chirurgie orthopédique et traumatologique. Masson, Paris

132. Honton HL, LeRebeller A, Legroux P, Ragni R, Tramond P (1978) Luxations traumatiques du genou. Rev Chir Orthop 64:213–219

133. Hsieh HH, Walker PS (1976) Stabilizing mechanism of the loaded and unloaded knee joint. J Bone Joint Surg [Am] 58:87–93

134. Hughston JC (1962) Acute knee injuries in athletes. Clin Orthop 23:114–133

135. Hughston JC (1973) Surgical approach to the medial and posterior ligaments of the knee. Clin Orthop 91:29–33

136. Hughston JC, Eilers AF (1973) The role of the posterior oblique ligament in repairs of acute medial (collateral) ligament tears of the knee. J Bone Joint Surg [Am] 55:923–940

136a. Hughston JC, Cross MJ, Andrews JR (1974) Clinical evaluation of knee ligament stability. In:Ingwersen OS, van Linge B, van Rens T, Rosingh G, Veraart B, Levay D (eds) (1974) The knee joint. Recent advances in basic research and clinical aspects. 126–130 Excerpta Medica, Amsterdam; American Elsevier, New York

137. Hughston JC, Andrews JR, Cross MJ, Moschi A (1976) Classification of knee ligament instabilities. Part I: The medial compartment and cruciate ligaments. Part II: The lateral compartment. J Bone Joint Surg [Am] 58:159–179

138. Hughston JC, Bowden JA, Andrews JR, Norwood LA (1980) Acute tears of the posterior cruciate ligament. J Bone Joint Surg [Am] 62:438–450

139. Huson A (1974) Biomechanische Probleme des Kniegelenks. Orthopaede 3:119–126

140. Ingwersen OS, van Linge B, van Rens T, Rosingh G, Veraart B, Levay D (eds) (1974) The knee joint. Recent advances in basic research and clinical aspects. Excerpta Medica, Amsterdam; American Elsevier, New York

141. Insall J (1971) A midline approach to the knee. J Bone Joint Surg [Am] 53:1584–1586

142. Insall J, Salvati E (1971) Patella position in the normal knee joint. Radiology 101:101–104

143. Insall J, Goldberg V, Salvati E (1972) Recurrent dislocation and the high-riding patella. Clin Orthop 88:67–69

144. Insall J, Falvo KA, Wise DW (1976) Chondromalacia patellae. J Bone Joint Surg [Am] 58:1–8

145. Ireland J, Trickey EL (1980) McIntosh tenodesis for anterolateral instability of the knee. J Bone Joint Surg [Br] 62:340–345

146. Jacobsen K (1976) Stress radiographical measurement of the anteroposterior, medial and lateral stability of the knee joint. Acta Orthop Scand 47:335–344

147. Jacobsen K (1977) Stress radiographical measurement of post traumatic knee instability. Acta Orthop Scand 48:301–310

148. Jäger M (1973) Abgrenzungen und Möglichkeiten der Wiederherstellung des Band- und Streckapparates des Kniegelenkes mit homologen Gewebsimplantaten. Z Orthop 111:375–377

149. Jäger M (1975) Die Möglichkeiten zur Verwendung von Dura bei Bandverletzungen des Kniegelenkes. Hefte Unfallheilkd 125:124–128

150. Jäger M, Wirth CJ (1975) Die anbehandelte "unhappy triad". Hefte Unfallheilkd 125:69–79

151. Jäger M, Wirth CJ (1978) Kapselbandläsionen. Biomechanik, Diagnostik, Therapie. Thieme, Stuttgart

152. Jaffrès R (1975) Les kystes méniscaux, considérations thérapeutiques et pathogéniques. Rev Rhum Mal Osteoartic 42:519–526

153. Jakob RP (im Druck) Die Diagnose der Kniebandinstabilitäten des lateralen Kompartimentes. Hauptverband der gewerblichen Berufsgenossenschaft (Hrsg), Bonn

154. Jakob RP, Noesberger B (1976) Das Pivot-shift Phaenomen, ein neues Zeichen der Ruptur des vorderen Kreuzbandes und die spezifische laterale Rekonstruktion. Helv Chir Acta 43:451–456

155. Jakob RP, Noesberger B, Saxer U (1977) Der Wert des Pivot-shift-Phänomens und der lateralen Rekonstruktion; zur Diagnose und Therapie der vorderen Kreuzbandruptur. Schweiz Z Sportmed 2:69–84

156. James SL (1978) Reconstruction of chronic medial ligament instability. In: Schultz KP, Krahl H, Stein WH (eds) Late reconstructions of injured ligaments of the knee. Springer, Berlin Heidelberg New York, pp 78–86

157. Jenkins DHR (1978) The repair of cruciate ligaments with flexible carbon fibre. J Bone Joint Surg [Br] 60:520–522

158. Jenkins DHR, Forster IW, McKibbin B, Rális ZA (1977) Induction of tendon and ligament formation by carbon implants. J Bone Joint Surg [Br] 59:53–57

159. Jenny G, Glaesener R, Jaeger JH, Kempf I (1975) L'instabilité rotatoire externe du genou. J Chir (Paris) 109:177–190

160. Jonasch E (1958) Zerreissung des äusseren und inneren Knieseitenbandes. Hefte Unfallheilkd 59:1–88

161. Jonasch E (1964) Das Kniegelenk. de Gryter, Berlin

162. Jones KG (1963) Reconstruction of the anterior cruciate ligament. J Bone Joint Surg [Am] 45:925–932

163. Jones KG (1970) Reconstruction of the anterior cruciate ligament using the central one-third of the patellar ligament. J Bone Joint Surg [Am] 52:1302–1308

164. Kapandji IA (1970) The physiology of the joints, vol II. Churchill Livingstone, Edinburgh London

165. Kaplan EB (1955) Iliotibial band. Morphology. Function. Anat Rec 121:319

166. Kaplan EB (1957) Surgical approach to the lateral (peroneal) side of the knee joint. Surg Gynecol Obstet 104:346–356

167. Kaplan EB (1957) Factors responsible for the stability of the knee joint. Bull Hosp Joint Dis 17:51–59

168. Kaplan EB (1958) The iliotibial tract. J Bone Joint Surg [Am] 40:817–832

169. Kaplan EB (1961) The fabello-fibular and short lateral ligaments of the knee joint. J Bone Joint Surg [Am] 43:169–179

170. Kaplan EB (1962) Some aspects of functional anatomy of the human knee joint. Clin Orthop 23:18–29

171. Kappakas GS, Brown TD, Goodman MA, Kikuike A, McMaster JH (1978) Delayed surgical repair of ruptured ligaments. Clin Orthop 135:281–286

172. Kennedy JC, Fowler PJ (1971) Medial and anterior instability of the knee. J Bone Joint Surg [Am] 53:1257–1270

173. Kennedy J, Willis RB (1976) Synthetic cruciate ligaments – preliminary report. J Bone Joint Surg [Br] 58:142

174. Kennedy JC, Weinberg MW, Wilson AS (1974) The anatomy and function of the anterior cruciate ligament. J Bone Joint Surg [Am] 56:223–235

175. Kennedy JC, Hawkins RJ, Willis RB, Danylchuk KD (1976) Tension studies of human knee ligaments. J Bone Joint Surg [Am] 58:350–355

176. Kennedy JC, Stewart R, Walker DM (1978) Anterolateral rotary instability of the knee joint. J Bone Joint Surg [A-] 60:–1031–1039

177. Kettelkamp DB (1973) Clinical implications of knee biomechanics. Arch Surg 107:406–410

178. Kettelkamp DB, Thompson C (1975) Development of a knee scoring scale. Clin Orthop 107:93–99

179. Khasigan HA, Evanski PM, Waugh TR (1978) Body type and rational laxity of the knee. Clin Orthop 130:228–232

180. Kieser C, Rüttimann A (1976) Die Arthroskopie des Kniegelenks. Schweiz Med Wochenschr 106:1631–1637

181. Klein-Vogelbach S (1976) Funktionelle Bewegungslehre. Springer, Berlin Heidelberg New York

182. Knese KH (1950) Kinematik des Kniegelenkes. Z Anat Entwicklungsgesch 115:287–322

183. Kostuik JP (1977) Anterior cruciate reconstruction by the McIntosh techniques. J Bone Joint Surg [Br] 59:511

184. Kostuik JP, Schmidt O, Harris WR, Wooldridge C (1975) A study of weight transmission through the knee joint with applied varus and valgus loads. Clin Orthop 108:95–98

185. Kouvalchouk JF, Seguin P, Rainant JJ, Cédard C, Padovani P (1973) Lésions anciennes du ligament croisé postérieur. Rev Chir Orthop 59:69–76

186. Krause WR, Pope MH, Johnson RJ, Wilder DG (1976) Mechanical changes in the knee after meniscectomy. J Bone Joint Surg [Am] 58:599–604

187. Lahlaidi A (1971) Valeur morphologique des insertions postérieures du ménisque externe dans le genou humain. Rev Chir Orthop 57:593–600

188. Lam SJS (1968) Reconstruction of the anterior cruciate ligament using the Jones procedure and its Guy's Hospital modification. J Bone Joint Surg [Am] 50:1213–1224

189. Lancourt JE, Cristini JA (1975) Patella alta and patella infera. J Bone Joint Surg [Am] 57:1112–1115

190. Lange M (1951) Orthopädisch-chirurgische Operationslehre. Bergmann, München, S 660–664

191. Lange M (1968) Orthopädisch-chirurgische Operationslehre. Ergänzungsband: Neueste Operationsverfahren. Bergmann, München

192. Lanz von T, Wachsmuth W (1972) Praktische Anatomie, Bd 1, Teil 4. Springer, Berlin Heidelberg New York

193. Larson RL (1978) Knee injuries in sports. Hosp Med 57–75

194. Larson RL, DeHaven K, Godfrey J, Kennedy JC, Eriksson E (1978) Sport injuries to the knee. Contemp Surg 12:42–56

195. Laurin CA, Beauchamp P (1977) The real challenge of cruciate ligament substitution. J Bone Joint Surg [Br] 59:511

196. Laurin CA, Lévesque HP, Dussault R, Labeille H, Peides JP (1978) The abnormal lateral patellofemoral angle. J Bone Joint Surg [Am] 60:55–60

197. Leach RE, Gegg T, Siber FJ (1970) Weight-bearing radiography in osteoarthritis of the knee. Radiology 97:265–268

198. Lemaire M (1975) Instabilité chronique du genou. J Chir (Paris) 110:281–294

199. Lerat JL, Bost J, Lecuire F, Chambat P, Weissbrod R, Dejour H, Trillat A (1977) Les ruptures ligamentaires récentes du compartiment externe du genou. Lyon Chir 73:401–405

200. Lindemann K (1950) Über den plastischen Ersatz der Kreuzbänder durch gestielte Sehnenverpflanzungen. Z Orthop 79:316–334

201. Losee RE, Johnson TR, Southwick WO (1978) Anterior subluxation of the lateral tibial plateau. J Bone Joint Surg [Am] 60:1015–1030

202. Madigan R, Wissinger HA, Donaldson WF (1975) Preliminary experience with a method of quadriceps plasty in recurrent subluxation of the patella. J Bone Joint Surg [Am] 57:600–607

203. Mann RA, Hagy JL (1977) The popliteus muscle. J Bone Joint Surg [Am] 59:924–927

204. Mansat C (1976) Traitement chirurgical des laxités anciennes antérointernes du genou. Rev Chir Orthop 62:321–336

205. Maquet PGJ (1976) Biomechanics of the knee. Springer, Berlin Heidelberg New York

206. Markolf KL, Graff-Radford A, Amstutz HC (1978) In vivo knee stability. J Bone Joint Surg [Am] 60:664–674

207. Marshall JL (1977) Knee ligament injuries. Orthop Clin North Am 8:641–648

208. Marshall JL, Olsson SE (1971) Instability of the knee. A longterm experimental study in dogs. J Bone Joint Surg [Am] 53:1561–1570

209. Marshall JL, Girgis FG, Zelko RR (1972) The biceps femoris tendon and its functional significance. J Bone Joint Surg [Am] 54:1444–1450

210. Marshall JL, Warren RF, Fleiss DJ (1975) Ligamentous injuries of the knee in skiing. Clin Orthop 108:196–199

211. Marshall JL, Fetto JF, Botero PM (1977) Knee ligament injuries, a standardized evaluation method. Clin Orthop 123:115–130

212. Mauck HP (1936) A new operative procedure for instability of the knee. J Bone Joint Surg 18:984–990

213. McCormick WC, Bagg RJ, Kennedy CW, Leukens CA (1976) Reconstruction of the posterior cruciate ligament. Clin Orthop 118:30–34

214. McDevitt C, Gilbertson E, Muir H (1977) An experimental model of osteoarthritis; early morphological and biomechanical changes. J Bone Joint Surg [Br] 59:24–35

215. McIntosh DL, Darby TA (1976) Lateral substitution reconstruction. J Bone Joint Surg [Br] 58:142

216. McIntosh DL, Tregonning RJA (1977) A follow-up study and evaluation of "over the top" repair of acute tears of the anterior cruciate ligament. J Bone Joint Surg [Br] 59:511

217. McMaster WC (1975) Isolated posterior cruciate ligament injury: Literature review and case reports. J Trauma 15:1025–1029

218. McMaster JM, Weinert CR, Scranton P (1974) Diagnosis and management of isolated anterior cruciate ligament tears. J Trauma 14:230–235

219. Menschik A (1974) Mechanik des Kniegelenkes, Teil 1. Z Orthop 112:481–495

220. Menschik A (1974) Mechanik des Kniegelenks, Teil 3, Sailer, Wien

220a. Menschik A (1977) The basic kinematic principle of the collateral ligaments, demonstrated on the knee joint. In: Chapchal G (ed) Injuries of the ligaments and their repair. Thieme, Stuttgart pp 9–16

221. Menschik A (1975) Mechanik des Kniegelenks, Teil 2. Z Orthop 113:388–400

222. Merchant AC, Mercer RL, Jacobsen RM, Cool CR (1974) Roentgenographic analysis of patello femoral congruence. J Bone Joint Surg [Am] 56:1391–1396

223. Mercier-Guyon J (1975) L'examen programmé du genou. Association Amicale des Etudiants en Pharmacie de Lyon, Lyon

224. Merke F, Eha M (1947) Nachuntersuchungen an Wackelknien infolge Kreuz- und Seitenbandverletzungen. Z Unfallmed Berufskr 40:262–291

225. Merkulowa RI (1973) Management of fresh isolated and combined injuries to the lateral ligaments of the knee joint in sportsmen (Russian). Ortop Traumatol Protez 12:20–24

226. Meyer H (1-53) Die Mechanik des Kniegelenks. Arch Anat Physiol Wiss Med 497–547

227. Meyer MH (1975) Isolated avulsion of the tibial attachment of the posterior cruciate ligament of the knee. J Bone Joint Surg [Am] 57:669–672

228. Mittelmeier H (1973) Meniskusverletzungen. Z Orthop 111:386–394

229. Montmollin B de (1951) Chondromalacia de la rotule. Rev Orthop 37:41–51

230. Montmollin B de, Le Coeur P (1980) La rupture isolée fraîche du ligament croisé antérieur du genou. Rev Chir Orthop 66:367–371

230a. Morscher E (1971) Cartilage-bone lesions of the knee joint following injury. Reconstr Surg Traumatol 12:2–26

230b. Morscher E (1974) Mikrotrauma und traumatische Knorpelschäden als Arthroseursache. Z Unfallmed Berufskr 4:220–231

230c. Morscher E (1976) Traumatische Knorpelimpression an den Femurcondylen. Hefte Unfallheilkd 127:71–78

230d. Morscher E (1978) Posttraumatic Cartilage impression of the femoral condyles. In: The knee: Ligament and articular cartilage injuries. Progress in orthopaedic surgery, Vol 3 pp 105–111. Springer, Berlin Heidelberg New York

231. Morscher E (1978) Osteotomy of the patella in chondromalacia. Arch Orthop Traumat Surg 92:139–147

232. Morscher E (1979) Traumatische Knorpelläsionen am Kniegelenk. Chirurg 50:599–604

233. Morscher E (Hrsg) (1977) Funktionelle Diagnostik in der Orthopädie. Enke, Stuttgart

234. Morscher E, Müller W (1974) Verletzungen des Kniegelenkes. Ther Umsch 31:227–235

235. Müller J, Willenegger D, Terbrüggen D (1975) Freie, autologe Transplantate in der Behandlung des instabilen Knies. Hefte Unfallheilkd 125:109–116

236. Müller W (1974) Das Kniegelenk des Fußballers. Orthopaede 3:193–200

237. Müller W (1974) Beitrag zur Frage der Entstehung der Meniskuszysten. Z Unfallmed Berufskr 3/4:115–120

238. Müller W (1975) Die Rotationsinstabilität am Kniegelenk. Unfallheilkunde 125:51–68

239. Müller W (1976) Die verschiedenen Typen von Meniskusläsionen und ihre Entstehungsmechanismen. Unfallheilkunde 128:39–50

240. Müller W (1977) Rehabilitation nach Kniegelenksoperationen. Z Phys Med [Suppl] 153–163

241. Müller W (1977) Verletzungen der Kreuzbänder. Zentralbl Chir 102:974–981

242. Müller W (1977) Sporttraumatologie des Kniegelenkes. Schweiz Z Sportmed 25:5–23

243. Müller W (1977) Neuere Aspekte der funktionellen Anatomie des Kniegelenkes. Unfallheilkunde 192:131–138

244. Müller W (1977) The knee joint of the soccer player. Prog Orthop Surg 1:117–129

245. Müller W (1977) Ligamentous lesions of the knee joint. In: Chapchal G (ed) Injuries of the ligaments and their repair. Thieme, Stuttgart, pp 55–62

246. Müller W (1977) Functional anatomy related to rotatory stability of the knee joint. In: Chapchal G (ed) Injuries of the ligaments and their repair. Thieme, Stuttgart, pp 39–46

247. Müller W (1978) Rotational stability of the knee. Prog Orthop Surg 3:59–73

248. Müller W (1978) Osteochondrosis dissecans. Prog Orthop Surg 3:135–141

248a. Müller W (1980) Allgemeine Diagnostik und Soforttherapie bei Bandverletzungen am Kniegelenk. Unfallheilkunde 83:389–397

249. Müller W, Dolanc B (1977) Funktions- und Stabilitätsprobleme am Kniegelenk des Fußballers. Schweiz Z Sportmed 25:25–36

250. Müller W, Gächter A (1979) Das posttraumatisch instabile Kniegelenk. Chirurg 50:605–611

251. Nicholas JA (1970) Injuries to the knee ligaments. JAMA 212:2236–2239

252. Nicholas JA (19-3) The five-one reconstruction for anteromedial instability of the knee. J Bone Joint Surg [Am] 55:899–922

253. Nietert M (1975) Untersuchungen zur Kinematik des menschlichen Kniegelenkes im Hinblick auf ihre Approximation in der Prothetik. Dissertation, Technische Universität Berlin

254. Noble J (1975) Congenital absence of the anterior cruciate ligament associated with a ring-meniscus. J Bone Joint Surg [Am] 57:1165–1166

255. Noesberger B (1972) Der traumatische Gelenkerguß. Ther Umsch 29:424–427

256. Noesberger B, Paillot JM Biomécanique du genou. Film, Springer, Berlin Heidelberg New York

257. Noyes FR (1977) Functional properties of knee ligaments and alternations induced by immobilization. Clin Orthop 123:210–242

258. Noyes FR, Grood ES (1976) The strength of the anterior cruciate ligament in humans and rhesus monkeys. J Bone Joint Surg [Am] 58:1074–1082

259. Noyes FR, Sonstegard DA, Arbor A (1973) Biomechanical function of the pes anserinus of the knee and the effect of its transplantation. J Bone Joint Surg [Am] 55:1225–1241

260. Noyes FR, DeLucas J, Torvik PJ (1974) Biomechanics of anterior cruciate ligament failure: An analysis of strain-rate sensitivity and mechanism of failure in primates. J Bone Joint Surg [Am] 56:236–253

261. Noyes FR, Torvik PJ, Hyde WB, DeLucas JL (1974) Biomechanics of ligament failure. II. An analysis of immobilization, exercise and reconditioning effects in primates. J Bone Joint Surg [Am] 56:1406–1418

262. Noyes FR, Grood ES, Nussbaum NS, Cooper SM (1977) Effect of intra-articular corticosteroids on ligament properties. Clin Orthop 123:197–209

263. Nozawa S (1973) A comparative study on the methods of treatment of torn ligaments of the knee joint (Japanese). J Jpn Orthop Assoc 47:793–810

264. O'Connor RL (1974) Arthroscopy in the diagnosis and treatment of acute ligament injuries of the knee. J Bone Joint Surg [Am] 56:333–337

265. O'Donoghue DM (1950) Surgical treatment of fresh injuries to the major ligaments of the knee. J Bone Joint Surg [Am] 32:721–738

266. O'Donoghue DM (1955) An analysis of end results of surgical treatment of major injuries to the ligaments of the knee. J Bone Joint Surg [Am] 37:1–13

267. O'Donoghue DM (1963) A method for replacement of the anterior cruciate ligament of the knee. J Bone Joint Surg [Am] 45:905–924

268. O'Donoghue DM (1973) Reconstruction for medial instability of the knee. J Bone Joint Surg [Am] 55:941–955

269. O'Donoghue DM (1973) Treatment of acute ligamentous injuries of the knee. Orthop Clin North Am 4:617–645

270. O'Donoghue DM (1973) Treatment of injuries to athletes. Saunders, Philadelphia London Toronto

271. O'Donoghue DM, Rockwood CA, Zariczny B, Kenyon R (1961) Repair of knee ligaments in dogs. J Bone Joint Surg [Am] 43:1167–1178

272. O'Donoghue DM, Rockwood CA, Frank GR, Jack SC, Kenyon R (1966) Repair of the anterior cruciate ligament in dogs. J Bone Joint Surg [Am] 48:503–519

273. O'Donoghue DM, Frank GR, Jeter GL, Johnson W, Zeiders JW, Kenyon R (1971) Repair and reconstruction of the anterior cruciate ligament in dogs. J Bone Joint Surg [Am] 53:710–718

274. Ogden JA (1974) The anatomy and function of the proximal tibiofibular joint. Clin Orthop 101:186–191

275. Ogden JA (1974) Subluxation of the proximal tibiofibular joint. Clin Orthop 101:192–197

276. Ogden JA (1974) Subluxation and dislocation of the proximal tibiofibular joint. J Bone Joint Surg [Am] 56:145–154

277. Olsson SE, Marshall JL, Story E (1972) Osteophytosis of the knee joint in the dog: A sign of instability. Acta Radiol [Suppl] (Stockh) 319:165–167

278. Owen R (1968) Recurrent dislocation of the superior tibio-fibular joint. J Bone Joint Surg [Br] 50:342–345

279. Palmer I (1938) On the injuries to the ligaments of the knee joint: a clinical study. Acta Chir Scand Vol. 81 [Suppl] 53

280. Palmer I (1958) Pathophysiology of the medial ligament of the knee joint. Acta Chir Scand 115:312–318

281. Pauzat (1895) Etudes sur le functionnement des ménisques du genou. Rev Chir 95

282. Pellegrino J, Maupin JM, Casanova G, Esquirol E, Larroque C (1971) La luxation antérieure isolée de l'extrémité supérieure du péroné. Rev Chir Orthop 57:547–554

283. Perren SM (1980) Biomechanik und Histomorphologie. Dehnungstheorie als Grundlage der sekundären und primären Heilung. (pers. Mitteilung) 30. AO Kurs, Davos

284. Perry J, Fox JM, Boitano MA, Skinner SR, Barnes LA, Cerny K (1980) Functional evaluation of the pes anserinus transfer by electromyography and gait analysis. J Bone Joint Surg [Am] 62:973–980

285. Pfab B (1927) Zur Blutgefäßversorgung der Menisci und der Kreuzbänder. Dtsch Z Chir 205:258–264

286. Pickett JC, Altizer TJ (1971) Injuries of the ligaments of the knee. Clin Orthop 76:27–32

287. Price CT, Allen WC (1978) Ligament repair in the knee with preservation of the meniscus. J Bone Joint Surg [Am] 60:61–65

287 a. Pridie KH (1959) A method of resurfacing osteoarthritic knee joints. J Bone Joint Surg [Br] 41:618–619

288. Puhl W (1971) Rasterelektronenmikroskopische Untersuchungen zur Frage früher Knorpelschädigungen durch leukocytäre Enzyme. Arch Orthop Unfallchir 70:87–97

289. Puhl W, Dustmann HO, Schulitz KP (1971) Knorpelveränderungen bei experimentellen Hämarthros. Z Orthop 109:475–486

290. Ramadier JO, Benoit J (1972) Reconstruction des ligaments latéraux et croisés. Rev Chir Orthop [Suppl 1] 58:78–84

291. Rechenberg B von (1978) Experimentelle Untersuchung zur Fixation der Ligg. Collateralia Medialia mit Schrauben und Unterlagsscheiben. Dissertation, Universität Zürich

292. Refior HJ (1973) Die Brückner-Plastik zum Ersatz veralteter vorderer Kreuzbandrupturen – Technik und Ergebnisse. Z Orthop 111:372–375

293. Refior HJ (1976) Die Reaktionen des hyalinen Gelenkknorpels unter Druck, Immobilisation und Distraktion. Hefte Unfallheilkd 127:23–36

294. Refior HJ, Jaeger M (1973) Indikation und Technik bei der Verwendung homologer, lyophilisierter, Gamma-Strahlen sterilisierter Dura zum Ersatz von Sehnen und Ligamenten. Aktuel Traumatol 3:125–127

295. Refior HJ, Wirth CJ (1976) Der plastische Ersatz veralteter Kreuzbandrupturen. Z Orthop 114:913–922

296. Rehn J (1973) Bandverletzungen des Kniegelenkes. Z Orthop 111:359–363

297. Reilly DT, Martens M (1972) Experimental analysis of the quadriceps muscle force and patellofemoral joint reaction force for various activities. Acta Orthop Scand 43:126–137

298. Renne JW (1975) The iliotibial band friction syndrome. J Bone Joint Surg [Am] 57:1110–111

299. Ricklin P (1966) Diagnostik des verletzten Kniegelenks. Praxis 55:294–298

300. Ricklin P, Rüttimann A, DelBuono MS (1971) Meniscus lesions. Thieme, Stuttgart

301. Roaas A, Nilsson S (1977) Injuries of the knee ligaments (Norwegian). Tidssler Nor Laegeforen 97:22–24

302. Roberts J (1974) The surgical knee. Surg Clin North Am 54:1313–1326

303. Rogers LF, Jones S, Davis AR, Dietz G (1974) "Clipping injury" fracture of the epiphysis in the adolescent football-player: An occult lesion of the knee. A J R 121:69–78

304. Ross RF (1932) A quantitative study of rotation of the knee joint. Anat Rec 52:209–223

305. Rubin RM, Marshall JL, Wang J (1975) Prevention of knee instability. Experimental model for prosthetic anterior cruciate ligament. Clin Orthop 113:212–236

306. Ruetsch H, Morscher E (1977) Measurement of the rotatory stability of the knee joint. In: Chapchal G (ed) Injuries of the ligaments and their repair. Thieme, Stuttgart, pp 116–122

307. Salter RB (1980) The stimulating effects of continuous passive motion on the healing of intraarticular fractures. 29. AO-Kurs, Davos (Communication)

308. Schallock G (1939) Untersuchungen zur Morphologie der Kniegelenksmenisci an Hand von Messungen und histologischen Befunden. Virchows Arch [Pathol Anat] 304:559–590

309. Scheller S, Mårtenson L (1974) Traumatic dislocation of the patella. Acta Radiol [Suppl] (Stockh) 336:1–160

310. Schmitt O, Biehl G (1979) Quantitative Elektromyographie zur Beurteilung der Kniegelenksstabilität bei veralteter vorderer Kreuzbandruptur vor und nach Wiederherstellungsoperation. In: Morscher E (Hrsg) Funktionelle Diagnostik in der Orthopädie. Enke, Stuttgart, S 34–37

311. Schmitt O, Mittelmeier H (1978) Die Bedeutung des Musculus vastus medialis und -lateralis für die Biomechanik des Kniegelenks. Arch Orthop Traumat Surg 91:291–295

312. Schulitz KP, Krahl H, Stein WH (1978) Late reconstructions of injured ligaments of the knee. Springer, Berlin Heidelberg New York

313. Schvingt E, Weill D, Petit R (1970) Les lésions dysplasiques des ménisques externes. Rev Chir Orthop 56:283–284

314. Ségal P, Lallement JJ, Raquet M, Jacob M, Gérard Y (1980) Les lésions ostéo-cartilagineuses de la laxité antéro-interne du genou. Rev Chir Orthop 66:357–365

315. Segesser B (1978) Moderne Möglichkeiten der Muskelrehabilitation mit Dynatronic. Z Unfallmed Berufskr 2:85–91

316. Segond P (1879) Recherches cliniques et expérimentales sur les épanchements sanguins du genou par entorse. Prog Med 7:297–299, 319–321, 340–341, 379–381, 400–401, 419–421

317. Shaw JA, Eng M, Murray DG (1974) The longitudinal axis of the knee and the role of the cruciate ligaments in controlling transverse rotation. J Bone Joint Surg [Am] 56:1603–1606

318. Silverskiöld N (1938) Chondromalacia of the patella. Acta Orthop Scand 9:214–299

319. Simmons EH (1975) Late results of ligamentous injuries of the knee. J Bone Joint Surg [Br] 57:258

320. Simon L (1978) Genou et médecine de rééducation. Masson, Paris New York Barcelona Milan

321. Slany A (1941) Autoptische Reihenuntersuchungen an Kniegelenken mit besonderer Berücksichtigung der Meniscuspathologie. Arch Orthop Unfallchir 41:256–286

322. Slocum D (1972) Reconstruction ligamentaire interne tardive. Rev Chir Orthop 58:97–99

323. Slocaum D (1972) Traitement des laxités externes chroniques du genou. Rev Chir Orthop [Suppl 1] 58:93–96

324. Slocum DB, Larson RL (1968) Rotatory instability of the knee. J Bone Joint Surg [Am] 50:211–225

325. Slocum DB, Larson RL (1968) Pes anserinus transplantation. J Bone Joint Surg 50:226–242

326. Slocum DB, Larson RL, James SL (1974) Late reconstruction of ligamentous injuries of the medial compartment of the knee. Clin Orthop 100:23–55

327. Slocum DB, James SL, Larson RL, Singer KM (1976) Clinical test for anterolateral rotatory instability of the knee. Clin Orthop 118:63–69

328. Smillie IS (1962) Injuries of the knee joint. Williams & Wilkins, Baltimore (4th edn 1970) Livingstone, Edinburgh

329. Smillie IS (1974) Diseases of the knee joint. Livingstone, London Edinburgh

330. Southmayd W, Quigley TB (1978) The forgotten popliteus muscle. Clin Orthop 130:218–222

331. Steindler A (1955) Kinesiology of the human body under normal and pathological conditions. Thomas, Springfield

332. Stewart JPR, Erskine CA (1979) An experimental analysis of injuries to the menisci of the knee joint. Int Orthop 3:9–12

305

333. Stilwell DL (1957) The innervation of tendons and aponeuroses. Am J Anat 100:289–317

334. Stilwell DL (1957) Regional variations in the innervation of deep fasciae and aponeuroses. Anat Rec 127:635–653

335. Strande A (1967) Repair of the ruptured cranial cruciate ligament in the dog. Universitetsforlaget, Oslo; Williams & Wilkins, Baltimore

336. Strasser H (1917) Lehrbuch der Muskel- und Gelenkmechanik, Springer, Berlin

337. Tapper EM, Hoower NW (1969) Late result after meniscectomy. J Bone Joint Surg [Am] 51:517–526

338. Tauber C, Heim M, Horoszoski H, Farine I (1978) Tear of the anterior cruciate ligament as a late complication on meniscectomy. Injury 10:223–224

339. Tillberg B (1977) The late repair of torn cruciate ligaments using menisci. J Bone Joint Surg [Br] 59:15–19

340. Tillmann B (1974) Zur funktionellen Morphologie der Gelenkentwicklung. Orthop Prax 1210:691–697

341. Tongue JR (1978) Patellar ligament ruptures. Western Orthop Association Orthop Resident Program

342. Tongue JR, Taylor LW (1978) Patellar ligament ruptures. Amer Academy of Orthop Surgeons 45th Annual Meeting (Communication)

343. Torg JS, Conrad W, Kalen V (1976) Clinical diagnosis of anterior cruciate ligament instability in the athlete. Am J Sports Med 4:84–93

344. Torsiü T (1977) Isolated avulsion fracture of the tibial attachment of the posterior cruciate ligament. J Bone Joint Surg [Am] 59:68–72

345. Trickey EL (1968) Rupture of the posterior cruciate ligament of the knee. J Bone Joint Surg [Br] 50:334–341

346. Trickey EL (1977) Pathological anatomy of knee ligament injuries. In: Chapchal G (ed) Injuries of the ligaments and their repair. Thieme, Stuttgart, pp 37–39

347. Trillat A (1962) Lésions traumatiques du ménisque interne du genou. Rev. Chir Orthop 48:551–560

348. Trillat A (1971) Les lésions méniscales externes. Rev Chir Orthop 57:318

349. Trillat A (1971) Les lésions méniscales internes. Rev Chir Orthop 57:318

350. Trillat A (1971) La rupture ligamentaire récente. Rev Chir Orthop 57:318

351. Trillat A (1971) Les laxités chroniques du genou. Rev Chir Orthop 57:318–319

352. Trillat A (1974) Acute injuries of the knee ligaments. In: Ingwersen OS, van Linge B, van Reus T, Rosingh G, Veraart B, Levay D (eds) The knee joint. Excerpta Medica, Amsterdam; American Elsevier, New York pp 159–162

353. Trillat A, Dejour H, Bousquet G (1973) Chirurgie du genou. Premières Journées Lyonnaise Avril 1971. Simep, Villeurbanne

354. Trillat A, Ficat P (1972) Laxités post-traumatiques du genou. Rev. Chir Orthop [Suppl 1] 58:31–114

355. Trillat A, Mounier-Kuhn A (1963) Les lésions méniscales chez les sujets de plus de soixante ans. Rev Rhum Mal Osteoartic 30:280–287

356. Trillat A, Rainaut JJ (1959) Traitement des laxités ligamentaires posttraumatiques du genou. Rev Chir Orthop 45:97–98

357. Trillat A, Dejour H, Conette A (1964) Diagnostic et traitement des subluxations récidivantes de la rotule. Rev Chir Orthop 50:813–824

358. Trillat A, Dejour H, Bousquet G (1969) Laxité ancienne isolée du ligament croisé antérieure. Etudes des résultats de différentes méthodes reconstructives ou palliatives. Rev Chir Orthop 55:163

359. Trillat A, Dejour H, Bousquet G (1978) Chirurgie du genou. Troisième Jornées Lyonnaises Sept. 1977. Simep, Villeurbanne

360. Uhthoff H (1980) Stress-Entlastung und langfristiger Knochenverlust, Zeitpunkt der Implantatentfernung, Refraktur. 30. AO-Kurs, Davos

361. Unverferth LJ, Olix MI, Ketterer WF (1978) A clinical follow-up of the pes anserinus transplantation for chronic anteromedial rotatory instability of the knee. Clin Orthop 134:149–152

362. Vallois HV (1914) Etude anatomique de l'articulation du genou chez les primates. Abeille, Montpellier

363. Vandekerckhove JR (1964) Die Menisken des Kniegelenks. Dissertation, Universität Saarbrükken

364. Vidal J (1972) Résultats thérapeutiques dans les lésions récentes (du genou). Rev Chir Orthop 58:57–59

365. Vidal J, Buscayret C, Fassio B, Escare P (1977) Traitement chirurgical des entorses graves récentes du genou. Rev Chir Orthop 63:271–283

366. Vigliani F, Martinelli B, Tagliapietra EA (1975) The early surgical treatment of rupture of the tibial collateral ligament of the knee. Ital J Orthop Traumatol 1:151–161

367. Volkov VS (1973) Diagnosis of tears of ligaments of the knee joint (Russian). Vestn Khir 111:98–103

368. Voorhoeve A, Hierholzer G (1975) Ergebnisse bei Transplantation homologer und heterologer Sehnen als Bandersatz bei instabilem Knie. Hefte Unfallheilkd 125:117–123

369. Wagner H (1964) Operative Behandlung der Osteochondrosis dissecans des Kniegelenkes. Z Orthop 98:333–355

370. Wagner HJ (1976) Die Kollagenfaserarchitektur der Menisken des menschlichen Kniegelenkes. Z Mikrosk Anat Forsch 90:302–324

371. Wagner M, Schabus R (im Druck) Das laterale pivot shift Phänomen. Untersuchungen am Leichenknie nach artifiziellen Kapselbandläsionen. III. Münchner Symposium für experimentelle Orthopädie. Springer, Berlin Heidelberg New York

372. Walker PS, Erkmann MJ (1975) The role of the menisci in force transmission across the knee. Clin Orthop 109:184–192

373. Wang JB, Marshall JL (1975) Acute ligamentous injuries of the knee. Single contrast arthrography – a diagnostic aid. J Trauma 15:431–440

374. Wang JB, Rubin RM, Marshall JI (1975) A mechanism of isolated anterior cruciate ligament rupture. J Bone Joint Surg [Am] 57:411–413

375. Wang CJ, Walker PS, Wolf B (1973) The effects of flexion and rotation on the length patterns of the ligaments of the knee. J Biomech (Tokyo) 6:587–596

376. Wang CJ, Walker PS, Wolf B (1974) Rotatory laxity of the human knee joint. J Bone Joint Surg [Am] 56:161–170

377. Warren LF, Marshall JL (1978) Injuries of the anterior cruciate and medial collateral ligaments of the knee. – A retrospective analysis of clinical records. Part I. Clin Orthop. 136:191–197

378. Warren LF, Marshall JL (1978) Injuries of the anterior cruciate and medial collateral ligaments of the knee. – A long-term follow-up of 86 cases. Part II. Clin Orthop 136:198–211

379. Warren LF, Marshall JL (1979) The supporting structures and layers on the medial side of the knee. J Bone Joint Surg [Am] 61:56–62

380. Warren LF, Marshall JL, Girgis F (1974) The prime static stabilizer of the medial side of the knee. J Bone Joint Surg [Am] 56:665–674

381. Watson-Jones R (1976) Fractures and joint injuries, vols I, II. Livingstone, Edinburgh London New York

382. Weigert M (1973) Kniebandnaht und Kniebandersatz. Z Orthop 111:364–368

383. Weigert M, Gronert MJ (1972) Kniebandnaht – Kniebandplastik. Arch Orthop Unfallchir 72:253–271

384. Weiner B, Rosenberg N (1974) Discoid medial meniscus: Association with bone changes in the tibia. J Bone Joint Surg [Am] 56:171–173

385. Wiberg G (1941) Roentgenographic and anatomic studies on the femorapatellar joint. With special reference to chondromalacia patellae. Acta Orthop Scand 12:319–410

386. Wiles P, Andrews PS, Devas MB (1956) Chondromalacia of the patella. J Bone Joint Surg §Br] 38:95–113

387. Wilson N (1967) A diagnostic sign in osteochondritis dissecans of the knee. J Bone Joint Surg [Am] 49:477–480

388. Wirth CJ (1976) Die frische Kombinationsverletzung des Kniegelenkes – Diagnostik und Therapie. Arch Orthop Unfallchir 84:221–233

389. Wirth CJ, Artmann M (1974) Verhalten der Roll-Gleit-Bewegung des belasteten Kniegelenkes bei Verlust und Ersatz des vorderen Kreuzbandes. Arch Orthop Unfallchir 78:356–361

390. Wirth CJ, Jäger M (1976) Die veraltete anteromediale Kniegelenksinstabilität – Frühergebnisse der Operation nach Nicholas. Orthop Prax 12:807–808

391. Wirth CJ, Refior HJ (1976) Der plastische Ersatz veralteter Kreuzbandrupturen. II. Spätergebnisse. Z Orthop 114:922–930

392. Wirth CJ, Artmann M, Jäger M, Refior HJ (1974) Der plastische Ersatz veralteter vorderer Kreuzbandrupturen nach Brückner und seine Ergebnisse. Arch Orthop Unfallchir 78:362–373

393. Witt AN, Jäger M, Refior HJ, Wirth CJ (1977) Das instabile Kniegelenk – aktuelle Gesichtspunkte in Grundlagenforschung, Diagnostik und Therapie. Arch Orthop Unfallchir 88:49–63

394. Wittek A (1927) Zur Naht der Kreuzbandverletzung im Kniegelenk. Zentralbl Chir 54:1538–1541

395. Wittek A (1927) Über Verletzungen der Kreuzbänder des Kniegelenkes. Dtsch Z Chir 200:491–515

396. Wittek A (1935) Kreuzbandersatz aus dem lig. patellae (nach zur Verth). Schweiz Med Wochenschr 65:103–104

397. Zippel H (1973) Meniskusverletzungen und -schäden. Barth, Leipzig

398. Zippel H (1977) Meniskusverletzungen. Med Sport 17:79–88

399. Baumann JU (1979) Ganganalyse. In: Morscher E (Hrsg) Funktionelle Diagnostik in der Orthopädie. Enke, Stuttgart, S 53–55

400. Taillard W (1957) Les syndromes douloureux du genou associés à une lésion de la "fabella". Rev Chir Orthop 43:129–136

401. Henche HR, Künzi HU, Morscher E (1981) The areas of contact pressure in the patellofemoral joint. International Orthopaedics (SICOT) 4:279–281

402. Köppel M (1977) Nachuntersuchungen von 176 Operationen am Bandsystem des Kniegelenks von 1970–1977 bei frischen Verletzungen und veralteten Instabilitäten. Dissertation an der medizinischen Fakultät der Universität Basel

403. Cabot JR, Vilarrubias JM, Cabot Dalmau J (1979) Stabilisation simplifiée du genou dans les laxités antéro-médiales. Communication at: 1st Congress of the International Society of the knee, Lyon

404. Salter B, Simmonds DF, Malcolm BW, Rumble EJ, Macmichael D, Clements ND (1980) The biological effect of continous passive motion on the healing of fullthickness defects in articular cartilage. J Bone Joint Surg [Am] 62:1232–1251

Subject Index

Italicized numbers refer to Figures

313

P.G.J.Maquet

Biomechanics of the Knee

With Application to the Pathogenesis and the Surgical Treatment of Osteoarthritis
2nd edition, expanded and revised. 1984. 243 figures. XVIII, 306 pages
ISBN 3-540-12489-6

From the reviews:
"... Dr. Maquet and his publishers are to be congratulated on producing a book of considerable beauty. Its general layout and the clarity of what are often complicated photographs of stress-loading in photo-elastic models, anatomical specimens and radiographs set a standard of technical excellence ..."
Rheumatology and Rehabilitation

R.S.Laskin, R.A.Denham, A.G.Apley

Replacement of the Knee

1984. 323 figures. XII, 228 pages. ISBN 3-540-12943-X

Late Reconstructions of Injured Ligaments of the Knee

Editors: **K.-P.Schulitz, H.Krahl, W.H.Stein**
With contributions by M.E.Blazina, D.H.O'Donoghue, S.L.James, J.C.Kennedy, A.Trillat
1978. 42 figures, 21 tables. V, 120 pages. ISBN 3-540-08720-6

Arthritis of the Knee

Clinical Features and Surgical Management
Editor: **M.A.R.Freeman**
With contributions by numerous experts
1980. 206 figures, 50 tables. XIII, 282 pages. ISBN 3-540-09699-X

M.K.Dalinka

Arthrography

1980. 324 figures, 4 tables. XIV, 209 pages. (Comprehensive Manuals in Radiology). ISBN 3-540-90466-2

C.J.P.Thijn

Arthrography of the Knee Joint

Foreword by J.R.Blickman
1979. 173 figures in 209 separate illustrations, 11 tables. IX, 155 pages
ISBN 3-540-09129-7

H.R.Henche

Arthroscopy of the Knee Joint

With a Foreword by E.Morscher
Translated from the German by P.A.Casey
1980. 163 figures, most in colour, diagrams by F.Freuler, 1 table. XII, 85 pages
ISBN 3-540-09314-1

M.Watanabe, S.Takeda, H.Ikeuchi

Atlas of Arthroscopy

3rd edition. 1979. 226 figures, 11 tables. X, 156 pages. ISBN 3-540-07674-3

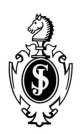

Springer-Verlag
Berlin
Heidelberg
New York
Tokyo

Springer AV Instruction Programme

Films/Videocassettes:

Theoretical and practical bases of internal fixation, results of experimental research:
Internal Fixation – Basic Principles and Modern Means
The Biomechanics of Internal Fixation
The Ligaments of the Knee Joint. Pathophysiology

Internal fixation of fractures and reconstructive bone surgery:
Internal Fixation of Forearm Fractures
Internal Fixation of Noninfected Diaphyseal Pseudarthroses
Internal Fixation of Malleolar Fractures
Internal Fixation of Patella Fractures
Medullary Nailing
Internal Fixation of the Distal End of the Humerus
Internal Fixation of Mandibular Fractures
Corrective Osteotomy of the Distal Tibia
Internal Fixation of Tibial Head Fractures (available in German only)

Joint replacement:
Total Hip Prostheses (3 parts)
Part 1: Instruments, Operation on Model
Part 2: Operative Technique
Part 3: Complications. Special Cases
Elbow-Arthroplasty with the New GSB-Prosthesis
Total Wrist Joint Replacement

Replantation surgery:
Microsurgery for Accidents

Slide Series:

ASIF-Technique for Internal Fixation of Fractures
Manual of Internal Fixation
Small Fragment Set Manual
Internal Fixation of Patella and Malleolar Fractures
Total Hip Prosteses
Operation on Model and in vivo, Complications and Special Cases

● Please ask for information material
● Order from:
Springer-Verlag Heidelberger Platz 3, D-1000 Berlin 33,
or Springer-Verlag New York Inc., 175 Fifth Avenue, New York,
NY 10010, USA

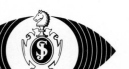

Springer-Verlag
Berlin
Heidelberg
New York
Tokyo